Public Policy in ALS/MND Care

Robert H. Blank
Jerome E. Kurent • David Oliver
Editors

Public Policy in ALS/MND Care

An International Perspective

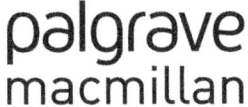

Editors
Robert H. Blank
University of Canterbury,
Christchurch, New Zealand

Jerome E. Kurent
Medical University of South Carolina
Charleston, SC, USA

David Oliver
University of Kent
Canterbury, UK

ISBN 978-981-15-5839-9   ISBN 978-981-15-5840-5   (eBook)
https://doi.org/10.1007/978-981-15-5840-5

Cover illustration: © Ed Reschke/Getty Images

This Palgrave Macmillan imprint is published by the registered company Springer Nature Singapore Pte Ltd.
The registered company address is: 152 Beach Road, #21-01/04 Gateway East, Singapore 189721, Singapore

FOREWORD

When I was a neuromuscular fellow back in 1980, I would observe how my mentors, Drs. Walter G. Bradley and Theodore L. Munsat, managed their ALS Clinic and early clinical trials. Because I was concentrating on basic research, I did not know the factors involved in running clinical programs. I have to admit I did not pay much attention to administration, as these issues were neither clinical nor scientific. A few years later when I wanted to start a multidisciplinary ALS Clinic, I struggled to learn how to do it successfully. This knowledge was clearly over my head.

When I wanted to conduct my first clinical trial with thyrotropin-releasing hormone (TRH), I would not have been able to accomplish this task without the support and assistance of my chairman Dr. John P. Conomy and his capable administrative assistant. I learned and started this process from scratch. In those days, public policies and the overall infrastructure for ALS was still in the early stages of development. I have to say that since then we have come a long way! We have many multidisciplinary ALS Clinics throughout many parts of the world. However, there are still some areas that lack these clinics. I often use the word, "ALS Community," which I believe includes people with ALS (PALS) and their family caregivers; doctors, clinicians, any scientists who are involved in the field; hospice and home care agencies; voluntary disease organizations and advocacy groups; investigator-initiated study groups; clinical trial consortia; the National ALS Registry; ALS-specific annual symposium organizers; funding agencies for research and patient care; federal health agencies; policy makers; regulatory agencies; pharmaceutical companies; and new biotech companies. All these stakeholders are working to improve ALS care and research to help combat this "intractable" disease.

In 2003, I was asked to assemble a new committee to promote excellence in end-of-life care among PALS by the Robert Wood Johnson Foundation and ALS Association. We published the committee's recommendations in 2005 and pointed to the need for improvement in public policies, more overall research in ALS, and the dissemination of key information (1). In 2011, I organized an international conference to promote clinical and patient-oriented research to identify the pathogenesis of ALS with the support of many funding agencies and pharmaceutical companies (ALS Community). Prof. Martin Turner and I published a conference supplement in 2013 in the journal *Amyotrophic Lateral Sclerosis and Frontotemporal Degeneration*. There were two articles that were devoted to discussing infrastructure and resources. Dr. Alexander V. Sherman and his colleagues reviewed public policies for funding agencies and discussed overall infrastructure resources for clinical research in ALS (2). Key infrastructure included ALS Clinics, brain banks, the National ALS Registry, and study consortia in the United States and Europe. Dr. David A. Chad also reviewed "Funding agencies and disease organizations: resources and recommendations to facilitate ALS clinical research" (3). Our efforts are still largely fragmented, and at times, I wonder if we may need to repeat our messages over and over again. It has now been ten years since the international conference. I must admit that management and care for PALS is much more complicated due to a multitude of health insurance companies, health care agencies, and palliative care and hospice providers. Movements such as "right to try" and "right to die" also require a great deal of knowledge. The number of ALS clinics has really grown in the United States, Canada, Europe, and Pan-Asian countries. These clinics have become more comprehensive, as they provide the best care for patients and conduct extensive clinical research including clinical trials.

Our ultimate goal is to find the cause and pathogenesis of ALS to develop a cure. In the meantime, we must develop medications to markedly slow down the disease. We also need to develop interventions to improve difficult symptoms in ALS, so PALS can maintain their quality of life for as long as possible. Again, the ALS Community as a whole is working toward these objectives. As I experienced many years ago, young energetic doctors and researchers are immediately confronted with a lack of knowledge on public policies and overall complex infrastructure even within the small world of ALS. I must admit knowledge of public policies in ALS health care has grown into a far more complicated web with an overwhelming amount of information. Some countries are more efficient and have great infrastructure, whereas other countries may not be as developed. Furthermore, effective implementation of this information is not easy. Some health agency workers or officials, government or non-government, may attempt to improve their policies and infrastructure for the benefits of PALS. Yet, if there are no data available, any improvement will be challenging. There are many ALS books on science and clinical care which have been published in the past, but there is a paucity of information on public policies and beyond, as well as the infrastructure for ALS care and research.

When I heard the plan for this book and its focus on public policies and infrastructure for the ALS Community (versus science or patient care), I was so excited, because I feel it is truly needed. The editors of this book include Dr. Robert Blank, a world expert on public policies and health care delivery systems; Dr. Jerome Kurent, a doctor who is most respected for compassion and humanistic care for PALS and their caregivers; and Dr. David Oliver, a doctor who introduced the concept of palliative care for PALS and successfully implemented it. The authors are among the world experts of ALS across 21 countries and provide commentary on their own countries' health policies and infrastructure for ALS. The title of the book is *Public Policies in ALS/MND Care*. Yet, I believe this book also covers broader issues that we need to know that go beyond research when treating PALS from diagnosis to end-of-life care.

One of the most important goals of this book is to provide the most comprehensive view possible of ALS/MND care and policy through commentary on different systems across 21 countries and beyond. When we face the impossible feat of finding the solution for ALS, we need to take a moment and critically evaluate the field. This book will give us the opportunity to really understand where the field stands and how we can move forward. The impact of this book will be wide-ranging, as it provides the most thorough and broad view of ALS/MND care and policy—not just locally but around the world. This is indeed the first book of its kind. I would like to provide my heartfelt congratulations to the editors and authors, who provided this crucial information and have addressed gaps in knowledge within the field. This is an essential book to read for any stakeholder in ALS.

Wesley J Howe Professor of Neurology (at CUIMC)   Hiroshi Mitsumoto
Columbia University Irving Medical Center
New York, NY
March, 2020

REFERENCES

Mitsumoto, H., M. Bromberg, W. Johnston, R. Tandan et al. (2005). Promoting excellence in end-of-life care in ALS. *Amyotrophic Lateral Sclerosis and Frontotemporal Degeneration* 6 (3): 145–54.

Sherman, A.V., A.K. Gubitz, A. Al-Chalabi, R. Bedlack et al. (2013). Infrastructure resources for clinical research in amyotrophic lateral sclerosis. *Amyotrophic Lateral Sclerosis and Frontotemporal Degeneration* 14 (Suppl 1): 53–61.

Chad, D.A., S. Bidichandani, L. Bruijn, J.D. Capra et al. (2013). Funding agencies and disease organizations: Resources and recommendations to facilitate ALS clinical research. *Amyotrophic Lateral Sclerosis and Frontotemporal Degeneration* 14 (Suppl 1): 62–66.

PREFACE

This book was first proposed by the three editors to be a co-authored volume on ALS/MND public policy in the United Kingdom and the United States. Thanks to an astute reviewer who suggested involving additional countries, we decided to develop an edited multi-authored volume which includes a broad range of contributors from across the globe. We were soon encouraged by the enthusiasm of the many ALS/MND experts willing to participate in this project, including representation from countries often overlooked in comparative studies. Authors from twenty-one countries were requested to describe the current state of ALS/MND public policy as well as implications for patient care.

This book focuses on the public policy and ethical dimensions of ALS/MND care. Policy issues include adequacy of funding for patient care and research, payment policy and regulatory functions of public and private insurers, long-term services and caregiver support, access to genetic testing and assistive technologies, and ensuring a competent and adequate workforce, especially for hands-on caregivers. There also are numerous challenges related to providing palliative and hospice care for patients with ALS/MND, as well as use of advance directives and the highly controversial area of assisted suicide. These are matters that confront policy makers in almost all geographic regions and were addressed whenever possible by each author.

To provide a starting point for coverage and to facilitate evaluation of comparative data, chapter contributors were asked to address a series of questions and issues (these are enumerated in Chapter 1) that embody a wide range of policy issues. To avoid repetition while maintaining the primary focus on policy, authors were requested not to include general background coverage of ALS/MND since this is provided in the introductory chapter along with policy themes of the book. A concluding chapter written by the editors examines the collective findings from the disparate countries represented in this book. Hopefully, this discussion will serve to facilitate workable and humane ALS/MND public policy for patient care and caregiver support in the coming decades. Overall, we argue for approaches that are both multidisciplinary and international.

We are indebted to the more than fifty authors who provided their expertise and insights of ALS/MND in producing the chapters that made this book a reality. We especially thank Professor Hiroshi Mitsumoto of Columbia Presbyterian Hospital for his invaluable assistance on this project and for writing the Foreword. We also thank Mr. Anushangi Weerakoon at Palgrave Macmillan Publishing for his enthusiastic support of the book's concept and for his encouragement over the duration of this project.

We dedicate this book to patients with ALS/MND and their families across the globe, and to provide hope for the future of eventually conquering this group of tragic disorders.

Sarasota, FL   Robert H. Blank
Charleston, SC   Jerome E. Kurent
Canterbury, UK   David Oliver

CONTENTS

Notes on Contributors

Anna Adamczyk is a specialist in neurology and in palliative medicine. She is Head of the Department of Palliative Medicine at the University Hospital No. 1 in Clinical Hospital in Bydgoszcz and a lecturer at the Department of Palliative Care at the Ludwik Rydygier Collegium Medicum in Bydgoszcz of the Nicolaus Copernicus University in Toruń. She works within palliative medicine, and practices as a neurologist, with an interest in caring for patients with diseases of the nervous system, particularly amyotrophic lateral sclerosis, and in the treatment of neuropathic pain.

Arsalan Ahmad MBBS, MD (Neurology), is Professor of Neurology at Shifa International Hospital, Shifa Tameer-e-Millat University, Islamabad, Pakistan. He completed his MBBS from Dow Medical College in 1990 and Doctor of Medicine in Neurology in 2000. He joined Shifa International Hospital in 2003 and was Head of Neurology from 2005 to 2009 and 2012. He was President of Pakistan Society of Neurology from 2016–2018 and President of Movement Disorders Society Pakistan from 2018–2020. He has an interest in movement disorders, neuromuscular disorders and neurogenetics. He has over 100 publications and abstracts including two articles on familial ALS in *The Neurogenetics Journal.*

Alexandra S. Amaler is a final year postgraduate law student at the University of Cape Town, who completed her moot on the question of assisted dying with respect to ALS.

Samar Aoun is Professor of Palliative Care Research. She adopts a public health approach and a focus on under-served population groups such as people with MND and advocates for person-centred health and social care. Her research programs on supporting family caregivers at end of life and the Public Health Model of Bereavement Support have informed policy and practice at the national and international levels. She chairs the MND Association in Western Australia, is a director on the board of MND Australia and a member of the scientific committee of MND Research Institute Australia.

Babawale Arabambi is a neurologist and physician at the Lagos State University Teaching Hospital, Nigeria, with a keen interest in stroke neurology, movement disorders, and clinical neurophysiology. He also co-manages the hospital's neurophysiology laboratory, where he performs and interprets the relevant procedures. He is a recipient of the International Scholarship Award of the American Academy of Neurology for his work on non-motor symptoms of Parkinson's disease in Nigerian outpatients in 2019. He has also authored/co-authored several publications touching on various fields in neurology.

Tamerlan Babayev graduated from Imperial College London in 2011 before undertaking postgraduate clinical training in the UK. He moved to Japan in April 2017 to take up an assistant professorship in International University of Health and Welfare and pursue a passion for medical education and research. His contribution to this book stems from an interest in medical ethics and the interplay between culture and healthcare policy.

Carol Birks has worked with people living with MND for over 20 years. She worked initially as manager of support services at MND NSW before becoming CEO of MND Australia in 2006. Her work with MND Australia encompasses influencing government policy to address the complex care needs of people with MND. Birks was a board member of the International Alliance of ALS/MND Associations from 2010 to 2017, serving as Treasurer and President. Birks has supported new and emerging ALS/MND associations globally, particularly in the Asia Pacific region. Birks is a registered nurse with a graduate diploma in palliative care.

Robert H. Blank PhD, has been Professor of Public Policy at universities in New Zealand (Canterbury), Britain (Brunel) and the U.S. (Idaho and

Northern Illinois) and a frequent guest professor at Aarhus University in Denmark and National Taiwan University in Taiwan. Among the over forty books he published on comparative health policy, genetic and reproductive policy, and neuroscience policy are *Rationing Medicine* (Columbia University Press), *Brain Policy* (Georgetown University Press), *Intervention in the Brain* (MIT Press), *Comparative Health Policy*, 1st–5th eds. (Palgrave) and *End of Life Decision Making: A Comparative Study* (MIT Press).

Benjamin Rix Brooks MD, is Medical Director of the Carolinas Neuromuscular/ALS–MDA-Care-Center and the Atrium Health ALS Association Certified-Treatment-Center-of-Excellence (CTCE) at the Atrium Health Neurosciences Institute that received the first ever Joint Commission awarded Disease-Specific Care Certification in ALS, and Professor, Department of Neurology, University of North Carolina School of Medicine, Charlotte Campus. Brooks is a founding member of the World Federation of Neurology Research Group on Motor Neuron Diseases leading efforts to design the El Escorial criteria for diagnosis of ALS and the ALS-Functional-Rating-Scale-Revised (ALSFRS-R). In 2012, he received the Forbes Norris Award from The International Alliance of ALS/MND Associations.

L. V. Brylev graduated from the Medical Faculty of Lomonosov Moscow State University in 2004 and completed residency in the Research Center of Neurology RAMS in 2006. He is head of the Department of Neurology at the Buyanov City Hospital, and the Medical Director of "Live now", a charity foundation for people with ALS. He is team leader of ALS Center Moscow, part of the European Network to Cure ALS Network, and co-author of *Russian Clinical Guidelines on ALS*.

Andrea Calvo is Associate Professor of Neurology at the Department of Neurosciences 'Rita Levi Montalcini' of the University of Turin. He has been vice-director at Turin ALS Expert Centre since 1997. He is the Co-Chair of the EAN Scientific Panel for ALS and FTD from 2019 and Chair of the Italian Motoneuron Diseases Study Group of the Italian Society of Neurology (SIN). His research interests are in the neurological field, particularly related to ALS and other neuromuscular diseases—epidemiology, clinical genetics, neuroimaging, palliative care, and clinical trials—with 170 papers in international journals.

Efrat Carmi is the CEO of IsrALS—The Israeli ALS Research Association--and has been with IsrALS since 2007. IsrALS is the primary organization supporting ALS research and patient care in the country. Efrat got her Psychology degree from Tel Aviv University and her MBA from the University of Central Florida. Efrat is an active member in the ALS/MND International Alliance and has served as a board member of the Alliance for six years.

Lu Chen MD, is a physician in the Department of Neurology, Peking University Third Hospital. Chen got her medical degree from Peking University Health Science Center in 2014. She is focusing on the study of ALS and has published thirty-six peer-reviewed articles. Her representative articles include studies about the natural history and clinical features of patients with ALS in China (*JNNP* 2015), the prevalence and incidence of ALS in China (*JNNP* 2020), and the difference in clinical features between German and Chinese ALS patients (*J Neurol* 2019).

Maike F. Dohrn is a specialist for neuromuscular disorders with a scientific focus on neurogenetics. She collaborated in the neuromuscular outpatient clinic of the RWTH Aachen University hospital as a student before she undertook her resident clinical training in 2015. She has conducted several studies on Charcot-Marie-Tooth disease, hereditary transthyretin amyloidosis, and small fiber neuropathies. Dohrn worked as an intern at the Center for Genomics and Transcriptomics (CeGaT) in Tübingen, Germany, and at the University of Porto, Portugal. Currently, she has a research fellowship at the John P. Hussman Institute for Human Genomics at the University of Miami, Florida.

Dongsheng Fan MD, Professor and Director of the Neurological Department at PUTH, has focused on the study with the aim of curing ALS. Fan and his colleagues have made great efforts for Chinese ALS patients, including the establishment of the biggest follow-up database in China. Their current works include clinical trial studies, palliative and hospice care, and genetic investigations to find new genes that cause ALS in families. The Neurological Department of PUTH has therefore become a nationally recognized center for research and clinical care in ALS in China.

Marcondes C. França Jr. MD, PhD, is Associate Professor in the Department of Neurology at the School of Medical Sciences at the University of Campinas (UNICAMP), Campinas, Brazil. He is the director of the ALS outpatient clinic at UNICAMP hospital. His research group has been working in the search for neuroimaging biomarkers and in the characterization of the genetic epidemiology of ALS in Brazil. França is the former chair of the Neuromuscular section at the Brazilian Academy of Neurology. He serves on the board of the Brazilian Association of Amyotrophic Lateral Sclerosis (ABrELA).

Miriam Galvin is Associate Professor in Intersectional Research Methodology at the Academic Unit of Neurology, School of Medicine, TCD and Atlantic Senior Fellow for Equity in Brain Health, Global Brain Health Institute. She works across a range of health research projects, mixed methods and qualitative research tracking patient and caregiver journeys, interaction with the health services and the conceptualisation and assessment of quality of life and caregiving experiences. She has a multi-disciplinary academic background in human geography, population health and psychosocial studies, with interests in research methodologies, medical anthropology, and discourse.

Marc Gotkine received his medical degree from King's College, London. After moving to Israel, he completed his residency in Hadassah University Hospital, Jerusalem. He set up the Hadassah ALS clinic and he also heads the neuromuscular service and EMG lab. The Hadassah ALS clinic serves as an ALS research hub for the whole country both in basic science and clinical trials. He has a special interest in studying the genetics of ALS in Israel, with a focus on ALS in consanguineous families. His other research interests are the genetics and epidemiology of ALS, ALS biomarkers and the microbiome in ALS.

Riadh Gouider is the head of Department of Neurology at Razi University Hospital, the Clinical Investigation Centre (CIC), the Alzheimer's center and the Multiple Sclerosis Center. He is Trustee of the World Federation of Neurology and Member in the ALS research project and related syndromes in tropical zone (TROPALS). He is a fellow of the European Academy of Neurology as well as the American Academy of Neurology since 2019. He authored and co-authored many original papers or book chapters such as Epidemiology of ALS and Clinical Features of ALS in Africa.

A. B. Guekht is the director of the Moscow Research and Clinical Center for Neuropsychiatry and Professor of Neurology at the Russian National Research Medical University. She is the author of more than 200 publications, including more than 90 papers in international peer-reviewed journals and chapters in international textbooks. She is the Elected Trustee of the World Federation of Neurology, Secretary-General of the National Society of Neurologists and involved in collaborative projects with the World Health Organisation.

Roop Gursahani is a practicing clinical neurologist at P.D. Hinduja National Hospital in Mumbai. He finished formal training and certification in Internal Medicine and then in Neurology by 1988. His special interests include epilepsy and palliative neurology. His advocacy efforts concern end-of-life care in India and include working for appropriate legislation, professional training, and public awareness. He is a member of the steering committee of ELICIT, the interdisciplinary task force of intensivists, palliative care physicians and neurologists for End of Life Care in India.

Orla Hardiman is Professor of Neurology at Trinity College Dublin and Consultant Neurologist at Beaumont Hospital, where she is Director of the National Amyotrophic Lateral Sclerosis service. She is also the National Clinical Lead in Neurology. She is one of only five active clinicians elected to the Royal Irish Academy. She is Editor-in-Chief of the journal *Amyotrophic Lateral Sclerosis and the Frontotemporal Degenerations*. Her research interests are in clinical phenotyping, epidemiology, genomics, biomarker development and new therapeutics in ALS and related disorders.

Jeannine M. Heckmann MBChB, PhD, is a neurologist in the Division of Neurology at Groote Schuur Hospital and the University of Cape Town, South Africa. Her clinical expertise is in neuromuscular diseases. She established and heads the multi-disciplinary ALS clinic at Groote Schuur Hospital, as well as an ALS research group, which collaborates with international partners.

Anne Hogden is a Senior Lecturer and researcher with the Australian Institute of Health Service Management. Her research interests are in healthcare communication, patient-centred care and decision-making and interprofessional team processes, with an emphasis on people with life-limiting conditions. Anne's research includes developing web-based decision tools to support people living with ALS/MND to make difficult decisions for care and quality of life. Her teaching work is in convening and delivering healthcare safety and quality and research units for the Master of Health Service Management, and supervision of PhD students.

Wendy S. Johnston is Professor Medicine in the Division of Neurology at the Faculty of Medicine and Dentistry at the University of Alberta, Edmonton, Canada. As Medical Director of the University of Alberta Amyotrophic Lateral Sclerosis Programme she leads a multidisciplinary team dedicated to the care of patients with ALS and other motor neuron diseases. Her research encompasses both qualitative research in ALS as well as an active investigational drug trial programme. She serves on the Board of ALS Canada and is past-Chair of the Canadian ALS Clinical Research network.

Imen Kacem is the director of the ALS center in Department of Neurology at Razi University Hospital. She is member in the ALS research project and related syndromes in tropical zone (TROPALS). She won the International Scholarship Award of the American Academy of Neurology in 2017. She authored and co-authored many papers and book chapters about ALS and CMT, such as Epidemiology of ALS and Clinical Features of ALS in Africa.

Aqdas Kazi MBBS, MRCP, CCST (Palliative Medicine), is a consultant in Palliative Medicine at Shifa International Hospital, Islamabad. After MRCP and completion of four years of Specialized Registrar training, she received the Certificate of Completion of Specialized Training in Palliative Medicine from the Royal College of the Physicians of the UK. After working at Singapore General Hospital with the hospital based palliative care team, she established the Palliative Care Unit at Shifa and is the lead for Home Based Palliative care. She teaches medical staff and has been an active advocate for Palliative Care at the national level.

Satish Khadilkar is one of the first few Indian neurologists to pursue the subspecialty of neuromuscular disorders, nationally and internationally. He has been involved with a new clinical sign, sarcoglycanopathies and dysferlinopathies and the gene in calpainopahties. He has over 130 publications to his credit and has written six and edited one book on neurology. He has been trustee and secretary of the Muscular Dystrophy Society and National Vice President of Multiple Sclerosis Society of India. He was the president of the Indian Academy of Neurology in 2018 and is the treasurer of Asian Oceanian Myology Center, where he represents India.

Seung Hyun Kim MD, PhD is Professor of Neurology and Director of ALS Clinic and Cell Therapy Center at Hanyang University Medical Center, Seoul. He earned his M.D. degree in medicine and Ph.D. in neuroanatomy from Hanyang University. He has pursued the field of ALS and neurodegenerative disorders. He is conducting translational research in the development of personalized medicine. He received the Secret of Life Award, Award from Ministry of Science, ICT and Future Planning. He serves as a member of the National Academy of Medicine of Korea and Editorial member of Molecular Neurodegeneration.

Jerome E. Kurent MD, MPH, is Professor of Neurology and Medicine at the Medical University of South Carolina and director of the ALS Multidisciplinary Clinic at the Ralph H. Johnson Veterans Affairs Medical Center. He completed residencies in Neurology and Internal Medicine at the Johns Hopkins Hospital, followed by fellowships in neuromuscular diseases and electromyography at the National Institutes of Health. He was a founding member of the MUSC ALS Multidisciplinary Clinic and served on the National Hospice and Palliative Care Organization ALS Work Group. Kurent has served as chair of the American Academy of Neurology *Ethics Section,* and the AAN *Pain and Palliative Care Section.*

Stela Lefter MD, is a consultant neurologist with subspecialist interest in neuromuscular disorders. She received her specialist training in Neurology from the Royal College of Physicians of Ireland. She trained in neuromuscular diseases at the National Neuroscience Centres in Dublin and Cork, Ireland, and MRC Centre for Neuromuscular Diseases, National Hospital for Neurology and Neurosurgery, Queen Square, London. Lefter was conferred with an M.D. degree in 2015 for her thesis 'A Population-Based Epidemiologic Study of Adult Neuromuscular Disease in the Republic of Ireland'. Her specialist research interests include muscle diseases, ALS, and peripheral neuropathies.

Tauana Bernardes Leoni MD, is a neurologist in the Department of Neurology at the School of Medical Sciences at the University of Campinas (UNICAMP), Campinas, Brazil. She supervises the clinical care of patients at the ALS outpatient clinic at UNICAMP hospital. Leoni is pursuing her PhD working in a research project devoted to characterizing the genotypes, phenotypes and imaging signatures of familial ALS in Brazil. She is a fellow of the Brazilian Academy of Neurology.

Wojciech Leppert is involved in the palliative care of patients at outpatient clinic, home hospice, and in consultations of patients in different units in hospitals. He has experience in oncology and his main area of research is pain and quality of life of patients and families in supportive and palliative care. He is Editor-in-Chief of an international journal *Palliative Medicine in Practice*, was elected in 2018 as a President of the Polish Association for Palliative Care, and was appointed in 2019 as National Consultant in palliative medicine in Poland to the Ministry of Health.

Westerly Luth is a research associate at the University of Alberta, working on projects under Wendy Johnston's qualitative research program. Her background is in psychology and public health.

Susan Mathers is a neurologist at Monash Health, Adjunct Senior Lecturer, School of Clinical Sciences, Monash University and Clinical Director of Neurology at Calvary Health Care Bethlehem, Melbourne. Her clinical and research interests focus on the management of progressive neurological diseases and models of care. She is a member of the scientific committee of the Motor Neurone Disease Research Institute of Australia, the Fight MND CURE Sub-Committee and a founding member of the Australian Motor Neurone Disease Registry and Victorian MND research tissue bank.

Christopher McDermott received his medical degree at the University in Leeds. He undertook the Wellcome Trust Research Training PhD Fellowship and completed his Specialist Training in Neurology at the University of Sheffield, becoming a Consultant Neurologist in 2006. McDermott is now the Professor of Translational Neurology at SITraN and a Consultant Neurologist at the Sheffield Teaching Hospitals Foundation NHS Trust, regularly undertaking specialist MND and neuromuscular clinics in Sheffield. He aims to develop the evidence base for delivering supportive and symptomatic care for patients living with MND. He is chair of the NIHR UK MND Clinical Studies Group.

Hiroshi Mitsumoto MD, DSc, is the Wesley J. Howe Professor of Neurology at Columbia University at The Neurological Institute of New York and New York-Presbyterian Hospital/Columbia University Medical Center. Mitsumoto has devoted his clinical and research effort to the investigation of ALS in both animal models and clinical trials in patients with ALS. He has written and lectured extensively on the topic of ALS. He served as Chair of the ALSA Medical Advisory Board until 1999 and is now a member of the MDA Medical Advisory Board, ALS CARE Board of Directors, and Neurology editorial board.

Amina Nasri is Assistant Professor of Neurology in the Department of Neurology, Razi Hospital. She is investigator in the Clinical Investigation Centre (CIC), member of the Tunisian Neurology Society since 2011 and fellow of the European Board of Neurology since 2015. She is member of the Movement Disorder Society since 2014. She won the International Scholarship Award of the American Academy of Neurology in 2020. She authored and co-authored many original papers or book chapters about movement disorder and Alzheimer disease as well as ALS.

D. V. Nevzorova graduated from Medical University in Ryazan in 1998. She entered the First Moscow Hospice in 2004 as head of department and in 2012 she was appointed to the position of Chief Medical Officer. In 2015 she became the Head of Federal Research and Clinical Center for Palliative Care at Sechenov First Moscow State Medical University. She is the chief specialist in palliative medicine in Russia and co-author of *Clinical Guidelines on Chronic Pain in Palliative Care Patients.*

Asfandyar Khan Niazi MBBS, MRCP, MPH, is the academic chief resident (PGY 5) in the Department of Neurology at Shifa International Hospital, Islamabad, Pakistan. He graduated from Shifa College of Medicine in 2014. He holds membership of the Royal College of Physicians (MRCP) of the UK and a Specialty Certificate Examination in neurology. He also has a background in public health with an MPH from the University of London. He has a keen interest in neurodegenerative and neuroinflammatory diseases.

Mieko Ogino MD, PhD, MMA, is board certified Neurologist and board-certified home care physician. She was a post-doctoral research fellow at Columbia University for four years, and was awarded a PhD degree from Kitasato University in 1994; she received the Master of Medical

Administration from Tokyo Medical and Dental University in 2008. She also finished a course at the Center for Biomedical Ethics and Law (CBEL) in Tokyo University 2005 and became a specialist in clinical ethics. She is the advocate for palliative care for non-cancer patients, especially neurological diseases. She is a director of various academic societies and member of several national associations.

Yomi Ogun BSc (Hons); MBChB; MPH (London), is Professor of Internal Medicine/Neurology and Consultant Physician/Neurologist at Lagos State University College of Medicine Teaching Hospital. With over 90 publications, he is a leading practicing neurologist in Nigeria and an authority on NeuroHIV, Stroke and Neurophysiology (EMG/NCS). Ogun is a Fellow of the Association of British-Council Fellows and the Royal Society of Tropical Medicine/Hygiene (U.K), and has been a member of the AAN-International Subcommittee 2019 and the WHO Stroke Rehabilitation-Program Interventions 2019, President of the African Academy of Neurology (2017–2019), President of the NSO, and President of NSNS/PANS.

Kiwook Oh MD, PhD, is an associate professor in the Department of Neurology, College of Medicine, Hanyang University, Seoul, Korea. He received his M.D. and Ph.D. degrees from Hanyang University. Since his early career, he is committed to patients with neurodegenerative diseases. His work focuses specifically on clinical genetics and clinical trials of ALS and neurodegenerative disease. His current project is 'Genetic architecture and clinical characteristics of Korean patients with motor neuron disease'.

David Oliver has recently retired from his full-time position as Consultant Physician in Palliative Medicine at the Wisdom Hospice in Rochester, Kent and is an Honorary Professor at the Tizard Centre at the University of Kent. He has lectured and published widely on neurological palliative care, particularly on the care of people with motor neuron disease. He was the Chair for the UK National Institute for Health and Care Excellence Guidelines on MND, released in February 2016. He is principal editor of "Palliative Care of Amyotrophic Lateral Sclerosis—from diagnosis to bereavement".

Evy Reviers is the daughter of an ALS patient, which is her motivation to serve as a representative of pALS at the national and international level. She is CEO of ALS Liga Belgium, focusing on stimulating and financing scientific research on ALS, contacts with ALS researchers, collaborations with university hospitals, and defending the rights of pALS at governmental institutions and agencies. As Chairperson of the European Organization for Professionals and Patients with ALS (EUpALS), she is particularly involved in regulatory aspects of ALS clinical trials and advocates the same rights for access to trials and future medicines for all pALS worldwide.

Ildefonso Rodriguez-Leyva MD, MSc, PhD, is head of the Neurology Program of the Faculty of Medicine of the Autonomous University of San Luis Potosí and is the Head of the Neurology Service of the Central Hospital "Dr. Ignacio Morones Prieto" from San Luis Potosi, SLP, Mexico. He has dedicated himself to educate physicians and improve the quality of Neurology in his country, by advancing the relationship of Mexican Neurology with the American Academy of Neurology, American Neurological Association, American Epilepsy Society, Movement Disorders Society, and the World Federation of Neurology.

Roman Rolke is Director of the Department of Palliative Medicine at RWTH Aachen University, Germany, since 2014. He is co-speaker of the Neuropalliative Working Group of the German Neurological Society and co-speaker of all physicians of the German Palliative Care Association. His research interests include assessment of pain profiles using quantitative sensory testing and late-stage neurological disorders. He is editor of several books on pain and palliative medicine. Rolke is Associate Editor of the *German Journal of Palliative Medicine.*

Ikram Sghaier has a BSc degree in analytical and experimental biology, M.Sc. degree in microbiology and molecular epidemiology, Specialist in immuno-genetics and virology. She won the Award for best participation in 2012 and 2015 from "STGE" during her PhD. She is Post-doc in the neuro-genetics laboratory, neurology department in RAZI Hospital Tunisia and the Clinical investigation centre (CIC) and is focusing in Amyotrophic lateral sclerosis disease (genetic background and atypical clinical features)

Bugyeong Son RN, is a nurse coordinator at the Cell Therapy Center, Hanyang University Medical Center, Seoul, Korea. She earned her bachelor's degree in science of nursing from Hanyang University. She has clinical nursing experience in the oncology department and has been involved with ALS/MND since joining Cell Therapy Center. She became a Director of International Cooperation in Korean ALS Association in 2019 and is now a second-year master's student at Hanyang University.

Ludo Van Den Bosch is a scientist investigating the molecular mechanisms involved in different neurodegenerative diseases, including ALS. In addition, he develops new therapeutic strategies for these diseases. He is full professor of Neuroscience at the University of Leuven and group leader at the VIB-Center for Brain & Disease Research. He is head of the Laboratory of Neurobiology and scientific founder of Augustine Therapeutics, a spin-off of VIB developing therapeutic strategies for neurodegenerative disorders.

Philip Van Damme is a neurologist at the University Hospital Leuven. During his neurology training, he undertook a PhD on the role of excitotoxicity in ALS. Afterwards he continued to focus on the neuromuscular disorder ALS. He is Professor of Neuroscience at the University of Leuven and is currently directing the Neuromuscular Reference Center, which coordinates the care of ALS patients. His research activities focus on translational ALS research including fundamental studies to understand the causes and disease mechanisms of ALS, clinical studies on biomarkers of the disease and prodromal disease stages, and clinical trials with novel treatments for ALS.

Ludo Vanopdenbosch is a private neurologist with subspecialty interests in neuro-oncology and multiple sclerosis. He is also director of palliative care and head of the ethics committee at AZ Sint Jan Brugge. His research interest is palliative care in neurology. At present he is co-chair of the scientific panel on palliative care of the European Academy of neurology. He is guest professor at the University of Leuven and the Free University of Brussels.

Simone Veronese MD, PhD is a consultant in palliative care, head of research at Fondazione FARO, Turin, Italy. He is a member of the Italian Society for Palliative Care (SICP), of the Group of Study for Bioethics and Palliative Care of the Italian Society of Neurology (SIN), and of the Reference Group for Neurology of the European Association of Palliative Care (EAPC). He is the author of several articles on the role of palliative care in neurodegenerative conditions, and on quality of life and outcome measurements.

M. N. Zakharova graduated from Sechenov Medical Institute in 1979. She started to work in the Research Center of Neurology as a resident and now she is head of the department. She is a professor on the Medical Faculty of Moscow State University and author of more than 200 articles and book chapters. She is co-author of the *Clinical Guidelines on Multiple Sclerosis and Amyotrophic Lateral Sclerosis.*

LIST OF FIGURES

LIST OF TABLES

CHAPTER 1

Introduction to Public Policy of ALS/MND

Jerome E. Kurent, David Oliver, and Robert H. Blank

Abstract This chapter outlines the framework and goals of this cross-national study of amyotrophic lateral sclerosis/motor neuron disease (ALS/MND) policy. It also describes the key features of ALS/MND and discusses criteria and associated challenges in making the diagnosis and the importance of excluding ALS/MND mimics. Epidemiology, genetics and possible environmental risk factors for ALS/MND are reviewed. Management of symptoms, challenges confronting caregivers, including access to palliative care and hospice during the end-of-life, and the broad range of ethical issues surrounding ALS/MND care are highlighted. This chapter examines the often-ignored public policy context and the importance of cultural and religious factors in understanding policy differences which exist across countries. Finally, this chapter introduces the countries

J. E. Kurent
Medical University of South Carolina, Charleston, SC, USA
e-mail: kurentje@musc.edu

D. Oliver
University of Kent, Canterbury, UK
e-mail: drdjoliver@gmail.com

R. H. Blank (✉)
University of Canterbury, Christchurch, New Zealand
e-mail: rblank24601@hotmail.com

© The Author(s) 2021
R. H. Blank et al. (eds.), *Public Policy in ALS/MND Care*,
https://doi.org/10.1007/978-981-15-5840-5_1

1

selected for this study and summarizes the key topics of importance the authors were asked to address in their chapters.

Keywords ALS • MND • Public policy • Cross-national studies • Multidisciplinary teams • Palliative care • End-of-life decisions

INTRODUCTION

Incurable progressive neurological disorders cause immense pain and suffering for their victims and their families. The associated huge economic and indirect costs to society are often difficult to calculate. A rapidly growing aging population in many regions of the world is strongly associated with the increased incidence of neurodegenerative disease and has major public policy implications. Amyotrophic lateral sclerosis/motor neuron disease (ALS/MND) may be the prime example of a devastating rapidly progressive neurodegenerative disease for which there is no cure or significant disease-modifying therapy. Although there are three approved drugs used for the treatment of ALS/MND, their benefits are limited, and most other treatment options are limited primarily to symptom management.

There is a clear need for effective public policy and research focused on ensuring optimal clinical care of patients with ALS/MND and provision of adequate supportive services. Increased research funding focused on an enhanced understanding of the etiology(ies) and pathophysiology of ALS/MND and mechanisms of motor neuron cell death is expected to lead to development of additional disease-modifying agents and ultimately to a cure. There is also the potential that insights gained from the study of ALS/MND may provide clues to other enigmatic neurodegenerative diseases, including dementia, that plague our societies.

A primary goal of this book is to develop a compendium of public policy summaries representative of many different countries across the globe. It discusses a range of ALS/MND policy elements and perspectives while providing a framework for understanding ALS/MND as it affects patients and their families, professional caregivers and researchers. The book should be of interest to those involved in health care policy and public health as well as for ALS clinicians including neurologists, nurses, nurse practitioners, allied health professionals and physicians' assistants involved in the complex range of issues related to ALS/MND. Additional stakeholders who should find this book of interest include social workers, ALS clinic coordinators and administrators and members of ALS and MND private foundations and public agencies dedicated to the optimum treatment of patients with ALS/MND—including the goal of its ultimate defeat. The book may also serve as a useful reference for organizations providing durable medical equipment such as wheelchairs, communication devices, beds and other assistive equipment utilized in the management of patients with progressive disability.

WHAT IS ALS/MND?

ALS is a progressive fatal neuromuscular disease first described by Charcot in 1869 which primarily affects spinal cord and brainstem motor neurons and the upper motor neuron system. ALS may be regarded as a syndrome rather than a specific disease entity. There is increasing evidence of wider neuronal involvement, including the frontal lobes, and cortical and subcortical regions (Westeneng et al. 2016). ALS is also known as Lou Gehrig's disease in the United States, named after the famous major league baseball player who succumbed to this illness in 1941, whereas in the United Kingdom, motor neuron disease is used to designate ALS. Within the classification ICD-9 (code 335.2), the term motor neuron disease is also indistinguishable from ALS. It has been suggested that the term motor neuron diseases be used to include both ALS and its clinical subtypes. Thus, ALS/MND as used here encompasses:

- ALS/MND, with both upper and lower motor neuron involvement, leading to a mixed picture of weakness associated with spasticity and flaccidity, muscle wasting, fasciculation and extensor plantar responses; average longevity three to five years; more than 90 percent of people with limb onset develop bulbar symptoms;
- Progressive bulbar palsy affects about 20 percent of patients in which there is involvement of the bulbar motor neurons, affecting speech and swallowing;
- Progressive muscular atrophy (PMA) affects about 5 percent, with predominantly lower motor neuron involvement leading to muscular weakness and wasting, particularly of the legs and arms. The prognosis is longer and may be five to ten years;
- Primary lateral sclerosis (PLS) which affects 1–2 percent with predominantly upper motor neuron involvement, including spasticity,

stiffness, increased deep tendon reflexes and extensor plantar response. It has a longer prognosis often greater than ten years

The most common clinical presentation of ALS/MND is spinal-onset and involves slowly progressive painless weakness and atrophy of a distal upper or lower extremity. Weakness typically progresses to involve the contralateral limb and then to other areas of the body including bulbar and respiratory muscles. Rarely—less than 5 percent—do patients first present with respiratory failure that requires ventilator support. The average age of onset is 55 to 57 years, with a male to female ratio of 1.7:1, except 1:1 having onset after 65 to 70 years of age. Death typically occurs within three to five years from respiratory muscle failure, although 25 percent of patients survive for five years and 10 percent are alive at ten years (Shaw et al. 2014).

Frontotemporal dementia (FTD) occurs in up to 15 percent of patients (McKhann et al. 2001). More subtle frontal lobe dysfunction may occur in another 20 to 25 percent of patients (Lomen-Hoerth et al. 2003; Strong et al. 2009; Phukan 2012). There are patients with FTD who later develop ALS/MND with a spectrum from pure ALS to pure FTD—often related to the *C9orf72* genetic abnormality (Couratier et al. 2017). An estimated 90 to 95 percent of patients have sporadic ALS (sALS) which occurs in the absence of a clear family history. Five to 10 percent of ALS patients have familial ALS (fALS) usually inherited as a Mendelian autosomal dominant gene. Reduced penetrance is not uncommon.

MAKING THE DIAGNOSIS OF ALS/MND: A DIAGNOSIS OF EXCLUSION

The neurologist must take a careful history and perform a meticulous neurological examination to determine if an alternative cause of the patient's symptoms can be identified. Depending on localizing signs and symptoms, MRI imaging of the spine is often necessary to rule out structural lesions, such as cervical or lumbar stenosis, herniated disc with foraminal encroachment and spinal cord compression, meningioma and other spinal cord pathology. Although there are no specific biomarkers currently available to confirm the diagnosis or to monitor the clinical course of ALS/MND, efforts are underway to identify biomarkers.

Table 1.1   Conditions that can mimic ALS/MND

Spinal cord pathology that causes spinal cord and/or nerve root compression
(myeloradiculopathy) includes but is not limited to cervical spondylosis and meningioma
Autoimmune neuropathies—including multifocal motor neuropathy
Spinobulbar muscular atrophy (Kennedy's disease)
Multiple sclerosis
Hereditary spastic paraplegia
Benign fasciculation syndrome
Myopathies—inclusion body myositis
Diabetic amyotrophy
Thyrotoxicosis
Hyperparathyroidism

As illustrated in Table 1.1, there are many conditions that can mimic ALS/MND. A second independent opinion from a neuromuscular specialist having special expertise in ALS/MND is often requested by the first neurologist suspecting ALS/MND in order to confirm the diagnosis of what many consider to be a "death sentence." Muscle biopsy and spinal fluid examination are not considered necessary for routine evaluation of patients suspected of having ALS/MND, but they may be helpful in diagnosing a suspected alternative condition or ALS mimic.

Criteria have been developed to assist with the diagnosis and management of ALS. These include the modified El Escorial criteria (Brooks et al. 2000), which are particularly relevant when considering clinical drug trials. The criteria suggest that for a diagnosis of ALS/MND, there should be progressive upper and lower motor neuron deficits in at least one limb or region of the human body (meeting the revised El Escorial criteria for possible ALS) or lower motor neuron deficits as defined by clinical examination (one region) and/or by EMG in two body regions (defined as bulbar, cervical, thoracic, lumbosacral). There must be progressive changes, fasciculations and near normal motor nerve conduction and no sensory abnormalities. There should be no abnormalities of the sensory nervous system, no impairment of the visual or autonomic nervous system and no sphincter involvement.

The Awaji criteria were subsequently developed and are based on the expanded role of the electrophysiological diagnosis of ALS/MND (Chen et al. 2010; Costa et al. 2012). Electromyography is a critical component of diagnosing ALS/MND. Diffuse denervation should be present in three different anatomical regions to meet electrophysiological criteria for the diagnosis of ALS/MND. Fibrillations and positive waves consistent with active denervation are typically present and are usually seen in association with high amplitude, prolonged duration motor unit potentials consistent with chronic denervation/re-innervation. Fasciculation potentials are often present. It is imperative that ALS/MND mimics have been ruled out.

EPIDEMIOLOGY OF ALS/MND

The incidence of ALS/MND across the world is unclear. A systematic review suggests that the incidence in Europe is 2–3/100,000 with a prevalence of 5–7/100,000 population (Chio et al. 2013), while the incidence of ALS in the United States is approximately 3–5/100,000. It is unclear if the differences across countries relate to the design of studies, the ability of patients to receive medical attention or differences in defining ALS/MND.

Although considered a rare disease, the incidence of ALS/MND is approximately one-half that of multiple sclerosis (MS). However, public perception and general awareness of MS is much greater than that of ALS/MND primarily due to the marked contrast in life expectancy for victims of these two disorders. Although patients with MS face a reduction in life expectancy of seven to twelve years (Magyari and Sorensen 2019), most patients with ALS/MND will not survive more than three to five years after diagnosis. The incidence of ALS/MND in the non-Caucasian population and individuals of mixed ethnicity is considered less than whites of European ancestry.

In the Western Pacific the incidence of ALS among the indigenous Chamorros in Guam had occurred at rates 50 to 100 times that noted elsewhere around the world (Armon 2013). ALS often co-existed with Parkinson-dementia complex. The incidence of Guamanian ALS has dramatically dropped since World War II, and it is suspected that dietary toxins present in cycad seed, which were used as a primary source of dietary flour, along with a possible genetic predisposition, may have been at least in part responsible for this phenomenon. Genetic susceptibility may have contributed to an increased incidence of ALS in the Kii Peninsula of Japan, which also represents a well-known, but poorly understood, ALS cluster.

GENETICS OF ALS/MND

The genetics of ALS/MND has become increasingly complex. The first ALS gene mutation—*SOD1*—was reported in 1993 (Rosen et al. 1993). There are now more than twenty different genes known to cause ALS. The majority of familial ALS is transmitted as a Mendelian autosomal dominant gene, but penetrance may be incomplete. The most common genes are:

- *SOD1*—accounting for 10–20 percent of fALS and 1 percent of sALS
- *C9orf72* hexanucleotide repeat—accounting for 40 percent of fALS in many countries, but less than 10 percent in Asia, found in 10–20 percent of sporadic ALS in Europe
- *TDP-43*—accounting for 4 percent of fALS and less than 1 percent of sALS
- *FUS/TLS*—accounting for 4 percent of fALS and more rare in sALS
- *Ataxin 2*—accounting for 4 percent of fALS and 1 percent of sALS
- *VCP*—accounting for 1–2 percent of fALS (Corcia et al. 2017)

Reviews have described in detail the rapidly evolving body of knowledge related to the genetics of ALS/MND and their contribution to advancing our understanding of the underlying basis for this disorder and means to develop effective therapies (Andersen and Al-Chalabi 2011; Brown and Al-Chalabi 2017). The investigation of these genetic mutations is providing some insights into mechanisms of motor neuron cell damage and death. Until recently, numerous clinical trials with humans affected with ALS/MND have not been able to duplicate positive results reported in animal studies (Benatar et al. 2009). However, the development of gene-specific therapies for ALS/MND may indeed be realized in the case of the *SOD1* mutant gene and *C9orf72*. The development of antisense oligonucleotides is well underway along with early-stage clinical trials for individuals having the *SOD1* genetic variant and *C9orf72* (Ly and Miller 2018; Miller et al. 2020). *SOD1* suppression with adeno-associated virus and microRNA was also recently reported (Mueller et al. 2020).

There is the underlying assumption that patients with sALS have a genetic predisposition for developing ALS/MND. The presumed genetic predisposition alone is considered insufficient, but in conjunction with other factors including environmental influences, it can trigger a process resulting in clinical ALS/MND. It has been suggested that a six-step process occurring over the life of an individual may converge with a genetic predisposition to initiate the cascade of motor neuron damage and cell death, resulting in ALS/MND (Al-Chalabi et al. 2014; Chio et al. 2018). Identical twin studies have failed to demonstrate an increased risk of developing ALS in the unaffected sibling (Al Chalabi et al. 2010; Xi et al. 2014; Tarr et al. 2019), perhaps supporting the suspected role of environmental factors and epigenetics.

Environmental Risk Factors

The suspected role of environmental factors as they relate to genetics in ALS has been discussed in detail (Al-Chalabi and Hardiman 2013). Numerous toxins and other insults as well as nutritional deficiencies have been considered. The role of physical trauma and emotional stress has also been studied, but without demonstrating a clear relationship to causality. More recent observations related to a suspected increased risk of ALS and other neurodegenerative diseases in US National Football League (NFL) professional athletes have been highlighted. The possible role of chronic traumatic encephalopathy (CTE) in a subgroup of patients with ALS has been suggested (McKee et al. 2010), although other reports have questioned this relationship (Bedlack et al. 2011; Armon and Miller 2011).

Toxins and other environmental agents which have been investigated include smoking, alcohol, heavy metals like lead and mercury, pesticides and electric shock. Smoking has been associated with ALS/MND risk in several studies, although its precise role in susceptibility has not been defined. Inhalation of other environmental toxins associated with urban pollution is also being investigated (Malek et al. 2013; Seelen et al. 2017). There is also renewed interest in toxins associated with cyanobacteria, which have ubiquitous presence in the environment. Viral infections including reverse transcriptase agents have been studied, but without definitive proof of causality. Patients with HIV/AIDS have developed ALS, but their neurological disability has not responded to antiviral therapy

In the United States, ALS has been declared a military service-connected disability based on several epidemiological studies (Horner et al. 2003; Weisskopf et al. 2005), suggesting a two-fold increase in risk for developing ALS by deployed veterans. An increased risk was first described for veterans deployed to Iraq, and subsequently for those involved in earlier conflicts and wars dating back to World War II. Numerous factors related to military service have been considered, but without demonstrating a direct causal link to ALS. These factors include burning oil fields, as in Iraq, multiple immunizations, concussion and other physical and emotional stressors, as well as nerve toxin antidotes, such as pyridostigmine. Italian soccer players have also experienced a significantly increased risk of developing ALS, but for unknown reasons. Occasional clustering of patients with ALS/MND has been reported, suggesting possible common environmental exposures, but with inconclusive findings.

MANAGEMENT OF SYMPTOMS

Multidisciplinary ALS clinics are considered the gold standard for providing comprehensive care (NICE 2016; Miller et al. 2009) and are widely accessible through most of North America, the United Kingdom, Europe and many countries around the globe. Their implementation has been associated with improved quality of life and possibly extension of the natural history of ALS/MND (Aridegbe et al. 2013; Rooney et al. 2015). The ALS Functional Rating Scale-Revised (ALS-FRS-R) is a tool routinely utilized in multidisciplinary clinics to monitor overall clinical status of the patient and is a reliable measure of clinical progression and loss of function (Cedarbaum et al. 1999). Numerous excellent resources are available to guide the clinical management of patients with ALS/MND (Miller et al. 1999; Miller et al. 2009; Bedlack and Mitsumoto 2013).

Most patients with ALS/MND will die of respiratory failure secondary to weakness and atrophy of diaphragmatic and accessory muscles of respiration. Patients will experience a wide range of disabling symptoms over the course of their illness including dyspnea, weakness and atrophy, muscle cramps, dysarthria, dysphagia, weight loss, pathological laughter and crying (pseudobulbar affect), drooling, pain, sleep disturbance and constipation (see Table 1.2). Multidisciplinary ALS clinics provide a wide range of professional expertise required to assist with management of these symptoms while providing comprehensive care for the patient and support for family caregivers.

Table 1.2 Symptom management

Symptom		Management
Pain	Muscle spasm Musculoskeletal Skin pressure	Muscle relaxants Nonsteroidal anti-inflammatory Analgesics/opioids
Cramps	Fasciculations Spastic muscles	Quinine sulfate (not available in US) Baclofen Gabapentin Tizanidine
Spasticity	Muscle spasm	Baclofen Tizanidine Gabapentin Physiotherapy
Sialorrhea	Reduced swallowing	Atropine/scopolamine Botulinum toxin injections Radiotherapy to salivary glands
Thick secretions		N-acetylcysteine Grape fruit juices Nebulized water
Laryngospasm		Sublingual lorazepam
Insomnia	Anxiety Respiratory failure Depression	Anxiolytics Noninvasive ventilation Antidepressants
Pseudobulbar affect	Uncontrolled laughter/crying	Amitriptyline, Dextromethorphan/quinidine sulfate
Dyspnea	Respiratory muscle weakness and respiratory failure	Noninvasive ventilation Opioids Tracheostomy ventilation
Dysarthria	Speech and language therapy assessment	Communication aids
Dysphagia	Speech and language therapy and dietitian assessment	Modified consistency of food Consider gastrostomy
Cognitive issues	Frontal lobe dysfunction Frontotemporal dementia Language/loss of empathy/ executive function loss/ memory loss	Psychological assessment Advice and support for caregivers
Constipation	Poor diet/anticholinergic medication side effects	Fluid and fiber Laxatives
Gastroesophageal reflux disease	Lower esophageal sphincter weakness	Meals while upright H-2 blockers Proton pump inhibitors

Palliative Care, Hospice and End-of-Life Care

As there is no curative treatment for ALS/MND, the approach is often palliative. The World Health Organization (WHO) defines palliative care as "the total active care of patients whose disease is not responsive to curative treatment. The goal of palliative care is the achievement of the best quality of life for patients and their families." The involvement of specialist palliative care/hospice care for ALS/MND started first at St Christopher's Hospice in London, UK, in 1967 and has spread across the world. Many guidelines have recommended palliative care including the American Academy of Neurology Ethics and Humanities Committee Position Statement (Carver 1996) which highlighted the urgency that neurologists understand and apply principles of palliative care in the management of their patients. The American Academy of Neurology Practice Parameter (Miller et al. 2009) and the EFNS Guidelines (Andersen et al. 2012) further supported this approach.

A palliative care approach considers the whole patient in the context of their family and caregivers—assessing the physical, psychological, social and spiritual aspects of care. It encompasses a multidisciplinary approach, and it has been recommended that the multidisciplinary team (MDT) for ALS/MND should include palliative care expertise (NICE 2016; Miller et al. 2009; Robert Wood Johnson Foundation 2004).

Ethical Issues in ALS/MND Care

Numerous challenging ethical issues often arise while caring for the patient with progressive neurodegenerative diseases, including ALS/MND. Table 1.3 illustrates some of these issues related to the management of patients with ALS/MND, beginning with communicating the bad news of the recent diagnosis of ALS/MND to a patient. A comprehensive description of the ethical issues and their resolution as they occur in neurology practice has been provided by Bernat (2008).

The subject of breaking the news to the patient with newly diagnosed ALS/MND is a matter of compassion and empathy and should include discussion of the possible available treatments, anticipated future needs, avoidances and preferences of the patient. The National Institute for Health and Care Excellence (NICE) Guidance gives clear recommendations (NICE 2016). The newly diagnosed patient may, or may not, suspect the seriousness of his neurological condition at the time of meeting

Table 1.3 Selected ethical issues and controversies

- Breaking bad news
- Abandonment
- Enrollment in clinical trials
- Genetic testing of patients
- Genetic testing of family members
- Use of feeding tube and option to withdraw once initiated
- Use of tracheostomy and mechanical ventilation
- Palliative sedation
- Physician-assisted suicide
- Euthanasia
- Organ donation by living patient with ALS
- Organ donation by deceased patient with ALS
- "Right to Try" legislation
- Treatment with unproven and potentially dangerous agents
- Charlatans and quacks offering ineffective or unproven therapies
- Role of public policy in addressing these issues

to summarize results of diagnostic testing with his or her neurologist. It is vitally important for the physician to break the bad news in-person and to allow adequate time for the patient to begin to process this life-changing information. Excellent resources are available to help guide this discussion (Johnston et al. 1996; Sloan and Borasio 2014).

The expression "Diagnose and Adios" has been used to characterize some neurologists' interactions with patients and suggests the lack of adequate empathic connection. This suggests that the neurologist may possibly be more intent on making the correct diagnosis than on caring for the patient. This approach is changing as the neurologist provides ongoing care, often as part of a multidisciplinary team (Gursahani 2016; NICE 2016). In the past, physicians sometimes tried to protect the patient from the bad news of a life-limiting diagnosis by using terms such as a "disease of the motor system" or simply delaying the diagnosis. There is no justification for withholding or downplaying the significance of diagnostic information considered essential to prepare for advance planning and for getting one's personal and business affairs in order.

The ethical principle of truth-telling requires that patients be provided honest and accurate information related to their illness. Most patients expect full disclosure of facts related to the diagnosis of serious illness. Prognosis and related discussions may be provided over a series of meetings at a pace comfortable to the patient since some patients may be overwhelmed with too much information provided at one time (Seeber et al. 2019). However, it is important to allow these discussions whenever the patient and family wish to facilitate discussion and to plan for the future (NICE 2016). The responses of patients with newly diagnosed ALS/MND can be variable (Johnston et al. 1996; Sloan and Borasio 2014). Some patients have a relatively positive response, "At least I know what I have," while others can express feelings of despair. There is a delicate balance between the neurologist providing immediate and full disclosure and communicating in a caring and empathic manner. Communication should be tailored to the unique needs of the patient to the extent this can be determined. Cultures vary to the extent to which critical information is expected to be communicated either directly to the patient, or sometimes preferably to family members. Many patients explore the Internet to seek out information related to their symptoms and suspected diagnosis.

It is usually helpful to ask the patient what he/she understands about their condition. Most patients have little knowledge about ALS/MND, although this is changing with the increased use of the Internet. A blunt approach used to provide the diagnosis in an abrupt manner is strongly discouraged and can be devastating to the patient and family. It is also reasonable to leave some room for hope, although this may be challenging. Clinical trials may offer optimism for some patients.

Medical paternalism, in which the patient is "protected" from bad news, is no longer accepted in most Western cultures. A direct and forthright discussion with the patient is expected. However, some cultures around the world expect that unfavorable information pertaining to a serious diagnosis be provided to family members of the patient rather than to the patient. These cultural norms should be respected by the physician and should be known in advance of the discussion if possible.

Patients with ALS have sometimes expressed a sense of physical or emotional abandonment by their physicians as their illness progressed. *Non-abandonment* of the patient is a key ethical obligation shared by all professionals involved in the care of patients with ALS/MND. Abandonment of the patient by a physician can be either physical or emotional. Following the diagnosis of ALS/MND, professional caregivers including physicians

Table 1.4   Triggers for initiating discussion about end-of-life issues in ALS/MND

- The patient or family asks, or "opens the door," for end-of-life information and/or possible interventions
- Severe psychological and/or social or spiritual distress or suffering
- Pain or other symptoms requiring higher than normal dosages of medications
- Dysphagia requiring a feeding tube
- Dyspnea or symptoms of hypoventilation, usually with reduced forced vital capacity of 50 percent or less
- Loss of function in two body regions (bulbar, arms or legs)

Modified from Robert Wood Johnson Foundation (2004)

may feel uncomfortable in following up the patient with an incurable disease. Increasingly, the ongoing care is shared within a multidisciplinary team, which shares the load and allows all aspects of care to be considered, often with an improvement of quality and even length of life (Aridegbe et al. 2013).

Professional caregivers may have a basic discomfort with death and dying, including fear of death, a sense of failure as well as challenges in confronting one's own mortality. However, there remains an obligation to discuss end-of-life care issues with the patient having advanced ALS/MND including the need for advance care planning. Table 1.4 lists six triggers for initiating a discussion about end-of-life care decision-making for the patient with ALS.

Clinical Trials

ALS/MND clinical trials offer hope for patients, and many are eager to participate. Clinical trial participation should be strongly encouraged. Although most patients appear to fully understand that participation in clinical trials will most likely not be of direct benefit to them, it is important that they have this clear understanding prior to enrollment in the interest of truth-telling and informed consent.

Genetic Testing

The genetics of ALS/MND have provided critical insights into molecular mechanisms of motor neuron cell damage and death and offer hope that meaningful therapies focused on specific gene defects can be developed. Availability of genetic testing for ALS/MND varies greatly around the world. There are numerous medical-ethical dilemmas arising from the availability of genetic testing for ALS/MND. Continued acquisition of new knowledge related to understanding and ultimately curing ALS/ MND will depend to a great extent on identifying additional genes. A recommendation for routine genetic testing of patients with sporadic ALS has been made, but this raises the challenging issue of the testing of unaffected individuals who are at potential risk of developing ALS/ MND. There also may be issues of payment by insurance companies and restricted resources and availability of genetic counseling and testing in many parts of the world.

Genetic testing for clinically unaffected family members at-risk and related to a patient with clinical ALS/MND having a strong family history has been a subject of discussion. Testing of individuals at-risk for developing ALS/MND can provide the opportunity to arrange for family planning in addition to making other key decisions involving employment and the acquisition of medical and life insurance. Genetic counseling prior to and following testing is obligatory whether the individual tests positive or negative for the gene. It has been questioned whether there is an ethical obligation to disclose positive results of gene testing to other family members even though they are not actively participating. Clinically unaffected individuals, although not suspecting that they might be carrying a mutant gene, could potentially benefit from this information. However, even if legislation exists to protect individuals having a genetic mutation, discrimination by insurance companies and employers might still occur, posing serious implications for the economic well-being of clinically unaffected patients who test positive for a deleterious ALS/MND gene.

Withholding and Withdrawal of Care

There are many ethical and legal issues at the end of life particularly concerning the withholding and withdrawing of care. In many countries there is no ethical or legal distinction between withholding and withdrawing of care, such as the placement or use of a feeding tube or the use of invasive ventilation. Such interventions can be either withheld altogether, or withdrawn once in place. These decisions are typically at the direction of a patient having decision-making capacity or his/her legal surrogate decision-maker. In some countries it is not legally permissible to withdraw treatment, such as invasive ventilation, once it has been initiated. These approaches vary by country and often have strong cultural underpinnings, which form the basis for law and public policy. Therefore, careful discussion is necessary before any consideration of these interventions, so that a clear decision is made; the implications of the intervention, such as the continued deterioration of the disease after ventilatory support has started, are discussed; and plans for future care, including the possible withdrawal of treatment (NICE 2016; Oliver and Turner 2010), are considered. If withdrawal is not possible within a country, these discussions are even more crucial so that a truly autonomous decision can be made.

There is increasing awareness of frontotemporal dementia and related cognitive change which can occur in ALS/MND, and a consideration of mental capacity to make decisions and advance care planning is important. There may be opportunities earlier in the disease progression when the person can make decisions and make their wishes for their future care known. If these are recorded clearly, as advance directives or defining a proxy to make decisions on their behalf, the person's wishes can be respected. However, it may be difficult to have these discussions, and patients and families may be resistant to looking ahead, but this may be the only opportunity as cognition and communication may be lost in the future (Goldstein 2014).

Palliative Sedation and Assisted Dying

At the end of life some patients experience significant distress. The aim of palliative care is to minimize suffering, and with good symptom management, a distressing death is considered rare (Neudert et al. 2001). However, on some occasions the patient may remain distressed—physically, emotionally or spiritually. In certain circumstances therapeutic/palliative sedation may be necessary. The European Association for Palliative Care framework has suggested that "Therapeutic/palliative sedation in the context of palliative medicine is the monitored use of medications intended to induce a state of decreased or absent awareness (unconsciousness) in order to relieve the burden of otherwise intractable suffering in a manner that is ethically acceptable to the patient, family and health-care providers" (Cherny et al. 2009). Morphine and benzodiazepine medications are typically used in a closely monitored clinical environment to sedate in order to relieve suffering.

The National Hospice and Palliative Care Organization (2010) has provided guidelines for the implementation of palliative sedation in the rare instance that it may be required. This includes the recommendation that patient caregivers as well as the patient, if capable, participate in a detailed discussion with hospice or palliative care professionals caring for the patient. This discussion should include the potential for premature death of the terminally ill patient even though this is considered unlikely. The US Supreme Court has also expressed support for palliative sedation.

The *Principle of Double Effect* justifies the morality of a single act that has the potential of causing two morally opposite effects (Bernat 2008). Although the intent is to relieve suffering, the potential to cause the premature death of the patient is acknowledged. Palliative sedation is ethical and legal in many, but not all, countries and should only be considered in the relatively rare instance when all other measures have failed to control the intractable pain and other symptoms not manageable by usually effective therapies. On occasions this may continue until death, but sometimes the level of sedation can be reduced if the patient remains comfortable.

Palliative sedation should not be confused with physician-assisted suicide (PAS) or euthanasia/medical aid in dying. Although there appears to be an increasing acceptance of PAS, this varies considerably by country. The patient desiring PAS must be diagnosed with a terminal illness and is provided a prescription by a participating physician for a lethal dose of one or more medications such as a barbiturate. The patient may choose to take the lethal dose of medication at a time and place of his/her choosing. The primary ethical dilemma focuses on patient autonomy and the right to make decisions concerning the fate of one's body versus the physician's duty to cause no harm and to preserve life. Euthanasia occurs when a doctor intentionally kills a person by the administration of drugs at that person's voluntary and competent request (Radbruch et al. 2016). This has been offered only in limited countries where it is legal and to someone with full capacity and autonomy. Euthanasia will always be controversial, even where legal.

As discussed in more detail in country chapters, assisted dying is now available in many countries, with varying legal regulations. Euthanasia and PAS are legal in Belgium, the Netherlands, Luxembourg, Canada, Colombia and the states of Victoria and Western Australia in Australia. In the United States, PAS is legal in nine states and the District of Columbia. Assisted dying is allowed in Switzerland. Patients with ALS/MND are often overrepresented in the people receiving assisted dying. In the Netherlands in 2010, 1.8 percent of all deaths were a result of either euthanasia or PAS. Twenty percent of MND patients received an assisted death compared with 5 percent of cancer patients and 0.5 percent of people with heart failure (Maessen et al. 2010).

Some patients with ALS/MND have expressed an interest in being organ donors after time of death. There is reluctance to accept organs from patients with ALS/MND out of concern that the potential for a transmissible agent being present in tissues represents an unacceptable risk to a would-be donor recipient. Ethical concerns relate to weighing organ recipient's safety versus depriving patients of potentially life-saving organs, albeit from patients with ALS/MND. On rare occasions, patients with ALS have petitioned to donate organs while still alive, and it has been reported that following euthanasia, the organs were donated (Bollen et al. 2016a, b).

Right to Try

The "Right to Try" movement offers the potential for patients having incurable diseases to have access to unlicensed drugs and other therapeutic interventions not presently available. There are ethical concerns related to patient safety versus the desire to allow the patient to exercise his/her free will and self-determination regarding personal choice related to risks and potential benefits of unproven therapies. Again, the following chapters show considerable variation across countries.

Not surprisingly, charlatans and "quacks" prey on patients with incurable diseases such as ALS/MND. There is a long history of patients with ALS/MND being taken advantage of by such individuals. Useless and potentially harmful potions and concoctions, having no scientific basis, have been taken by patients at considerable personal risk and economic cost. The violation of ethical principles is obvious, but is very difficult to contain.

PUBLIC POLICY CONTEXT

Embedded in many of these ethical concerns are legal and public policy issues. Moreover, funding of ALS/MND research and care must compete for public attention and political support for its share of societal resources, not only with non-health areas but also with more visible causes like cancer and AIDS and even other neurological diseases such as Alzheimer's disease, Parkinson's disease and MS. The move of ALS/MND to the policy domain also brings to the forefront political deliberations and divisions and places the resolution of issues in the milieu of interest group politics. Given the high economic, social and personal stakes surrounding ALS/

MND, conflict is unavoidable because each group has its own demands for attention and resources.

As noted earlier, the impact of ALS/MND goes well beyond the health care needs of the person affected. As the impact of ALS/MND progresses, the patient becomes increasingly dependent on others for basic daily care and routine tasks, a physically safe environment and protection from exploitation or abuse. Addressing the diverse medical and social care needs of ALS/MND patients requires the adoption of a multifaceted policy framework and agenda that explicitly acknowledge their complex and unique needs and the impact it has on caregivers and society at large. Public policies related to social service agencies that provide housing and financial and legal services must complement other policies. These include research funding, prevention and risk reduction, symptom management, access to assistive technologies and efficient health care delivery. Although there are many books on ALS/MND, none to date provides a major focus on these areas. This book is offered as a first step in filling this void.

Funding policies are critical for research to determine the cause(s) of ALS/MND, how to prevent it, diagnose it early and accurately and how to slow its progression, if not cure it. At present, funding levels for ALS/MND research are low, even on a per-patient level, as compared to cancer, heart disease and AIDS. Furthermore, long-term services and support are critical for ALS/MND patients. Payment policy for both home and institutional care and strategies to support community living are fundamental for those with late-stage ALS/MND. An increasing proportion of patients is likely to spend some time in long-term care facilities at some point in their life. Critically important to support for those who remain in their homes are services such as caregiver support, respite care centers and, at some stage, palliative and hospice care services.

Considerably more resources are needed to better understand the impact of environmental factors on ALS/MND and develop more effective preventive strategies. Although to date the public health/preventive dimension of ALS/MND has been constrained, as more is known about its causes, this will become more relevant. Addressing healthy lifestyle and risk factors where they are known as well as community readiness are important for a population approach to managing the growing burden. Related to this is the need for regulation of the marketing of untested natural supplements and other products for ALS/MND patients.

Policies must be put in place to address the challenge of ensuring a competent and adequate workforce, especially for hands-on caregivers, such as personal care assistants and home health aides. At present much care is informal by family and friends, but this is changing in many countries. A shift to paid caregivers raises questions as to whether they need to be regulated through licensing or other mechanisms. Here again the comparative approach is valuable in how best to develop compensation mechanisms for family caregivers of patients with chronic incurable illnesses. There is also a need to provide protection from potential exploitation, abuse and neglect. Although there is little evidence of abuse of ALS/MND patients by formal or informal caregivers, it is a well-documented problem with Alzheimer's patients and others in long-term care.

Basic policy questions relate to what institutional services exist for the care of ALS/MND patients; how, where and by whom these patients are treated; how aggressive and costly the treatment regime is (e.g. what is the availability of intensive care units?); who makes the final decisions as to level of care given; and who pays the escalating costs? What types of hospice operate and what level of palliative care and pain management are accessible to patients with ALS/MND? More specific questions regarding the end of life relate to availability of medical specialists and adequate pain management, palliative care and hospice services. Control of pain, of other symptoms and of psychological, social and spiritual problems is paramount to provide the best possible quality of life for patients and their families.

Accompanying the medical dimensions of policy-making at the end of life are the social and legal aspects. In many Western countries, considerable emphasis in recent decades has been directed toward empowerment of the patient or patient autonomy. A wide variety of legal mechanisms have been created toward this end. Prominent among these advance directives (ADs) are the living will and the durable power of attorney for health care. The stated goal of ADs is to return to the individual the ability to control the dying process, by expressing avoidances and preferences often related to life-extending interventions. However, they also include a resource allocation dimension and in most cases are designed to specify limits on continued treatments, but in some instances may include the directive to "do everything possible." A key policy question is how different countries define and deal with these challenging end-of-life issues.

Cross-cultural Studies

The cross-national policy context presented in this book is crucial in comparing how various countries are dealing with these issues and for learning what are the most effective policies to pursue. Although it is risky to uncritically apply policies that appear to work in one country to another, cross-national research is useful to generate the evidence necessary to consider the full array of policy options open to decision-makers. Exploring the experiences of their counterparts in other jurisdictions in dealing with similar problems can be invaluable. An examination of international experiences also illuminates both the difficulties faced by and the range of approaches available to policy-makers. Studying the issues surrounding ALS/MND across many country settings can elucidate the commonalities of problems and variables across countries and provide valuable strategies for framing policy.

Likewise, cultural factors and social values vary across countries and in some cases are most crucial for ALS/MND policy. Values dominant in the West such as individual rights, personal autonomy, truth-telling and the dependence on technology to fix problems, including death, are not universal, despite what much of the bioethics literature assumes. Moreover, there may be strong cultural and value divisions within each country that are important in understanding policy issues. For instance, religious beliefs are a particularly critical dimension for death-related policies, and perhaps the single most important factor in some countries. Moreover, social structures can be central to the care of the chronically and terminally ill and in setting the boundaries of such care. In many countries extended families and communities still have a central role to play, while in other countries even the nuclear family seems to play a limited role in caregiving.

COUNTRIES SELECTED

One of the goals of this book was to expand the scope of the study to include a diverse range of countries, especially low- and middle-income countries that are often neglected. The editors were successful in commissioning chapters from twenty-one countries across the globe. As illustrated in Table 1.5, they span six continents and are representative of large and small, younger and older populations, reflecting wide variations in growth rates and urbanization and a broad range of GDP and economic variables.

The health policy of any country is the product of a multitude of factors including the intrinsic social, cultural and political fabric of a country, its political institutions and traditions, the legal system and the characteristics of its health care community. For instance, policy-making authority might be highly centralized or widely dispersed across multiple levels. Moreover, in some countries, unions and/or corporate structures are strong factors in determining social policy and might, in effect, have a veto power over

Table 1.5 Country characteristics

Country	Population	Growth rate (%)	GDP/capita in USD	Median age	Urban pop (%)
Australia	25,088,636	1.28	50,400	38	90
Belgium	11,562,784	0.56	46,600	42	96
Brazil	212,392,717	0.72	15,600	33	86
Canada	37,279,811	0.88	48,400	41	83
China	1,420,062,022	0.35	16,700	39	60
Germany	82,438,639	0.18	50,800	47	76
India	1,368,737,513	1.08	7200	28	34
Ireland	4,847,139	0.90	73,200	39	65
Israel	8,424,904	1.49	36,400	30	92
Italy	59,216,525	−0.13	38,200	48	72
Japan	126,854,745	−0.26	42,900	48	94
Mexico	127,575,529	1.09	19,900	29	80
Nigeria	200,962,417	2.60	5900	18	52
Pakistan	204,596,442	1.88	5400	23	40
Poland	38,028,278	−0.20	29,600	42	61
Russia	143,895,551	−0.05	27,900	40	73
S. Korea	51,339,238	0.34	39,500	43	82
S. Africa	58,065,097	1.16	13,600	27	63
Tunisia	11,718,694	0.95	11,900	32	69
UK	66,959,016	0.58	44,300	41	81
US	329,093,110	0.71	59,800	38	84

Source: World Factbook (2020)

proposed policy changes made by the government. Likewise, the influence of the medical industry and medical and nursing associations varies widely, as does the power of insurance providers in shaping health policy.

In addition to the values and institutions of a country, health policy is shaped by the composition of its population and by demographic patterns. Heterogeneous, multicultural populations require more complex health systems than more homogeneous ones. Likewise, older populations have needs different from younger ones. Populations can also be stratified by class, economic status or other social groupings. The way in which medical resources are distributed also reflects the current state of medical technology and the public expectations and demands that accompany it. Population growth rates are also crucial because they point to future health needs and relate to the dynamic composition of the population. A high growth rate requires planning for expanded services, and depending on where the growth is coming from (e.g. births, immigration), a change in types of services is needed. In contrast, a low or negative growth rate might indicate difficulties in funding services even at the existing level.

Not surprisingly, health policy is influenced significantly by a country's financial resources. Studies across developed and developing countries find that the per capita income of a country is the single most important factor when explaining health expenditure variation. Some countries often have difficulties meeting even minimal health needs, much less the types and range of services needed by patients with ALS/MND. By including a wide range of countries on this measure, we should obtain a much more complete picture of existing ALS/MND policy as well as the policy challenges it raises.

SUMMARY OF INDIVIDUAL CHAPTER OBJECTIVES

Chapter authors were asked to discuss key aspects of public policy in their respective countries as it relates to ALS/MND funding, patient care and family caregiver support. One emphasis was on governmental agencies and actions, special reports pertaining to ALS/MND patient care and research support, as well as activities of private foundations and advocacy groups. Other foci included the location of care provided; access to assistive technologies; the availability of ALS/MND multidisciplinary clinics; use of advance directives; and the legal status of palliative sedation, withholding and withdrawing life-extending care, PAS and euthanasia. Authors were also asked what social and cultural factors unique to their country might help explain ALS/MND policy and what changes and improvements in policy could lead to enhanced patient care and research support for ALS/MND.

To address these concerns and provide a starting point for coverage and facilitate comparative data, chapter contributors were asked to address, where appropriate for their country, the below questions and issues. To avoid repetition, authors were asked not to include the background information on ALS/MND which has been provided in this chapter.

1. Incidence and prevalence and deaths of ALS/MND in their country.
2. What, if any, governmental action, reports, committees on ALS/MND exist?
3. Major governmental agencies involved in care—national, state, local.
4. The most active private ALS/MND organizations, associations, advocacy groups.

5. Policy associated with ALS/MND research and the relative contributions from the public versus private sectors.
6. How much public funding for research and care? Is it satisfactory?
7. Public/media/commercial perceptions of ALS/MND.
8. What proportion of ALS/MND patients live at home vs institutional care?
9. Composition of caregivers—informal, formal (paid). Any trends?
10. Governmental aid for family caregivers—financial or respite care?
11. Access to assistive technologies such as electronic communication devices?
12. Status of multidisciplinary team care and clinics.
13. "Right to try" legislation advocating for ALS/MND patients to be treated with drugs that have not yet been approved.
14. Genetic testing for ALS/MND. Who pays? What protections for confidentiality are provided for patients and blood relatives being tested?
15. What proportion dies at home, in nursing facility, hospital or hospice?
16. Access to palliative and hospice care, with estimate of percent of ALS/MND patients eventually enrolled in hospice care?
17. Legal status of advance directives and withholding or withdrawing mechanical ventilation and other life-extending interventions and mechanical support.
18. Legal status of palliative sedation, euthanasia and physician-assisted suicide.
19. What factors unique to the country (cultural, social, religious, economic, etc.) are critical for understanding decision-making in that country?
20. What, if any, changes in policy are needed to improve care of ALS/MND patients and support for family caregivers and to advance research support for the cure or development of disease-modifying treatments?

We thank the numerous authors who gave generously their time and collaborative efforts while providing insights and expertise necessary for the publication of this book. We hope those reading this volume will find it a useful guide to international perspectives on public policy for ALS/MND and will help facilitate the development of future collaboration and exchange of ideas across even more countries. The concluding chapter will discuss policy options and summarize how best to ensure workable and humane ALS policy for the coming decades. An underlying theme is that such a policy requires a cross-national, multidisciplinary effort.

REFERENCES

Al Chalabi, A., F. Fang, M.F. Hanby et al. (2010). An estimate of amyotrophic lateral sclerosis heritability using twin data. *Journal of Neurology, Neurosurgery and Psychiatry* 81: 1324–26.

Al-Chalabi, A. and O. Hardiman (2013). The epidemiology of ALS: A conspiracy of genes, environment and time. *Nature Reviews Neurology* 9: 617–28.

Al-Chalabi, A., A. Calvo, A. Chio et al. (2014). Analysis of amyotrophic lateral sclerosis as a multistep process: A population-based modelling system. *Lancet Neurology* 13: 1108–13.

Andersen, P.M. and A. Al-Chalabi (2011). Clinical genetics of amyotrophic lateral sclerosis: What do we really know? *Nature Reviews Neurology* 7: 603–15.

Andersen, P.M., S. Abrahams, G.D. Borasio et al. (2012). The efns task force on diagnosis and management of amyotrophic lateral sclerosis. EFNS Guidelines on the clinical management of amyotrophic lateral sclerosis (MALS)—revised report of an EFNS Task Force. *European Journal of Neurology* 19: 360–75.

Aridegbe, T., R. Kandler, S.J. Walters et al. (2013). The natural history of motor neuron disease: Assessing the impact of specialist care. *Amytrophic Lateral Sclerosis* 14: 13–19.

Armon, C. (2013). What is ALS? In R.S. Bedlack and H. Mitsumoto, eds., *Amyotrophic Lateral Sclerosis: A Patient Care Guide for Clinicians*. New York: Demos Medical Publishing.

Armon, C. and R.G. Miller (2011). Correspondence regarding TDP-43 proteinopathy and motor neuron disease in chronic traumatic encephalopathy. *Journal of Neuropathology and Experimental Neurology* 70: 97–98.

Bedlack, R.S. and H. Mitsumoto, eds. (2013). *Amyotrophic Lateral Sclerosis: A Patient Care Guide for Clinicians*. New York: Demos Medical Publishing.

Bedlack, R.S., A. Genge, A.A. Amato et al. (2011). Correspondence regarding TDP-43 proteinopathy and motor neuron disease in chronic traumatic encephalopathy. *Journal of Neuropathology and Experimental Neurology* 70: 96–97.

Benatar, M.G., J.E. Kurent, and D.H. Moore. (2009). Treatment for familial amyotrophic lateral sclerosis/motor neuron disease. *Cochrane Reviews* 21: CD006153. https://doi.org/10.1002/14651858.CD006153.pub2.abstract

Bernat, J.L. (2008). *Ethical Issues in Neurology*, 3rd edition. New York and London: American Academy of Neurology Press and Lippincott Williams & Wilkins.

Bollen, J., R. Ten Hoopen, D. Ysebaert et al. (2016a). Legal and ethical aspects of organ donation after euthanasia in Belgium and the Netherlands. *Journal of Medical Ethics* 42 (8): 486–89.

Bollen, J., W. de Jongh, J. Hagenaars et al. (2016b). Organ donation after euthanasia: A Dutch practical manual. *American Journal of Transplantation* 16: 1967–72.

Brooks, B., R. Miller, M. Swash, and T. Munsat (2000). Diseases WFoNRGoMN. El Escorialrevisited: Revised criteria for the diagnosis of amyotrophic lateral sclerosis. *Amyotrophic Lateral Sclerosis and other Motor Neuron Disorders* 1: 293–99.

Brown, R.H. and A. Al-Chalabi (2017). Amyotrophic lateral sclerosis. A review. *New England Journal of Medicine* 377: 162–72.

Carver, A.C. (1996). End-of-life care: A survey of US neurologists' attitudes, behavior and knowledge. *Neurology* 53: 284–93.

Cedarbaum, J.M., N. Stambler, E. Malta et al. (1999). The ALSFRS-R: A revised ALS functional rating scale that incorporates assessments of respiratory function. *Journal of Neurological Sciences* 169: 13–21.

Chen, A., L. Weimer, T. Brannagan et al. (2010). Experience with the Awaji Island modifications to the ALS diagnostic criteria. *Muscle and Nerve* 42: 831–32.

Cherny, N.I., L. Radbruch et al. (2009). European Association for Palliative Care (EAPC) recommended framework for the use of sedation in palliative care. *Palliative Medicine* 23: 581–93.

Chio, A., G. Logroscino, B.J. Traynor et al. (2013). Global epidemiology of amyotrophic lateral sclerosis: A systematic review of the published literature. *Neuroepidemiology* 41: 118–30.

Chio, A., L. Mazzini, S. D'Alfonso et al. (2018). The multistep hypothesis revisited—The role of genetic mutations. *Neurology* 91: e635–42.

Corcia, P., P. Couratier, H. Blaco et al. (2017). Genetics of amyotrophic lateral sclerosis. *Revue Neurologique* 173: 254–62.

Costa, J., M. Swash, and M. de Carvalho (2012). Awaji criteria for the diagnosis of amyotrophic lateral sclerosis: A systematic review. *Archives of Neurology* 69 (11): 1410–16.

Couratier, P., P. Corcia, G. Lautrette, M. Nicol, and B. Marin (2017). ALS and frontotemporal dementia belong to a common disease spectrum. *Review of Neurology (Paris)* 173: 273–79.

Goldstein, L.H. (2014). Control of symptoms: Cognitive dysfunction. In D. Oliver, G.D. Borasio, and W. Johnston, eds., *Palliative Care in Amyotrophic Lateral Sclerosis: From Diagnosis to Bereavement*, 3rd edition. Oxford: Oxford University Press, pp. 107–25.

Gursahani, R. (2016). Palliative care and the Indian neurologist. *Annals of Indian Academy of Neurology* 19 (Suppl 1): S40–44.

Horner, R.D., K.G. Kamins, J.R. Feussner et al. (2003). Occurrence of amyotrophic lateral sclerosis among Gulf War Veterans. *Neurology* 61: 742–49.

Johnston, M., L. Earll, E. Mitchell et al. (1996). Communicationg the diagnosis of motor neurone disease. *Palliative Medicine* 10: 23–34.

Lomen-Hoerth, C.J., S. Murphy, S. Langmore et al. (2003). Are amyotrophic lateral sclerosis patients cognitively normal? *Neurology* 60: 1094–97.

Ly, C.V. and T.M. Miller (2018). Emerging antisense oligonucleotide and viral therapies for amyotrophic lateral sclerosis. *Current Opinions Neurology* 31 (5): 648–54.

Maessen, M., J.H. Veldink, L.H. van den Berg et al. (2010). Requests for euthanasia: Origin of suffering in ALS, heart failure and cancer patients. *Journal of Neurology* 2010: 1192–98.

Magyari, M. and P.S. Sorensen (2019). The changing course of multiple sclerosis: Rising incidence, change in geographic distribution, disease course, and prognosis. *Current Opinions in Neurology* 32 (3): 320–36.

Malek, A., A. Barchowsky, R. Bowser et al. (2013). Exposure to hazardous air pollutants and the risk of amyotrophic lateral sclerosis. *Environmental Pollution* 197: 181–86.

McKee, A.C., B.E. Gavett, R.A. Stern et al. (2010). Correspondence regarding TDP-43 proteinopathy and motor neuron disease in chronic traumatic encephalopathy. *Journal of Neuropathology and Experimental Neurology* 42: 851–52.

McKhann, G.M., M.S. Albert, M. Grossman et al. (2001). Clinical and pathological diagnosis of frontotemporal dementia report of the work group on frontotemporal dementia and pick's disease. *Archives of Neurology* 58: 1803–9.

Miller, R.G., J.A. Rosenberg, D.F. Gelinas, H. Mitsumoto et al. (1999). The care of the patient with amyotrophic lateral sclerosis (an evidence-based review): Report of the quality standards subcommittee of the American Academy of Neurology: ALS practice parameters taskforce. *Neurology* 52: 1311–23.

Miller, R.G., C.E. Jackson, E.J. Karsarkis, J.D. England et al. (2009). Practice parameter update: The care of the patient with amyotrophic lateral sclerosis: Multidisciplinary care, symptom management, and cognitive/behavioural impairment (an evidence-based review). *Neurology* 73: 1227–33.

Miller, T., M. Cudkowicz, P.J. Shaw et al. (2020). Phase 1-2 trial of antisense oligonucleotide Tofersen for SOD1 ALS. *New England Journal of Medicine* 383: 109–19.

Mueller, C., J.D. Berry, D.M. McKenna-Yasek et al. (2020). SOD1 suppression with adeno-associated virus and microRNA in familial ALS. *New England Journal of Medicine* 383: 151–58.

National Hospice and Palliative Care Organization (2010). Position statement and commentary on imminently dying terminally ill patients. *Journal of Pain and Symptom Management* 2010: 914–23.

National Institute for Health and Care Excellence (2016). Motor neurone disease: Assessment and management. NICE Guideline NG 42. www.nice.org.uk/guidance/NG42

Neudert, C., D. Oliver, M. Wasner and G.D. Borasio (2001). The course of the terminal phase in patients with amyotrophic lateral sclerosis. *Journal of Neurology* 248: 612–16.

Oliver, D.J. and M.R. Turner (2010). Some difficult decisions in ALS/MND. *Amyotrophic Lateral Sclerosis* 11: 339–43

Phukan, J. (2012). The syndrome of cognitive impairment in amyotrophic lateral sclerosis: A population-based study. *Journal of Neuropathology and Experimental Neurology* 83: 102–08.

Radbruch, L., C. Leget, P. Bahr et al. (2016). Euthanasia and physician-assisted suicide: A white paper from the European Association for Palliative Care. *Palliative Medicine* 30: 104–16.

Robert Wood Johnson Foundation (2004). Completing the continuum of ALS care: A consensus document. https://www.promotingexcellence.org/als/als_report/

Rooney, J., S. Byrne, M. Heverin et al. (2015). A multidisciplinary clinic approach improves survival in ALS: A comparative study of ALS in Ireland and Northern Ireland. *Journal of Neurology, Neurosurgery and Psychiatry* 86: 496–503.

Rosen, D.R., T. Siddique, D. Patterson et al. (1993). Mutations in Cu/Zn super-oxide dismutase gene are associated with familial amyotrophic lateral sclerosis. *Nature* 362: 59–62.

Seeber, A.A., A.J. Pols, A. Hijdra et al. (2019). Experiences and reflections of patients with motor neuron disease on breaking the news in a two-tiered appointment: A qualitative study. *BMJ Support Palliative Care* 9 (1): e8. https://doi.org/10.1136/bmjspcare-2015-000977.

Seelen, M., R.A. Toro Campos, J.H. Veldink et al. (2017). Long-term air pollution exposure and amyotrophic lateral sclerosis in Netherlands: A population-based case-control study. *Environmental Health Perspectives* 125: 097023.

Shaw, C., A. Quinn and E. Daniel (2014). Amyotrophic lateral sclerosis/motor neuron disease. In D. Oliver, G.D. Borasio, and W. Johnston, eds., *Palliative Care in Amyotrophic Lateral Sclerosis: From Diagnosis to Bereavement*, 3rd edition. Oxford: Oxford University Press.

Sloan, R. and G.D. Borasio (2014). Communication: Breaking the news. In D. Oliver, G.D. Borasio, and W. Johnston, eds., *Palliative Care in Amyotrophic Lateral Sclerosis: From Diagnosis to Bereavement*, 3rd edition. Oxford: Oxford University Press.

Strong, M., G.M. Grace, M. Freedman et al. (2009). Consensus criteria for the diagnosis of frontotemporal cognitive and behavioral syndromes in amyo-trophic lateral sclerosis. *Amyotrophic Lateral Sclerosis* 10: 131–46.

Tarr, I.S., E.P. McCann, B. Benyami et al. (2019). Monozygotic twins and triplets discordant for amyotrophic lateral sclerosis display differential methylation and gene expression. *Scientific Reports* 9: 1–17.

Weisskopf, M.G., M.J. O'Reilly, M.L. McCullough et al. (2005). Prospective study of military service and mortality from ALS. *Neurology* 64: 32–37.

Westeneng, H.J., R. Walhout, M. Straathof et al. (2016). Widespread structural brain involvement in ALS is not limited to the *C9orf72* repeat expansion. *Journal of Neurology, Neurosurgery and Psychiatry* 87: 1354–60.

World Factbook (2020). https://www.cia.gov/library/publications/the-world-factbook/

Xi, Z., Y. Yunosova, M. Van Blitterswijk et al. (2014). Identical twins with the C9orf72 repeat expansion are discordant for ALS. *Neurology* 83: 1476–78.

CHAPTER 2

Public Policy in MND Care: The Australian Perspective

Samar Aoun, Carol Birks, Anne Hogden, and Susan Mathers

Abstract Financial support, access to respite care, 'in-home support' and assistive technologies and access to specialist palliative care for MND patients vary between and within the Australian states and the age groups of patients. While care takes place mainly at home, proportions dying at

S. Aoun (✉)
Perron Institute for Neurological and Translational Science, Perth, Australia
e-mail: dr.s.aoun@gmail.com

La Trobe University, Melbourne, Australia
e-mail: samar.aoun@perron.uwa.edu.au

C. Birks
MND Australia, Canberra, Australia
e-mail: carolb@mndaustralia.org.au

A. Hogden
University of Tasmania, Sydney, Australia
e-mail: anne.hogden@utas.edu.au

S. Mathers
Calvary Health Care Bethlehem and Monash University, Melbourne, Australia
e-mail: susan.mathers@calvarycare.org.au

© The Author(s) 2021
R. H. Blank et al. (eds.), *Public Policy in ALS/MND Care*,
https://doi.org/10.1007/978-981-15-5840-5_2

home vary between 25 and 34 percent. MND multidisciplinary clinics operate in the capital city of each mainland state. Most states have statutory Advance Health Directives, but voluntary assisted dying is only available in the states of Victoria and Western Australia to date. To improve care and advance research, improvements are needed at three levels: the government, the workforce and the community. Public services need to be delivered in a more timely, efficient, integrated and equitable manner. In order to inform future planning and policies for solutions to the growing demand for family/informal care and the associated challenges encountered by family carers, it is essential to integrate family carers' needs into service planning.

Keywords MND associations • Research funding • Multidisciplinary teams • Assistive technology • Genetic testing • Palliative care • Voluntary assisted dying • Integrated care • Funding models

Incidence, Prevalence and Deaths of MND in Australia

An accurate figure for the incidence of MND in Australia is difficult to ascertain as there are no official records of every person diagnosed nor mandatory reporting. In Australia, MND associations maintain a record of people with a confirmed diagnosis of MND who join as members. From July 2018 to June 2019, 756 people recently diagnosed with MND had joined a state MND association (Motor Neurone Disease Australia 2019). However, diagnosis may have taken some time or people may not have joined immediately following diagnosis. The Australian MND Registry also registers people with MND who are referred to a specialist MND clinic, however, this registry does not capture people diagnosed with MND who are not referred to these clinics or who cannot access them due to distance. A Deloitte Access Economics Report commissioned by MND Australia in 2015 estimated the mortality rate to be 3.14/100,000 across the entire population (Deloitte Access Economics 2015). It could be assumed that mortality rate and incidence rate are similar, which would indicate that based on the current population of Australia of 25,088,636, the incidence rate is approximately 788 persons per year.

The Deloitte Access Economics Report found that Australia has a relatively high level of prevalence in comparison to other countries, and it was estimated that there were 2094 Australians living with MND in 2015. Of that 60 percent were males and 40 percent were females. The highest prevalence rate was reported in males aged between 75 and 84. Based on the analysis undertaken in this report, the overall prevalence of MND in Australia is estimated to be 8.7/100,000 Australians, or 1 in 11,434 Australians.

Each year MND Australia makes a special request to the Australian Institute of Health and Welfare (AIHW) for data from the National Mortality Database on deaths with MND as underlying cause and deaths with MND as an associated cause. Adding both associated causes and underlying causes of death gives the total known deaths associated with MND in Australia. This data indicates that there were 755 known deaths of people with MND in 2018 due to any cause, of which 692 deaths were specifically due to MND (MND was listed as an underlying cause) (Motor Neurone Disease Australia 2018a).

Governmental Agencies Involved in Care

The complex and progressing nature of MND requires an interdisciplinary approach encompassing health, disability, community, aged, respite and carer support services.

The Australian healthcare system provides people with access to general practitioners (GPs), neurology, respiratory, gastroenterology, neuropsychology, rehabilitation, nursing, palliative care and allied health services to address their medical needs and to monitor progression. Universal access to healthcare is available through the national publicly funded Medicare system, supported (for some people) by private health insurance, with either local, state or federal governments being responsible for delivery of services.

Access to allied health can be complex with some allied health providers funded through the health system and others through the recently introduced National Disability Insurance Scheme (NDIS). The NDIS provides fully funded reasonable and necessary disability supports to Australians with a permanent disability who are aged 64 or younger when they enter the scheme (Carer Gateway 2019). The last few years have seen a national roll out of the NDIS with a full roll out completed on 1 July 2019. This scheme is a transformational change in the way disability supports are provided and funded in Australia. The scheme is funded by the Australian government and to date all sides of politics have pledged to fully fund the scheme.

For people aged 65 years or older when diagnosed with MND, their disability support must be accessed through the aged care system. Unlike the NDIS where anyone with a permanent disability, including people with MND, is entitled to access the scheme, older people with MND must be assessed as eligible to access an aged care community home care package. These packages are funded by the Australian government with a cap on the number of packages available, a means-tested co-payment and a limit on funds available to support assessed needs.

Access to assistive technology may be through a person's MND association, their NDIS plan or a state government-funded equipment service. Similarly, respite and carer support services may be accessed through or funded by MND associations, the NDIS or Australian government carer respite services.

Active MND Associations and Advocacy Groups

MND associations were established in each of the Australian states and the Australian Capital Territory (ACT) over 37 years ago to support people living with MND; their family, friends and carers; and the health and community providers involved in their care (Motor Neurone Disease Australia 2018b). The ACT association merged with MND New South Wales (NSW), and today the six state MND associations provide direct services and support through the National MND Support Service Model to people living with MND and their family and friends across Australia (Motor Neurone Disease Australia 2018c).

MND Australia was established in 1991 by the state MND associations to provide a national voice for MND. MND Australia is focused on improving the lives of all Australians impacted by MND by influencing policy through advocacy, providing and developing trusted information in various formats, raising awareness and understanding of MND nationally and promoting and funding the best research. MND Australia is committed to building partnerships and strategic alliances to more effectively liaise with government to ensure that policies support the interests of people living with MND. To advocate effectively, MND Australia works to co-advocate with related organizations in the research, medical and care sectors such as the Neurological Alliance Australia, Palliative Care

Australia, Carers Australia, Research Australia, Stem Cells Australia and Rare Voices Australia. MND Australia has been an active member of the International Alliance of ALS/MND associations for over 26 years. More recently, MND Australia has focused specifically on supporting collaborations and partnerships in the Asia Pacific region.

There are several other MND organizations in Australia. The MND and Me Foundation was established in 2010 in Queensland to provide additional support to Queenslanders impacted by MND and to fund vital research (MND and Me 2019). Fight MND (formerly known as Cure MND) was established in 2014 to raise awareness and funds for research, mainly clinical trials, and assistive technology (Fight MND 2019).

Funding for Research and Care

In Australia, funding for MND research is provided by a combination of government, private, non-government/not-for-profit and philanthropic sectors. Care is mostly funded through state and federal government agencies related to health, disability and aged care. The MND Research Australia (former name MNDRIA) is the research arm of MND Australia and has been funding MND research with the greatest chance of moving us closer to a world free of MND for over 30 years. A recent report *25 Million 25 Milestones: Changing the Future of MND* highlights the impact of MND Research Australia funding in Australia over this time (Motor Neurone Disease Australia 2017a). The ALS/MND community and the state-based MND associations have always been effective fundraisers, channeling funds to care, equipment, as well as research through MND Research Australia.

Since its inception in 2014, Fight MND has raised substantial funds (over $28.5 million to mid-2019) for research, thereby changing the research landscape in Australia through accelerating precision medicine and access to clinical trials. As well as funding competitive research grants through the National Health and Medical Research Council (NHMRC), the medical research future fund (MRFF) and other commonwealth agencies, the federal government in recent years has contributed funding to Fight MND to fund research focused on clinical trial pathways in Australia.

Although several specialist MND clinics have developed across Australia, this has largely been driven by local partnerships and small groups of motivated individuals. These groups are now working together at a national level to increase access to research and clinical trials for people with

MND. The sustainability of these alliances, however, still relies on piece-meal funding from competitive grants and philanthropy, despite education and research being part of the remit of state-funded tertiary and quaternary health services.

Proportion of Patients Who Live at Home vs. Institutional Care

The aim of care in Australia is to support people to live and die in the setting of their choice. Most people with MND prefer to remain at home and in their community to receive care and most people achieve this goal. Others may remain at home with support from family, friends and government-funded health and community home-based support and then choose to enter a hospice or hospital for end-of-life care. For Australians who do not have enough family and community support to stay at home, an admission to a residential aged care facility is then required. With the introduction of the NDIS, it is more likely that older people are in this situation. There are no accurate figures for people with MND living in residential aged care. However, according to deaths in Table 2.1, the proportion could be between 16% and 28% depending on the Australian state.

Composition and Support for Caregivers

The demographic information on informal caregivers is gleaned from a national survey undertaken in Australia to explore the experiences with receiving the diagnosis of MND (Aoun et al. 2017a). The mean age of responding family caregivers (n = 190) was 62.1 years (SD = 12.4, range 25–88): 67.2 percent were females, 93.8 percent were married, 82.8 percent were the spouses or partners of the person with MND, 11.7 percent

Table 2.1 Proportions in each place of death (percent) 2017–18

Place of death	Victoria	WA	NSW
Home	25	34	25
Hospital	23	28	24
Hospice/palliative care unit	22	17	21
Nursing home	28	16	18
Unknown	2	4	11

were their adult children and 52.9 percent of family caregivers were retirees. Although there is no official information on the composition of paid caregivers in the MND setting, they are employed under two government-funded schemes, the NDIS for the group under 65 years and the My Aged Care packages for the group 65 years and over.

Australia has a national strategy for supporting family caregivers (Carer Recognition Act 2010) and National Palliative Care Strategy (2018) (Carer Recognition Act 2010 (Austl.); Australian Government 2018). Government financial support exists for people with significant disability including those with terminal illness that indirectly benefits carers; however, direct support is generally income and asset tested. A carer payment provides income support for inability to work because of the demands of caregiving. There is also a carer allowance which is a smaller income supplement for daily caregiving to those aged or with severe disability. Support for out-of-pocket costs such as travel and accommodation is available for patients, but not their caregivers, and there is a subsidy for patients living more than 100 km from a healthcare provider. There are concessions for carers traveling with a disabled person in the form of carer's card or companion card for those with significant and permanent disability (WA Companion Card 2016). The Taxi User's Subsidy Scheme (TUSS) is another resource that can be accessed at a reduced rate (Department of Transport 2019).

Respite care provision is poor and the NDIS can provide planned respite. There is a work and care charter which promotes flexible working hours and flexible leave for caregivers, but it is voluntary with no obligations from employers. Carers of those with a disability may be eligible for reduced tax on income and for pension supplement for those receiving an existing carer's payment. However, forms to access carers' allowance and payments are generally aimed at long-term disability, not shorter, quicker deterioration as is the case with most MND cases. Furthermore, there are two energy-related schemes to help people in certain circumstances meet their energy needs: The Energy Concession Extension Scheme and the Thermoregulatory Dysfunction Energy Subsidy Scheme (www.finance.wa.gov.au).

ACCESS TO ASSISTIVE TECHNOLOGIES

According to a Deloitte Access Economics Report (Deloitte Access Economics 2015) commissioned by MND Australia in 2015, aids and equipment comprise one of the highest per-person costs. The often-rapid rate of progression requires *fast-track* access to a wide range of equipment since items need to be available as soon as a need arises and may only be required for a short period of time. The report states that aids and equipment cost $31,598 per person in 2015 and confirmed the MND association equipment loan service as a cost-effective model in providing equipment to maintain independence and communication.

For people living with MND, the full range of assistive technology may include aids and equipment to support comfort, independence and daily living, communication technology and non-invasive ventilation to support breathing, and quality and length of life. Non-invasive ventilation improves survival by 13 months on average (Berlowitz et al. 2016). Under the NDIS, people living with MND aged 64 and under are entitled to "reasonable and necessary" assistive technology to meet their needs. Where available and appropriate, a person's NDIS plan includes funding to cover hire or rental costs to enable fast-track access to individual items or a bundle of assistive technology provided by the MND association. In addition, it includes funding for reasonable and necessary home modifications and specialized individualized assistive technology.

People aged 65 or older when diagnosed with MND access assistive technology through state government assistive technology loan services, which often entail long waiting times. MND associations in Australia have built assistive technology loan pools or equipment libraries through funding received from donors, state government funding and philanthropic grants. This vital service helps people living with MND to access assistive technology in a timely manner. The range of technology available from MND associations does vary, and therefore timely access to government-funded assistive technology schemes continues to be a focus for advocacy.

People living with MND must undergo an assessment by an appropriate allied health professional, and a referral made before assistive technology is supplied by an MND association or a government-funded scheme. This professional will then train the person with MND and their carer in the correct use of the technology. Specialized respiratory support is usually provided through the person's MND clinic or health service, but access varies by state. From 1 October 2019, the NDIS has started to fund health-related supports if they are a regular part of the participant's life and a result of their disability. This includes respiratory and nutritional support.

STATUS OF MULTIDISCIPLINARY TEAM CARE AND CLINICS

Specialist neurology-led MND multidisciplinary clinics operate in Sydney, Melbourne, Brisbane, Adelaide, Canberra and Perth. Most of these clinics work out of public hospitals. In some regional and rural communities, local health practitioners have established MND-specific multidisciplinary models of care to support a coordinated approach to people living with MND in their community. Some MND multidisciplinary clinics offer e-Health (or telehealth) services to support patients and families in non-metropolitan areas, linking with local service providers where possible (Henderson et al. 2014; James et al. 2018).

"RIGHT TO TRY" LEGISLATION FOR ALS/MND PATIENTS

There is no legislation regarding right to try in Australia; however, after discussion with their neurologist, individuals may be able to apply to access products that have not yet been approved in Australia through a Special Access Scheme (SAS). There are three SAS pathways that a health practitioner may use to access an unapproved therapeutic good for an individual patient on a case-by-case basis. Category A is a notification pathway (for a patient defined as seriously ill) that may be accessed by a prescribing medical practitioner; Category B is an application pathway that can be accessed by health practitioners (usually medical or dental practitioners) if patients do not fit the Category A definition; Category C is a notification pathway that allows certain types of health practitioners to supply therapeutic goods that are deemed to have an established history of use (Motor Neurone Disease Australia 2017b).

GENETIC TESTING OF PATIENTS WITH MND

Costs for genetic testing vary considerably in Australia. Cost depends on the type of testing being conducted (diagnostic, predictive or confirmatory), the genes being tested and the type of genetics service that is accessed. For example, the cost of testing a single gene, most commonly *SOD1* or *C9orf72*, varies according to which gene is being tested. Similarly, the cost of testing a panel of genes is considerably higher than for a single gene. Moreover, the cost of predictive genetic testing in a family member with an identified gene mutation is less expensive than for diagnostic testing for that family (Crook et al. 2017). Some public hospital genetic testing services provide subsidized or free testing for MND-related genes, particularly for patients or relatives who are from a family with a history of MND. However, private genetic testing services will vary in what they charge. These costs are not covered by Medicare, the national government health insurance scheme. Genetic testing for research purposes entails no cost to the patients or family members who agree to participate in the research.

The decision to have genetic testing is voluntary, and the results are confidential, as with any medical intervention. Although an appointment with a genetic counselor is not required when the results are given, genetic counseling is recommended with pre- and post-testing (Hogden and Crook 2017). When family members are treated at the same time, the results are typically given individually to preserve confidentiality. Even so, family members may choose to have each other present for support. Testing results cannot be shared without the express consent of the person being tested, except as required by law. This includes sharing with health professionals and other family members. If testing is conducted for research, confidentiality is protected through research processes approved by a human ethics research committee. Further information about genetic testing is available for people with MND and their families from MND Australia (Motor Neurone Disease Australia 2018d).

PLACE OF DEATH: AT HOME, IN NURSING FACILITY, HOSPITAL OR HOSPICE

Recent mortality data (2017–18) obtained from three MND associations (personal communication), two large ones on the east coast (Victoria and New South Wales [NSW]) and one small on the west coast (Western Australia [WA]), suggest a total of 892 MND deaths in the past two years in the three Australian states. Looking at the proportions in Table 2.1, more deaths occurred at home and in hospital in Western Australia compared to Victoria and NSW where more deaths occurred in a nursing home or in a hospice. This reflects differences in access to and/or availability of inpatient and community services in each state.

ACCESS TO PALLIATIVE AND HOSPICE CARE

In a recent national survey of bereaved people, more people with cancer (64%) had received palliative care services in comparison to other non-malignant illnesses (4–10%), with non-malignant diseases still under-represented in palliative care in Australia (Aoun et al. 2017c). There is a very short period of a median of one month that patients were under a specialist palliative care service.

There is increasing evidence that palliative care integrated in a multidisciplinary approach to care leads to improved symptoms and quality of life of people with MND and their families (Oliver et al. 2016). It is recommended that a palliative approach be integrated into the care plan from the time of diagnosis to optimize quality of life by relieving symptoms; providing emotional, psychological and spiritual support pre-bereavement; minimizing barriers to a good death and supporting the family post-bereavement. These outcomes can only be achieved if palliative care knowledge and expertise is extended beyond the domain of specialist palliative care services to include the full scope of health and community-based services providing care, mostly at home, in order to meet the extensive range of needs of people with MND and their family carers from diagnosis to bereavement (Aoun 2018).

In Western Australia, MND patients are usually accepted into a specialist palliative care service only in the last three months of life, if they need ongoing treatment for significant unrelieved symptoms such as breathlessness, secretion management, pain and non-invasive ventilation. They are discharged if their condition improves or remains stable. People with MND in nursing homes will usually end up at hospice to receive palliative care, while those who remain at home will receive some palliative care toward the end, but only after this is arranged by their referring GP, neurologist or respiratory physician. Therefore, in line with improving the palliative approach to care and because palliative care has become synonymous with service provision in the last months or weeks of life, the MND association in Western Australia has embarked on state-wide educational program for health and community-based services at the start of 2019, which has received very positive feedback.

Palliative care is supported in Victoria by MND Palliative Care Shared Care Workers, one funded in each region. They are the "go to person" in palliative care regarding MND and they work closely with MND association advisors. Palliative care is supported by additional funding for inpatient and community-based services to recognize the extended services that may be required by people with MND, including top-up funding (Victorian Government 2008).

LEGAL STATUS OF ADVANCE DIRECTIVES AND WITHHOLDING OR WITHDRAWING LIFE-EXTENDING INTERVENTIONS AND MECHANICAL SUPPORT

The legal status of Advance Health Directives (AHD) is complicated by differences between state and territory laws. Advance Care Planning (ACP) is supported in Australia by both statute law and common law (Advance Care Planning Australia 2018). However, the laws and legislative frameworks vary from state to state. All states and territories have statutory Advance Care Directives (ACDs), excepting New South Wales and Tasmania. In these states, ACDs are recognized as valid in common law. All ACDs in Australia can include refusal of specific, or all, treatments (except palliative care) and withdrawal of life-extending measures. Most states and territories recognize ACDs of other states and territories, except the Australian Capital Territory and Tasmania. This has implications for people with MND intending to visit, receive services or relocate interstate. However, according to a recent national survey of bereaved people, the uptake of such AHD and ACP documents is still low in Australia at about 10 percent, although those who received palliative care were two to three times more likely to have an ACP or AHD in place (Aoun et al. 2017c).

LEGAL STATUS OF EUTHANASIA AND PHYSICIAN-ASSISTED SUICIDE

Euthanasia is illegal in Australia, but Victoria and Western Australia are the only two states to recently enact similar voluntary assisted dying laws. From June 2019, Victorians who are suffering from an incurable, advanced and progressive disease, illness or medical condition, and who are experiencing intolerable suffering, are eligible (Health Victoria 2019). The condition must be assessed by two medical practitioners as being expected to cause death within six months. Exceptions are for people suffering from a neurodegenerative condition, such as MND or multiple sclerosis, where the condition must be expected to cause death within 12 months.

Voluntary assisted dying is only available to people over the age of 18 who have lived in Victoria for at least 12 months and who have decision-making capacity. To be eligible, people must be experiencing suffering that cannot be relieved in a manner the person considers tolerable. In the

Victorian model, the responsibility of assisted dying lies with the patient. However if the patient is physically incapable of self-administering, the doctor needs to apply for a practitioner administration permit.

The voluntary assisted dying laws for Western Australia were passed on 10 December 2019 with an 18-month implementation period. Voluntary assisted dying in WA may be through self-administration or practitioner administration of the dying substance. The death certificate must not include any reference to voluntary assisted dying.

CRITICAL FACTORS FOR UNDERSTANDING POLICY MAKING IN AUSTRALIA

Healthcare Structure and Funding Arrangements

The Australian healthcare system has a complex structure dominated by the constitutional boundary between federal and state responsibilities. The major responsibilities of the Australian government include health service funding, regulation of health products, services and workforce, primary and aged care and veteran's affairs. The federal government has responsibility for the universal public health insurance scheme, Medicare (including subsidizing medical services and providing funding for primary health networks).

The Australian government partially funds eight state and territory health systems.

These systems are primarily responsible for the delivery and management of public health services, including public hospitals, community health and public dental care, and the regulation of healthcare providers and private health facilities. Public hospitals, for example, are licensed, regulated and funded by the Australian, state and territory governments, but managed by state and territory governments. Local governments fund and deliver some health services such as environmental health programs.

The Australian healthcare system is a combination of both public and private health organizations and individual providers. Australia provides universal healthcare to the population regardless of geographical location or financial capacity. This includes access to emergency medical care via ambulance/paramedicine services, emergency departments and intensive care units. However, these systems are now underpinned by co-payment arrangements, whereby patients in many instances contribute directly—through private health insurance or payments for medicines, tests or specialists—and indirectly—via taxation arrangements—to fund the care they receive (Australian Institute of Health and Welfare 2016).

Geography

Australia's vast geography combined with a relatively small population that is concentrated around coastal areas has a significant impact on how easily Australians can access the health services they need (Hogden et al. 2017). This is particularly so for people with MND in accessing specialized MND and palliative care services. Specialized MND multidisciplinary clinics exist in only six metropolitan areas, meaning that people living in regional or rural areas may have to travel long distances (hours or even days) to receive services. This puts regional and rural patients at a disadvantage if fatigue and mobility problems restrict them.

While telehealth offers a solution for many therapeutic interventions, palliative care, particularly at the end-of-life, requires hands-on service (Henderson et al. 2014; James et al. 2018). The training of local health providers in an integrated palliative approach may go a long way toward reducing the tyranny of distance (Hogden et al. 2018).

Cultural Diversity

Australia is culturally diverse: one in four Australians was born overseas, identifying with more than 270 ancestries; and 20 percent of Australians speak a language other than English at home (Australian Human Rights Commission 2015). Over 200 languages are spoken in this multicultural society. MND occurs in all populations; therefore, services for people with MND and their families also need to provide for a range of languages, health literacy abilities and cultural beliefs. Health services increasingly have become more tailored to the characteristics of the local community. For example, specialized services are provided for aboriginal health by members of the indigenous community. Service providers need an understanding of the end-of-life considerations of their local communities, including chaplaincy, attitudes to information-sharing, death customs (including preparation of the body and timing of burial after death) and Australian laws and procedures (which differ from state to state).

POLICY CHANGES NEEDED TO IMPROVE MND CARE AND ADVANCE RESEARCH SUPPORT

For over two decades, the policies of both federal and state levels of government in Australia have promoted an integrated, patient-centered approach to service delivery. Despite this, care is still seen as fragmented by many consumers and care providers. According to the Productivity Commission (2017):

> progress towards an Australia-wide integrated system of care across primary, hospital and other sectors has been poor, hampered by weak information flows and coordination, inadequate attention to the experiences of patients and flawed incentives and inadequate governance arrangements (in large part created by the Commonwealth/State divide in funding arrangements).

What are the barriers, then, to a functioning system, capable of meeting the needs and preferences of people living with MND on a day-to-day basis? Barriers exist in at least three different but interacting domains: government, workforce and community.

Government and the Bureaucracy

The public contributes financially and, through the ballot box, philosophically to how the health and welfare systems run. It is ironic, perhaps tellingly so, that a government trying to deliver the wide range of necessary public services to citizens, in an efficient and equitable manner, should itself have a dichotomous structure, separating federal and state jurisdictions, as well as authority over health and disability funding and reporting. An "all of government" approach is needed to meet an expectation that reasonable health, disability and social needs will be met in future. Such an overarching authority could use algorithms to fast-track people diagnosed with rapidly changing diseases like MND through the bureaucracies when employment, financial, family and domestic well-being are threatened by a progressive, life-limiting illness. With the current roll-out of the National Disability Insurance Scheme (NDIS), there is a growing acknowledgment that living well with a chronic disease is not all about healthcare and that planning disability supports must anticipate the changing needs related to disease trajectories. It remains inequitable that people with MND under the age of 65 years receive vastly superior levels of disability support through the NDIS compared to those diagnosed after 65 years through the aged care system.

Government and the Workforce

Team-Based, Multidisciplinary Care

Multidisciplinary, team-based care is beneficial to people living with MND, improving symptom management, quality of life and survival (Hogden et al. 2017; Oliver et al. 2016), yet there is no government-driven integration of care delivery across sectors and no targeted funding for this model of care. "Medicare does not provide care which is coordinated and integrated around the needs of patients; and it does not help the people providing the care to do this" (Health 2040. Victorian Government discussion paper).

Funding Models for Innovation

Funding models need to support innovation in the workforce to allow the system to operate in a more unified way. Local solutions and partnerships between motivated regional players have been shown to produce more successful collaborations and better flow of information (Goodwin et al. 2013). The current system also fails to identify a named care coordinator, who the patient can choose to manage all their services and improve communication across their care team. Most "coordinators" manage aspects of a patient's services (NDIS or aged care funding, healthcare, palliative care), but may lack the big picture view and the ability to advocate with certain providers.

Workforce Capability/Education

Studies have also shown that the workforce is often not trained or supported to function as a team and commonly fails to communicate outside of their own workplace (Banfield et al. 2013). The Neurological Alliance Australia, in a joint statement with Palliative Care Australia, called for improved access to palliative care services for people living with neurological conditions, but it also identified a need for education for palliative care staff to improve their knowledge, understanding and confidence in providing care to people with these conditions.

Workforce Deployment

Although the government has placed a greater emphasis on advance care planning in recent years, achieving the person's goals for management is often confounded when symptoms or contingencies occur out of hours when many GPs rely on locum services. It is therefore difficult for them to provide medical leadership in the care of patients who have chosen to die at home. Also, many palliative care services do not provide home visits after hours, relying on phone advice and the resources of families to administer drugs and monitor effect. Therefore, emergency departments become the default provider for managing symptoms or social break-down—swelling the number of people who, although they want to die at home, end up dying in hospital.

In Australia, there is poor integration of mental health services with neurological care for people with organic neurological illnesses. Addressing anxiety, mood and behavioral disturbance, which are often co-morbid with neurodegenerative conditions, should be indivisible from the management of the physical symptoms of the disease. Both require skilled care from knowledgeable staff working in partnership. Accommodating people when they require inpatient, respite or residential care also needs policy to promote a person- and family-centered approach to achieve age-appropriate settings, the right staff skill mix and least restrictive outcomes.

As chronic diseases are now the leading cause of death around the world, government policy should foster comprehensive care models that are sustainable around the clock and across distance from specialist centers. Increasingly, we see these types of models used in triage and acute intervention in stroke, trauma and the newborn, often supported by telemedicine. Because of their comprehensive knowledge base and multidisciplinary make-up, specialist MND services, if appropriately resourced and indemnified, could support other practitioners in the wider community, including assessment or advice in urgent situations.

Government and the Community

Health Literacy

According to the Australian Bureau of Statistics, almost 60 percent of adults in Australia have poor health literacy. This is associated with increased rates of hospitalization, emergency care and poor outcomes, as well as increased healthcare costs. Publicly funded campaigns to educate the general population about the risks of smoking or to raise awareness of

HIV/AIDS have been very successful in changing behavior. Educating people about their own bodies, disease prevention, supported decision-making and how their taxpayer-funded services work should be even easier with so many media platforms now available. Policy could also give focus to addressing the special needs of groups where social determinants of low health literacy are already known (poor health status, high use of health services, low socio-economic status, less educated and older age).

Shared Information Systems
The lack of shared information systems also impairs communication and fosters fragmented care decisions. An opt-out, national e-health record (My Health Record) is being launched and could be beneficial if patients and providers are trained in its use. Ideally, the patient should be able to consent to some or all the content being shared with their care team. My Health Record has also been suggested as a conduit for accessible health information and prompts. Surveys and data-linkage could also assess individual health literacy, patient experiences and other health metrics.

With the financial support of an NHMRC Partnership grant, a consortium of MND clinicians, researchers and MND associations in Australia are working toward effective data-linkage of current registries and databases. Patients, carers and providers will also be able to input their own data and access information and resources through a consumer-controlled App or Website.

Although assistive technologies help people with MND overcome verbal or written communication difficulties, hospital systems and bureaucracies still usually communicate by phone or letter. Email and texting are viable alternatives for people with these disabilities and should be encouraged, especially if secure platforms are provided.

Sustaining the Natural Resilience of Families and the Socio-economic Benefits of Informal Care
Family carers of people with MND often describe their caring experiences as unrelenting due to the progressive nature of the disease and the hopelessness of recovery. Studies have reported that family carers suffer from anxiety, depression, fatigue, impaired quality of life and reduced social contacts. While the management of physical symptoms in MND is paramount, attending to such family carers' psychosocial factors is crucial to prevent deterioration in health outcomes. Most individuals with MND live at home, where their psychosocial functioning is intimately connected to the extent and quality of support they receive from family members.

Notwithstanding the physical, psychological and emotional burden of the disease on family carers, the Deloitte Access Economic Report has quantified the economic disadvantage on families supporting people with MND, who provide an estimate of 7.5 hours of informal care per day. The productivity loss due to such informal care in Australia was estimated to be $68.5 million in 2015, or $32,728 per person, with individuals shouldering most of these costs ($44 million) and government bearing the rest ($24.5 million) (Deloitte Access Economics 2015). Therefore, it is important to design and evaluate effective models of care and find ways to deliver them to families living and caring for someone with MND (Aoun et al. 2017b). Models of care with practical and emotional benefits already provided by MND associations have not been well investigated (Aoun et al. 2018). In order to inform future planning and policies for solutions to the growing demand for family care and the associated challenges encountered by family carers, it is essential to integrate family carers' needs into service planning.

Acknowledgments We acknowledge the contribution of Ashley Crook to the genetic testing section, and Leanne Jiang for assistance in formatting the references.

References

Advance Care Planning Australia (2018). Advance care planning and the law. https://www.advancecareplanning.org.au/for-health-and-care-workers/legal-requirements

Aoun, S.M. (2018). The palliative approach to caring for motor neurone disease: From diagnosis to bereavement. *European Journal for Person Centered Healthcare* 6 (4): 675–84.

Aoun, S.M., L.J. Breen, D. Oliver, R.D. Henderson et al. (2017a). Family carers' experiences of receiving the news of a diagnosis of Motor Neurone Disease: A national survey. *Journal of the Neurological Sciences* 372: 144–51.

Aoun, S.M., K. Deas, L.J. Kristjanson, and D.W. Kissane (2017b). Identifying and addressing the support needs of family caregivers of people with motor neurone disease using the Carer Support Needs Assessment Tool. *Palliative and Supportive Care* 15 (1): 32–43.

Aoun, S. M., B. Rumbold, D. Howting, A. Bolleter, and L.J. Breen (2017c). Bereavement support for family caregivers: The gap between guidelines and practice in palliative care. *PLoS One* 12 (10): e0184750.

Aoun, S.M., A. Hogden, and L.K. Kho (2018). "Until there is a cure, there is care": A person-centered approach to supporting the wellbeing of people with Motor Neurone Disease and their family carers. *European Journal for Person Centered Healthcare* 6 (2): 320–28.

Australian Government (2018). National Palliative Care Strategy 2018. https://
    www.health.gov.au/internet/main/publishing.nsf/Content/EF57056B
    DB047E2FCA257BF000206168/$File/12291_PC-Strategy.pdf
Australian Human Rights Commission (2015). Face the facts: Cultural diversity.
    https://www.humanrights.gov.au/our-work/education/face-facts-cultural-
    diversity
Australian Institute of Health and Welfare (2016). Australia's health 2016.
    Australia's health series no. 15. Cat. no. AUS 199. Canberra: AIHW. https://
    www.aihw.gov.au/getmedia/f2ae1191-bbf2-47b6-a9d4-1b2ca65553a1/
    ah16-2-1-how-does-australias-health-system-work.pdf.aspx
Banfield, M., K. Gardner, I. McRae, J. Gillespie et al. (2013). Unlocking informa-
    tion for coordination of care in Australia: A qualitative study of information
    continuity in four primary health care models. *BMC Family Practice* 14 (1): 34.
Berlowitz, D.J., M.E. Howard, J.F. Fiore, S. Vander Hoorn et al. (2016).
    Identifying who will benefit from non-invasive ventilation in amyotrophic lat-
    eral sclerosis/motor neurone disease in a clinical cohort. *Journal of Neurology,
    Neurosurgery and Psychiatry* 87 (3): 280–86.
Carer Gateway (2019). What is respite. https://www.carergateway.gov.au/
    respite/what-respite
Carer Recognition Act (2010). (Cth) (Austl.).
Crook, A., K. Williams, L. Adams, I. Blair, and D.B. Rowe (2017). Predictive
    genetic testing for amyotrophic lateral sclerosis and frontotemporal dementia:
    Genetic counselling considerations. *Amyotrophic Lateral Sclerosis and
    Frontotemporal Degeneration* 18 (7–8): 475–85.
Department of Transport (2019). Application for the Taxi Users' Subsidy Scheme.
    www.transport.wa.gov.au/mediaFiles/taxis/ODT_F_App_TUSS.pdf
Economics, D.A. (2015). Economic analysis of motor neurone disease in Australia
    Motor Neurone Disease, (November).
Fight MND (2019). FightMND. https://fightmnd.org.au/
Goodwin, N., L. Sonola, V. Thiel, and D.L. Kodner (2013). Co-ordinated care for
    people with complex chronic conditions: Key lessons and markers for success.
    The King's Fund UK. ISBN 978-1-909029-19-4.
Government, V (2008). Motor neurone disease and palliative care report on the
    project MND pathway.
Health Victoria Government (2019). Voluntary assisted dying. https://www2.
    health.vic.gov.au/hospitals-and-health-services/patient-care/end-of-life-
    care/voluntary-assisted-dying
Henderson, R.D., N. Hutchinson, J.A. Douglas, and C. Douglas (2014).
    Telehealth for motor neurone disease. *The Medical Journal of Australia*
    201 (1): 31.
Hogden, A. and A. Crook (2017). Patient-centered decision making in amyo-
    trophic lateral sclerosis: Where are we? *Neurodegenerative Disease Management*
    7 (6): 377–86.

Hogden, A., S.M. Aoun, and P.L. Silbert (2018). Palliative care in neurology: Integrating a palliative approach to amyotrophic lateral sclerosis care. *European Journal of Neurology* 6 (1): 68–76.

Hogden, A., G. Foley, R.D. Henderson, N. James, and S.M. Aoun (2017). Amyotrophic lateral sclerosis: Improving care with a multidisciplinary approach. *Journal of Multidisciplinary Healthcare* 10: 205.

James, N., E. Power, A. Hogden, and S. Vucic (2018). Patients' perspectives of multidisciplinary home-based e-Health service delivery for motor neurone disease. *Disability and Rehabilitation Assistive Technology* 14 (7): 1–7.

MND and Me (2019). MND and me. http://www.mndandme.com.au/

Motor Neurone Disease Australia (2017a). $25 million, 25 milestones: Changing the future of MND. https://www.mndaust.asn.au/Discover-our-research/$25-Million,-25-Milestones-Changing-the-future-o.aspx

Motor Neurone Disease Australia (2017b). Position statement: Development and approval of drugs to treat motor neurone disease. https://www.mndaust.asn.au/About-us/Policies-and-position-statement/National-policies-and-position-statements/Development-and-approval-of-MND-drugs.aspx

Motor Neurone Disease Australia (2018a). MND death statistics. https://www.mndaust.asn.au/Discover-our-research/Latest-research/Statistics.aspx

Motor Neurone Disease Australia (2018b). Until there is a cure, there is care. https://www.mndaust.asn.au/News-and-media/State-Association-facts-and-figures.aspx

Motor Neurone Disease Australia (2018c). MND support service model. https://www.mndaust.asn.au/About-us/Policies-and-position-statement/National-policies-and-position-statements/MND-Support-Service-Model-2018.aspx

Motor Neurone Disease Australia (2018d). MND Australia familial MND and genetic testing. http://www.mndaust.asn.au/Documents/Information-resources/MND-Australia-Familial-MND-and-genetic-testing-201.aspx

Motor Neurone Disease Australia (2019). Support from state MND associations. https://www.mndaust.asn.au/Find-help/Support-from-state-MND-associations.aspx

Oliver, D.J., G.D. Borasio, A. Caraceni, M. de Visser et al. (2016). A consensus review on the development of palliative care for patients with chronic and progressive neurological disease. *European Journal of Neurology* 23 (1): 30–38.

Productivity Commission (2017). Integrated care, shifting the dial: 5-year productivity review, supporting paper No. 5, Canberra.

WA Companion Card (2016). Homepage. http://www.wacompanioncard.org.au/

CHAPTER 3

Public Policy in ALD/MND Care: The Belgian Perspective

Evy Reviers, Ludo Vanopdenbosch, Ludo Van Den Bosch, and Philip Van Damme

Abstract Belgium has a population of 11 million people, which means that there should be 110–220 ALS cases per year and that there are 440 to 880 people living with ALS. There is no population-based national registry for ALS, but a national database for neuromuscular diseases exists.

Document note organization ALS Liga Belgium is available on www.ALS.be
All information on the European Organization for Professionals and Patients with ALS EUpALS is available on www.ALS.eu

E. Reviers
ALS Liga Belgium, Leuven, Belgium
e-mail: Evy@als.be

L. Vanopdenbosch
AZ Sint Jan Brugge Oostende, Brugge, Belgium
e-mail: Ludo.vanopdenbosch@azsintjan.be

L. Van Den Bosch • P. Van Damme (✉)
KU Leuven, Leuven, Belgium
e-mail: ludo.vandenbosch@kuleuven.vib.be; philip.vandamme@uzleuven.be

© The Author(s) 2021
R. H. Blank et al. (eds.), *Public Policy in ALS/MND Care*,
https://doi.org/10.1007/978-981-15-5840-5_3

The multidisciplinary care for patients with ALS and their families is orga-nized in neuromuscular reference centers. Most patients stay at home even in the terminal stages of the disease, thanks to a generous care budget which can be used by patients for home care. Euthanasia is legal in Belgium, and about 25 percent of patients with ALS are thought to plan their end of life this way, mostly at home in a terminal disease stage. ALS Liga Belgium is a very well-organized and active organization, which plays an important role in the care for patients living with ALS, in the public awareness of the disease, in fund raising for research and in defending the rights of ALS patients and their families.

Keywords ALS • Neuromuscular reference center • Care budget • ALS Liga • Euthanasia • Palliative sedation

Incidence, Prevalence and Deaths of ALS/MND in Belgium

In Belgium, there is no national registry for ALS/MND. However, a national database for neuromuscular disorders exists, that is, the Belgian Neuromuscular Disease Registry (BNMDR, https://www.sciensano.be/en/belgian-neuromuscular-disease-registry-bnmdr) (Roy et al. 2015). This database is operated by Sciensano, a national institute for science and health, which also is responsible for health and disease monitoring in Belgium. The database was commissioned in 2008 and continues to grow. Data from pediatric and adult patients with neuromuscular conditions fol-lowed in one of the seven Neuromuscular Reference Centers in Belgium are collected in this database. The capture of patients continues to grow. According to this database, the prevalence amounts to 8–12/100,000 in the districts with the highest capture rate. The number of new patients is estimated to be around 220 per year, and a similar number of patients die of the disease every year. A recent study reported even slightly higher mor-tality numbers per year (Maetens et al. 2019). Due to improved multidis-ciplinary care with nutritional and non-invasive respiratory support, the median survival has increased with a few months over the last decade (Fig. 3.1).

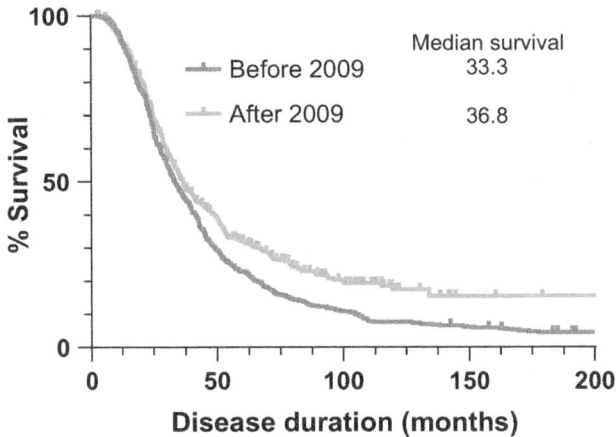

Fig. 3.1 Kaplan-Meier curve of patients seen at the University Hospitals Leuven before 2009 (n = 474) and after 2009 (n = 726)

GOVERNMENTAL AGENCIES INVOLVED IN CARE

There are no governmental committees on ALS/MND in Belgium. Although several benefits for patients with ALS are available, they are not exclusive for ALS patients. Patients living with a rapidly progressive condition can apply for a care budget using a fast-track procedure. Such patients are also supported by assistive goods for mobility and communication by respective agencies of the regions they are living in.

The care for patients with neuromuscular disorders, including patients with ALS/MND, is organized through neuromuscular reference centers (NMRCs). There are seven neuromuscular reference centers in Belgium, in Antwerp, Gent/Brugge, Leuven, three in Brussels and one in Liège. The NMRC with the largest cohort of ALS patients is in Leuven (University Hospitals Leuven). It sees about 100 new cases per year, follows about 300 patients and is actively involved in ALS research. NMRCs have multi-disciplinary teams typically consisting of administrative workers, specialized nurses, social workers, physiotherapists, occupational therapists, dieticians, speech therapists, psychologists, rehabilitation physicians, pulmonologists and neurologists.

The cost of the care is covered by the government. The centers receive a fixed fee per patient, which allows them to organize high-quality care for patients and their families. The initiation of non-invasive ventilation is only possible in neuromuscular reference centers. Home care, however, is not supported through this system. Although this network of multidisciplinary reference centers is well-established, probably about one-third of patients stay with their local neurologist and opt not to be offered the possibility of non-invasive ventilation and multidisciplinary care.

Private ALS/MND Organizations and Advocacy Groups

ALS Liga Belgium is a non-profit organization founded in 1995, managed by patients and patients' relatives only. It offers patients with ALS/MND, their families and friends, a diversified service, based upon four pillars:

- Stimulating and financing scientific research on ALS.
- Informing and providing direct support to patients with ALS/MND and their families.
- Defending the rights of patients with ALS/MND at governments and agencies.
- Providing free-of-charge high-tech aid goods for mobility and communication.

In addition to a national role, the ALS Liga Belgium also plays a prominent role at the international level. It has initiated several international projects, both within and outside Europe, and cooperates actively with the International Alliance of ALS/MND Associations.

The ALS Liga Belgium also established EUpALS, the European Organization for Professionals and Patients with ALS. EUpALS takes the interest of European patients with ALS/MND to heart. It creates equal rights for all European ALS/MND patients by providing them better access to research and according information. It especially focuses on harmonizing the European legislation related to research and optimizing the quality of life to the benefit of patients with ALS/MND.

Policy Associated with ALS/MND Research

There is no national funding body specifically devoted to ALS/MND research in Belgium. Research applications can be submitted to general funding agencies such as the Fund for Scientific Research. Typically, such applications will be reviewed by international reviewers, and the final decision will be taken by a panel with expertise in neurological disorders. The amount of public funding for ALS research is therefore not fixed and entirely depends on the quality of the research proposals submitted. The relative contribution from the private sector has increased over the years. Ten years ago it was less than 5 percent of total research budgets, but currently it exceeds 30 percent.

The care budget is allocated to neuromuscular reference centers (NMRCs) by the government in the same way as for other patients with neuromuscular conditions. A fixed fee per patient in multidisciplinary follow-up is provided to the hospital in order to cover the costs of the in-hospital care teams. The care at home is not covered through this system, but through direct financial support to patients with high care needs.

Since 2014, the Belgian government also has funded ALS/MND care by providing a fixed yearly budget of 120,000 euros (US$133,000) for two full time equivalent liaison workers. They support patients with ALS/MND in their homes. In particular, the liaison workers coordinate home care by interacting with all stakeholders especially in acute situations. This service is free of charge for the patients.

Fundraising from the general public at the national level is done by ALS Liga Belgium, with multiple fundraising campaigns and initiatives, often local initiatives, but sometimes also in collaboration with other European countries in international events. At the local level at the University of Leuven, there are three ALS funds that raise money locally for research purposes.

Public and Media Perceptions of ALS/MND

The knowledge of the general public about ALS/MND has increased over the last years. The Ice Bucket Challenge contributed to this awareness as well as the continuous efforts of ALS Liga Belgium. For instance, close collaboration of ALS Liga Belgium with the production team of the soap series THUIS recently resulted in a character that was suffering from

ALS/MND. In this way, the general public became aware of ALS/MND in the TV season in 2018–19.

CARE OF ALS/MND PATIENTS IN BELGIUM

The default pathway for the organization of care for patients with ALS is home care, organized by the patients and their families. The multidisciplinary teams have an advisory role and help with the organization of the care. Most patients stay at home throughout their disease trajectory. By using a home care budget (see later in the chapter), many patients can organize their care at home even in the later stages of the disease when they are completely dependent on the help of others. Less than 10 percent of patients are cared for in hospices, usually as care needs have become too high at home. Patients without family, or patients with care demands that exceed the capacity of the local caregivers, can be admitted to institutional care. However, most hospices are not equipped to handle patients on non-invasive or invasive ventilation and typically have a population of elderly people.

The use of non-invasive ventilation is usually not hampered by a lack of care at home. So long as patients have supervision 24 hours a day from caregivers that have had training on the use of non-invasive ventilation, the option to start non-invasive ventilation is available. Invasive ventilation is rarely initiated for several reasons, such as personal preferences and cultural reasons, but also because of the burden of the home care. The patient is responsible to organize the home care for invasive ventilation, and this requires medically trained caregivers 24 hours per day. As this is not reimbursed in Belgium, many patients do not undergo tracheostomy, and probably less than 1 percent of patients eventually become invasively ventilated.

There are no dedicated homes for people living with ALS. In the framework of a National Convention, however, some hospices have dedicated beds for patients that have high care needs, for example, those that require ventilation when home care is no longer possible. In the final stage of the disease, the role of the general practitioner becomes very important because patients often are no longer able to travel to the multidisciplinary clinics. Palliative care, palliative sedation and euthanasia are possible at home under the supervision of the general practitioner. As a result, few patients die in hospitals in neurology wards or in palliative care units.

Composition of Caregivers: Informal, Formal (Paid)

The team of caregivers can be composed of informal and formal members. In many cases, close relatives take part in the care of the patients. There are legal systems that allow working part-time to care for a close family member. Patients can also rely on formal home nurses for help with washing, clothing, wound-care, tube feeding and so forth. Such home nurses can come for brief visits one to three times per day, but there are challenges to have the visits organized at fixed time points. These formal caregivers can be hired through the home care budget (see later). Apart from these systems, there are local initiatives to support ill people at home.

Despite the different care options, the organization of care can be quite challenging for patients in later stages of the disease when they need a permanent caregiver. Once the patient depends on a caregiver at night, such as for pressure area care or to cope with aspiration or the relief of cramps, the burden increases. In practice, the search for informal or formal caregivers working at night is difficult.

Governmental Aid for Family Caregivers

In Belgium, governmental aid for family caregivers is provided by respective agencies from the region in which they live, each with distinct regulations. In Flanders, the Flemish Agency for Persons with a Disability (VAPH) introduced a personal budget (PVB) that amounts to 60,778 € (US$75,400) per year for persons with a progressive degenerative disorder. Patients with ALS/MND can apply via a fast-track procedure. The personal budget can be used to organize the needed care and support by, amongst others, the family caregivers.

Inhabitants of Flanders who are not eligible to receive this personal budget can apply at their health insurance fund for a premium for family care of 130 € (US$145) per month. In Wallonia, the Walloon Agency for Persons with a Disability (AVIQ) also provides personal budgets (BAP) to persons with a disability, which is set between 1000 € (US$1100) and 35,000 € (US$ 39,000) per year. In the German community, the agency Dienststelle für Selbestimmtes Leben informs patients with ALS/MND about the financial aid and respite care that is available to their citizens.

Access to Assistive Technologies

Patients with ALS/MND in Belgium have access to assistive technologies through specific procedures and conditions depending on the region in which they live. In Flanders, from January 2019 a new leasing system is in place via the Vlaamse Sociale Bescherming (VSB; Flemish Social Protection) for mobility aids such as walkers, manual or power wheelchairs and scooters. Persons with a progressive degenerative disease, including ALS/MND, can apply by a fast-track procedure. For a (partial) refund of purchases of other aid goods (transportation tools, electric beds, communication devices) as well as adaptations of their home, persons living in the Flemish Region can under certain conditions apply at the agency VAPH. In Wallonia and the capital city Brussels, the respective agencies AVIQ and PHARE provide a system of reimbursements of purchases of assistive technologies. However, no fast-track procedures are available for people with ALS/MND.

Finally, ALS Liga Belgium has the specific service ALS Mobility & Digitalk (ALS M&D) dedicated to rent assistive technologies for mobility and communication to patients with ALS/MND. This lending service is free of charge and open to those patients who do not qualify to obtain the assistive goods via the systems set up by the respective regional agencies.

STATUS OF MULTIDISCIPLINARY TEAM CARE AND CLINICS

The multidisciplinary teams (neuromuscular reference centers) are funded by the state. The teams will receive a fixed sum per annum to organize the care for the patients in an ambulant setting. Home visits are possible, especially by occupational therapists, to advise on the use of aids and to advise on refurbishments to the home needed to make the care at home feasible. Home visits on a regular basis, by a specialized nurse, unfortunately are not covered through the system of neuromuscular reference centers. The multidisciplinary teams are in close contact with the general practitioner and help to get the care at home organized. At the same time, they monitor nutritional and respiratory status and advise on the use of tube feeding, noninvasive ventilation and so forth. Typically, patients with ALS are seen every two to six months, depending on the rate of disease progression. Between visits, they are in regular contact with a specialized nurse for further questions. For non-medical support, patients can contact patient organization ALS Liga Belgium. A liaison person of ALS Liga Belgium supports patients with ALS/MND in their home situation in acute situations.

Right to Try Unapproved Drugs for ALS/ MND Patients

There is no national legislation that supports the right to try in Belgium. However, in Belgium (as in the rest of the European Union), laws supporting the use of experimental drugs in a compassionate use or named patient format prior to registration exist. For less expensive experimental drugs, any physician can prescribe drugs that are not as yet approved by EMA and that are not on the market in Belgium. However, experimental drugs with a high price are problematic unless the company is willing to provide the drug for free in an early access program. If this is not the case, it is deemed unethical by most physicians and ethics committees to let the patient cover the cost of the treatment.

There is no legal obligation for physicians to prescribe experimental drugs, and most patients understand that the use of experimental drugs outside the context of a clinical trial can be harmful. ALS centers and the ALS Liga Belgium attempt to communicate in a uniform manner about experimental therapies to avoid misunderstanding by patients and their caregivers. Participation in clinical trials is the preferred option to offer selected patients access to non-approved treatment in a safe manner. Off-label symptomatic medication is prescribed for some indications such as drooling.

Genetic Testing for ALS/MND

Many patients in Belgium are interested to know if they carry pathogenic mutations in known ALS genes. Also, in patients without a positive family history, gene testing is frequently offered. The genetic testing in Belgium is almost completely covered by the health care system. There are fixed tariffs for gene tests, and the proportion of the bill that is charged to the patient is small. For example, to get a diagnostic gene test for ALS, which currently includes testing for *C9orf72*, *SOD1*, *TARDBP* and *FUS*, the total cost is 570 € (US$ 630), but only 8.65 € (US$ 9.50) is charged to the patient. In familial cases, 55 percent have a *C9orf72* expansion, 20 percent a *SOD1* mutation and less than 5 percent a *TARDBP* or *FUS* mutations. In about 7 percent of sporadic patients, a *C9orf72* repeat expansion is found (Debray et al. 2013).

Whenever pathogenic mutations are found, family members of ALS patients are offered genetic counseling. Individuals over 18 years old can undergo a predictive gene test after genetic counseling, which is routinely provided. This is mostly carried out in people who are planning to have children. This gene test is performed in duplicate on two independent blood samples and costs 2 × 158.52 € (US\$ 175), of which 2 × 8.65 € (US\$ 19) is charged to the person that requests the test. Mutation carriers can opt to prevent transmission of disease-causing mutations by in vitro fertilization and pre-implantation genetic diagnostics. Up to six attempts are reimbursed by the health care system.

Access to Palliative and Hospice Care

Belgium has a variety of structures and services for palliative care that can be provided at home, in day centers and in palliative care units in hospitals and nursing homes. Although there is sufficient access to palliative care units and hospices, this option is not widely used in Belgium. As pointed out earlier, most patients receive palliative care at home and prefer to stay at home until the very end. If the care burden exceeds the capacity of the caregivers, a difficult decision to transfer the patient must be taken.

Patients with ALS all have access to the palliative status, which gives them additional rights for support. In Belgium, the palliative status is not only for the terminal disease stage. The term supportive care is preferred over palliative care as it enables support throughout all stages of the disease from diagnosis onwards. The percentage of patients enrolled in palliative care is influenced by the euthanasia law.

Although there are no reliable numbers on the actual percentage of patients who die at home in Belgium, it has been assumed to be high. A recent study, however, suggests that it is only around 40 percent (Maetens et al. 2019). Some patients are admitted to the hospital in the terminal disease stage with respiratory infections, respiratory failure or because the situation at home becomes too strenuous. Of those, estimated to be less than 15 percent, most will die in the neurology ward and a small proportion will be admitted to a palliative care unit.

Advance Directives and Withholding or Withdrawing Life-Extending Interventions

Advance directives (ADs) are an important part of the management of patients living with ALS. There is a legally binding possibility for patients to register the treatments they no longer want to receive and to describe their wishes in case of a sudden cardiac arrest, admission on intensive care, coma and so forth. The patient's ADs can be registered on a plastic card that is stored in their wallet. In addition, most hospitals have internal procedures for registering the ADs of patients. It is observed in Belgium that most patients in the later stages of the disease opt not to be resuscitated in case of an emergency, not to be intubated in case of respiratory failure and not to be transferred to an intensive care unit. Probably less than 2 percent of patients opt for invasive ventilation. Withdrawing unwanted life-extending interventions, including mechanical ventilation, is possible. Even when patients never indicated their wishes about invasive ventilation, it is possible to stop mechanical support after discussing this with the patient, or if this is no longer possible, with the close relatives.

Palliative Sedation and Euthanasia

In Belgium, palliative sedation and euthanasia are legal. In 2002, the euthanasia law was passed. Prior to passing the law by the federal parliament, the ALS Liga Belgium provided substantial input to the policymakers and made adaptations to the draft text. It states that under certain circumstances, physicians who carry out euthanasia will not be prosecuted. Legally, euthanasia is defined as the medical act to intentionally end the life of a patient at his or her request.

Patients can only submit a written request for euthanasia if they are conscious and mentally competent, if they have a medical condition that cannot be cured and if they have persistent unsupportable, untreatable physical or psychological suffering. The patient's decision should be taken freely, without pressure from their surroundings and after careful consideration. The physician should discuss other options, such as palliative care, and make sure that all conditions are fulfilled. If the patient is expected to die within a reasonable time, only one additional independent physician's advice is sought. If this is not the case, there should be a waiting period of at least one month between the request and the act of euthanasia, and the advice of a third independent physician is mandatory. The physician who carries out the euthanasia is obliged to report to a federal committee which checks if all requirements were fulfilled. Every two years, a report on the use of euthanasia is made available publicly. Between 2014 and 2017, on average 52 ALS patients per year died per year after euthanasia. This corresponds roughly to about 25 percent of the ALS deaths each year.

Because there is no obligation to report on the use of palliative care and palliative sedation, it is not clear what proportion of patients makes use of these possibilities.

Organ donation following euthanasia is possible, but only at the explicit request of the ALS patient. The euthanasia is then performed in hospital, followed by a time-out hands-off waiting time of five minutes after the cessation of heart beating, after which organs can be procured according to a non–heart-beating donor procedure. The ethical and practical difficulties are significant, and independence between the euthanasia team and the organ transplantation team is essential (Bollen et al. 2016).

Factors Unique to Belgium

In comparison with other European countries, the following trends are observed in Belgium: (1) many patients want gene testing to make sure that their children can make informed decisions about family planning, (2) many patients want to stay at home as long as possible, (3) very few opt for mechanical ventilation and (4) euthanasia is legal, and a considerable proportion of patients makes use of this possibility.

Factors that contribute to this unique situation are heterogeneous and cultural, social and economic in nature. The contribution of religious factors has decreased over the last decades. Patient autonomy, living with family and quality of life are typically highly valued. Most patients actively plan the end-of-life management themselves. Economic factors, such as reimbursement for genetic testing and personal care budgets, facilitate the use of gene testing (also in sporadic patients) and reduce the number of patients who are admitted in hospices for care.

The Belgian regions (Flanders, Wallonia, Brussels, the German community) differ somewhat in terms of culture, social cohesion, religion and economy. Therefore, national decision-making is often a compromise made among the regions, or made solely on a regional level. As a result, decision-making on the national level mostly takes more time than at the regional level.

Conclusions: ALS/MND Policy in Belgium

In Belgium, there are many options for the care of ALS/MND patients and support for their families. Some regulations are unique and therefore well appreciated, like fast-track application procedures.

However, the Belgian landscape of the organization of care is highly scattered over different agencies and institutions and is differently organized in the various regions of the country, and this makes it hard for patients to find their way. For many of the applications there is a huge administrative burden, sometimes long waiting lists and sometimes patients are not eligible due to age restrictions. The organization of care would benefit from a more harmonized system in which patients can address their questions and apply for support to a single agency or institute.

At the level of research, the situation in Belgium could improve if dedicated funding schemes for ALS research, including clinical research, would exist. Furthermore, the research foundation is geared toward more fundamental research, and it is difficult to receive a grant for more clinically oriented studies.

References

Bollen, J., R. Ten Hoopen, D. Ysebaert, W. van Mook, and E. van Heurn (2016). Legal and ethical aspects of organ donation after euthanasia in Belgium and the Netherlands. *Journal of Medical Ethics* 42: 486–89.

Debray, S., V. Race, V. Crabbe, S. Herdewyn, G. Matthijs, A. Goris, B. Dubois, V. Thijs, W. Robberecht, and P. Van Damme (2013). Frequency of C9orf72 repeat expansions in amyotrophic lateral sclerosis: A Belgian cohort study. *Neurobiol Aging* 34: 2890, e2897–2890, e2812.

Maetens, A., L. Deliens, J. De Bleecker, A. Caraceni, M. De Ridder, K. Beernaert, and J. Cohen (2019). Healthcare utilization at the end of life in people dying from amyotrophic lateral sclerosis: A retrospective cohort study using linked administrative data. *Journal of the Neurological Sciences* 406: 116444.

Roy, A.J., P. Van den Bergh, P. Van Damme, K. Doggen, V. Van Casteren, and B.S. Committee (2015). Early stages of building a rare disease registry, methods and 2010 data from the Belgian Neuromuscular Disease Registry (BNMDR). *Acta Neurologica Belgica* 115: 97–104.

CHAPTER 4

Amyotrophic Lateral Sclerosis in Brazil

Tauana Bernardes Leoni and Marcondes C. França Jr.

Abstract Brazil is a country of continental dimensions, with remarkable regional heterogeneity which greatly influences the distribution of ALS as well as the standards of care across the nation. The overall prevalence and phenotypic presentation of ALS in Brazil is like that of Europe and North America. However, the genetic basis of the illness seems to be different; mutations in *VAPB* indeed account for a high proportion of familial ALS in Brazil. The Brazilian public healthcare system has various policies for people with ALS that include dispensing riluzole, providing non-invasive ventilatory support and wheelchairs and enabling rehabilitation. Unfortunately, these are often not implemented in many regions of the country. Much work still needs to be done to improve the general care of patients with ALS across Brazil.

Keywords Amyotrophic lateral sclerosis • Brazil • Public healthcare • Epidemiology of ALS

T. B. Leoni • M. C. França Jr. (✉)
University of Campinas, Campinas, Brazil
e-mail: tbleoni@uol.com.br; mcfrancajr@uol.com.br

© The Author(s) 2021
R. H. Blank et al. (eds.), *Public Policy in ALS/MND Care*,
https://doi.org/10.1007/978-981-15-5840-5_4

INTRODUCTION

Brazil is a country of continental dimensions, with remarkable heterogeneity among regions, particularly in terms of socio-economic development and ethnic background. In general, southern Brazil has better social indicators, whereas the scenario in the northern and north-eastern parts of the country is worse. The Brazilian population results from a mixture of Caucasian, African, Japanese and Amerindian descendants. However, the relative proportions of each race are not the same in the different regions of the country. In the south, there was relatively recent immigration flux from Europe, mostly Italian and German, and in this region, there is a relatively higher contribution of people from Caucasian descent. In contrast, the influence of Africans and Amerindians is much higher in the north and north-eastern regions (Pena et al. 2009). We believe that readers must be familiar with these introductory concepts about Brazil in order to understand the epidemiology and the current standards of care of ALS across the country.

ALS IN BRAZIL: OVERVIEW

The general profile of Brazilian patients suffering from ALS is in many ways like that reported in European and North American series. However, recent publications have also highlighted some local specificities of the disease, particularly related to the genetic epidemiology (Chadi et al. 2017).

There are few published surveys devoted to the epidemiology of ALS in Brazil. Perhaps, the most comprehensive study was published by Moura et al. (2016). These authors looked at death certificates across the country to uncover ALS-related burden in the period between January 2004 and December 2013. They found that the ALS-related death rate in Brazil ranged from 0.36/100,000 in 2004 to 0.58/100,000 in 2013. Considering adjusted mortality rates, they were able to estimate the incidence of ALS in persons over 20 years of age to be 0.61 to 0.89/100,000 and that in persons above 45 years of age 1.77 to 2.3/100,000, with clear predominance in Caucasians. In this scenario, the odds ratio of dying due to ALS was almost three times higher in Caucasians than in all other races.

This seemingly Caucasian predominance is also reflected by the geographical distribution of ALS-related deaths, which is higher in the southeast and southern regions, with more than half of all ALS-related deaths occurring in these regions. Matos et al. used a similar approach—using death certificate data—to estimate ALS-related death rates in the largest city of Brazil (São Paulo). The estimates were like those previously found, ranging from 0.44 cases per 100,000 in 2002 to 0.76 per 100,000 in 2006 (Matos et al. 2011).

Another epidemiological study was performed by Linden-Junior et al. (2013) in the city of Porto Alegre, the capital of the southernmost state of Brazil. These authors contacted all active neurologists and neurosurgeons in the city to gather data about the ALS patients followed by each of them. Using this approach, they reached a prevalence of five cases per 100,000 residents in Porto Alegre, with similar distribution between men and women. In addition, prevalence was found to increase with age, reaching the peak values between 70 and 79 years (30.5/100,000).

Following a different approach, a group at the University of Campinas (UNICAMP) also obtained prevalence and incidence estimates regarding ALS. We analyzed riluzole dispensing data, which in Brazil is only approved to treat ALS and is only given by the public health system. We estimated in the city of Campinas an incidence of 1.49/100,000/year and a prevalence of 3.92/100,000 (Vicente dos Anjos and França Jr 2013).

Detailed phenotypic characterization of the published Brazilian cohorts is shown in Table 4.1. Overall, the clinical presentation of Brazilian patients with ALS is similar to that found in European/North American individuals (Loureiro et al. 2012). The only remarkable difference is the age at onset, which seems to be younger in Brazil. Cognitive and behavioral impairment have been recognized only recently in Brazil. Branco et al. found that only 5 percent of all patients met the criteria for

Table 4.1 Phenotypic characterization of Brazilian patients with ALS

Authors (year)	de Castro-Costa et al. (1999) Fortaleza (Northeastern)	Loureiro et al. (2012) Rio de Janeiro (Southeastern)
Number of subjects	78	227
Mean age at onset (years)	42.0	53.6
Men (%)	51 (65.4%)	84 (37%)
Spinal (classical)	93%	64.8%
Bulbar	2.2%	30.4%
Diplegic	–	1.3%
Hemiplegic	–	0.4%
Progressive lateral sclerosis	–	–
Pseudopolyneuritic	–	2.2%
Progressive muscular atrophy	2.2%	2.2%

frontotemporal dementia (FTD), but 20 percent had definite evidence of cognitive impairment (Branco et al. 2017).

Genetic aspects of ALS have gained much attention recently. Overall, 10 percent of all patients have familial ALS (fALS), which (often) segregates an autosomal dominant trait and is caused by pathogenic variants in approximately 20 genes (Renton et al. 2014). In European cohorts, mutations in *C9orf72* and *SOD1* account for the majority of fALS cases (Zou et al. 2017). The genetic epidemiology of fALS appears to be slightly different in Brazil. Chadi et al. evaluated 31 unrelated families from São Paulo and found that these two genes explained approximately 20 percent of them (Chadi et al. 2017). Interestingly, the p.Pro56Ser variant at *VAPB* was by far the most frequent genetic cause of ALS in this tertiary hospital-based sample from southeastern Brazil (46.3% of all cases). This specific subtype of the disease is named familial ALS type 8 and was first described in Brazilian families (Nishimura et al. 2004). Up until now, very few patients outside Brazil have been reported. It is characterized by predominant lower motor neuron involvement and relatively slow progression compared to other forms of fALS. Tremor and autonomic dysfunction are other conspicuous and distinctive manifestations associated to *VAPB*-related ALS (Marques et al. 2006).

Recently, in a large multicentric study devoted to investigating the frequency of *C9orf72* mutations in Brazilian patients with either ALS or FTD, Cintra et al. (2018) found that the highest frequency of *C9orf72* mutations occurred in the group that presented both FTD and ALS (50% of familial and 17.6% of sporadic cases). For patients with pure ALS, the frequency was 11.8 percent for familial and 3.6 percent of sporadic cases. These numbers are much smaller than those from northern Europe, and again indicate that the genetic underpinnings of ALS have geographical/ethnical differences.

ORGANIZATION OF THE HEALTHCARE SYSTEM IN BRAZIL

The healthcare system in Brazil includes both governmental and private institutions. The public healthcare system is known as Unified Health System (SUS, acronym in Portuguese). Prior to reforms accomplished in 1988, only citizens who contributed to the social security system were able to receive public healthcare services. Today, every Brazilian citizen has access to healthcare, which is considered a constitutional right. This is clearly expressed in the Federal Constitution of 1988, Article 196, which states that health is a "right of all" and a "duty of the State". This directive is regulated by Law 8.080/1990, which operationalizes public healthcare.

Public healthcare is based on three basic principles: universal access, equity and integrated care. This means that the system is designed to assist everyone, to provide the amount/type of care tailored for each individual need and to offer all types of medical care, such as mental care, rehabilitation, preventive services and complex surgeries. By June of 2019, there were 47,125,850 individuals with private healthcare insurance across the country, corresponding to 35.2 percent of the total population. The remaining 64.8 percent rely on the public system. There are variations within the country, but as a rule, private care is better than public care. The relative proportions are rather heterogeneous, and some states have a higher percentage of private insurance coverage than others. Notably, the poorer states from the north have less private coverage and depend largely on SUS (Agência Nacional de Saúde Suplementar 2019a, b; Instituto Brasileiro de Geografia e Estatística (IBGE) 2014, 2019).

Public Policies for ALS Patients in Brazil

The vast majority of the population depends entirely on public healthcare. The Ministry of Health has issued a document to guide diagnostic and therapeutic measures for ALS patients (the last updated version is from 2015), with riluzole, non-invasive ventilatory assistance and some homecare services available within the public system.

Currently, there are three FDA-approved drugs for ALS, two of them for disease-modifying treatment (riluzole and edaravone) and one for symptomatic treatment (Nuedexta for pseudobulbar affect). In Brazil, only riluzole is approved by the local regulatory agency ANVISA. This greatly limits access of the other two drugs for Brazilian patients in general. Rare patients are on edaravone by means of compassionate use; the high purchase and import costs, however, are major concerns. SUS provides riluzole free of charge to all patients that meet the criteria for definite or probable ALS (El Escorial). The only required documents are a medical prescription and the results of the medical tests that confirm the diagnosis of ALS—nerve conduction studies +EMG (Federal Act 1151, 11 November 2015). There is no clear definition about when and for which patients to stop the medication.

Several medicines for symptomatic relief (e.g., cramps, pain, sleep disorders) are available in the public system and easily accessible for patients once they have a medical prescription. As of 2008, the public healthcare system provides non-invasive ventilatory assistance in accordance to Federal Act 1370 of 3 July 2008 that established the Non-Invasive Ventilatory Assistance Program for Carriers of Neuromuscular Diseases. For ALS patients, the inclusion criteria for providing supportive ventilatory devices are the presence of clinical or laboratorial ($PaCO_2$ >45 mmHg and/or persistent SpO_2 <88% during arousal or sleep) signs of ventilatory failure (Ministry of Health 2008). However, assistive cough devices are not included in this policy. Another important device for daily life provided by SUS is the wheelchair. Some patients are entitled to request a motorized wheelchair depending on the extent and severity of disability (Table 4.2).

In contrast to these provisions, 24-hour multi-professional homecare is not provided in the public health system for persons with ALS, and most Brazilian patients on homecare are covered by private health insurance. Under SUS, there is still non-specific legislation and no guarantees about homecare services. Some patients only received this assistance from SUS after they appealed to lawsuits, which have not always been successful. Nevertheless, SUS can provide domiciliary healthcare, and since 2002 there has been legislation to regulate this (Law #10424, of 04/15/2002, which creates ammendments to Law #8080, of 09/19/1990). Since then, there have been some programs consisting of multidisciplinary teams that act at prevention, rehabilitation and therapeutic levels, including general practitioners, social workers, physiotherapists and nurses. In most cases, physiotherapists and nurses come twice a week, and doctors visit on a monthly basis. Patients must be referred by their primary doctors in order to be included in these programs. Each region has its own rules, and unfortunately, many small cities in the country do not offer such healthcare.

Despite these public policies, families very frequently must hire caregivers to help in the care of ALS patients. This is particularly true for those

Table 4.2 Items provided by Public Healthcare in Brazil for patients with ALS

Neurological care
Riluzole
Symptomatic medications
Non-invasive ventilatory support
Domiciliary healthcare
Enteral nutrition
Wheelchairs

patients in the late stages of the disease when help is needed for all daily activities. If the family can afford it, they can hire from specific agencies that are found in most large Brazilian cities. Many families hire an auxiliary nurse or someone trained as elderly caregiver. Some entities and associations that are committed to the ALS cause provide courses to train caregivers free of charge. In such training sessions, individuals are instructed on how to deal with ventilatory devices, cough assistance devices, gastrostomy management and other specific ALS-related issues.

According to the Brazilian law, patients diagnosed with ALS are entitled to obtain some taxation benefits. They can request immediate retirement due to the disability. In addition, since they require permanent assistance of another person for daily care, the earning value should be increased by 25 percent (art. 45 of Law 8.213/1991). These individuals are also exempted from the income tax. Public transportation fees are waived too—not only for them, but also for caregivers.

Palliative Care in Brazil

Palliative care is a rather new medical area in Brazil, and for that reason not yet well developed. Currently only three Brazilian centers offer in-patient palliative care. Even now this topic is often misunderstood by healthcare professionals and society in general. A general misconception holds the idea that palliative care means simply providing euthanasia for severely ill patients. Fortunately, increasing effort has taken place in order to develop and regulate palliative care in our country. This aspect of medical care has been lately addressed in recent official publications issued by the Ministry of Health.

In 1997 the Brazilian Association of Palliative Care (ABCP) was created, and in 2005 National Academy of Palliative Care (ANCP) started its activities. Today, we have 199 institutions, either public or private, offering palliative care over the Brazilian territory (https://paliativo.org.br/). There is a specific ALS clinic with combined direction of neurologists and palliative care specialists at the State University of São Paulo (UNESP). This is the first clinic with such focus in Brazil, and hopefully, it will help to disseminate appropriate palliative guidelines for this disease (Lopes et al. 2017).

END-OF-LIFE DECISION-MAKING

In 2006, the organization that regulates all medical activities in Brazil, the Federal Council of Medicine, published a resolution (Resolution CFM n° 1.805/2006) stating that in the terminal phase of serious and incurable diseases, the assisting physician is allowed to limit or withdraw procedures and treatments that prolong the patient's life (Conselho Federal de Medicina 2006). Obviously, it is necessary to ensure that care to alleviate the symptoms that lead to suffering is in place as part of comprehensive care, respecting the wishes of the patient or his legal representatives. This directive has been considered the very first legal guideline in the fight against dysthanasia in Brazil. Since then, an increasing proportion of patients with ALS have opted not to proceed with invasive procedures in the late phases of the illness.

According to the Brazilian penal code, euthanasia is considered a crime (Brazilian Penal Code, Article 121 and its paragraph 1). To avoid misconceptions, a Brazilian Palliative Care Manual emphasizes the difference between euthanasia and palliative sedation. It also defines when to start palliative care for ALS patients: reduced breathing capacity, need for help with all daily living activities, critical nutritional impairment and life-threatening infections (Tavares de Carvalho and Parsons 2012).

ALS ADVOCACY GROUPS IN BRAZIL

We have two large patient advocacy groups for ALS patients: ABrELA (an acronym for Brazilian Association of Amyotrophic Lateral Sclerosis) and the Paulo Gontijo Institute (IPG). ABrELA was founded in 1998 and, since then, has worked with a special focus in providing reliable medical information to assist patients and families. It is also responsible for the organization of the Annual Brazilian Symposium on ALS that targets both healthcare professionals and lay people.

The IPG is a private non-profit non-governmental organization created in 2005 three years after the physicist and civil engineer Paulo Gontijo died due to ALS. In his will, he gave instructions for the creation of a foundation directed to support research in ALS. IPG activities have a dual perspective—to provide support for patients and families and to foster scientific investigation. The assistance branch covers all national territory providing free access to health professionals, social workers and legal assistance to patients and families. The Institute offers psychological appointments as well. IPG has been also involved in the development of educational campaigns both for lay people and healthcare professionals as well as in creating manuals and guides to assist relatives. On the research area, the Institute has given scholarships to young investigators interested in ALS and has funded the Annual IPG research award that is given for talented scientists working with ALS.

ALS RESEARCH IN BRAZIL

Governmental agencies are the main sources for research funding in Brazil. Similarly, public universities account for virtually all scientific publications. There are some investigation groups with specific interest in ALS based at the University of São Paulo (USP), University of Campinas (UNICAMP), Federal University of Minas Gerais (UFMG) and Federal University of São Paulo (UNIFESP). Despite the scarce funding opportunities, these groups have contributed in the discovery of new genes for fALS, the investigation of novel imaging biomarkers and the phenotypic characterization of the disease in Brazil (Nishimura et al. 2004; Tavares de Andrade et al. 2018; Coatti et al. 2017).

Federal agencies have recently funded two large research initiatives directed to ALS in Brazil. The Ministry of Health released more than US$500,000 in March 2018 to establish a stem cell laboratory at the Federal University of Alagoas that will focus efforts in the treatment of ALS. The other study is based at USP and named Brazil ALS Project. It is focused on the design and execution of clinical trials using stem cells to treat ALS. In addition, authors will investigate novel potential markers for the disease.

UNMET NEEDS AND FUTURE PERSPECTIVES

We believe that the Brazilian public healthcare system already has many positive policies for ALS; however, they are often not implemented in many regions of the country. This occurs due to several reasons, such as insufficient funding and lack of qualified professionals particularly in remote parts of Brazil. Consequently, patients from different regions of the nation have distinct standards of care. This leads to delayed diagnosis and suboptimal care in some cities, particularly in the north and northeast areas. The mean diagnostic delay for ALS in Brazil is 28.1 months for spinal onset and 20.1 months for bulbar onset (Moura et al. 2017). This is more than double that of Europe, at around 10.1 months (Nzwalo et al. 2014).

Several measures are needed to overcome these problems. The most important is the availability of adequate funding and the training of professionals across the country as ALS is a relatively rare disease and even general neurologists may feel unfamiliar with the disease. In a similar way, finding physical and speech therapists experienced in the care of ALS is a challenging task in many small Brazilian towns. Combined efforts from the government, patient advocacy groups and the Brazilian Academy of Neurology could dramatically improve this scenario.

Due to the currently inexorable and fast progression of the disease, most people with ALS are interested in engaging in clinical trials. Unfortunately, very few therapeutic trials come to Brazil. The major reason for that is the bureaucracy involved with the ethical and regulatory approvals for this type of investigation. Although there are some large and well-organized ALS research centers in Brazil, many pharmaceutical companies simply do not consider coming here. There is a need to update the regulatory framework for clinical research, particularly for rare diseases, which would greatly improve the chance of having ALS-directed clinical trials in Brazil.

References

Agência Nacional de Saúde Suplementar. (2019a). Beneficiários de planos privados de saúde, por cobertura assistencial (Brasil—2009–2019). Retrieved from https://www.ans.gov.br/perfil-do-setor/dados-gerais.

Agência Nacional de Saúde Suplementar (2019b). Taxa de cobertura dos planos de assistência médica por Unidades da Federação (Brasil—Julho/2019). Retrieved from https://www.ans.gov.br/perfil-do-setor/dados-gerais.

Branco, L.M., T. Zanao, T.J. De Rezende, R.F. Casseb et al. (2017). Transcultural validation of the ALS-CBS Cognitive Section for the Brazilian population. *Amyotrophic Lateral Sclerosis and Frontotemporal Degeneration* 18 (1–2): 60-67.

Chadi, G., J.R. Maximino F.M.H. Jorge et al. (2017). Genetic analysis of patients with familial and sporadic amyotrophic lateral sclerosis in a Brazilian Research Center. *Amyotrophic Lateral Sclerosis and Frontotemporal Degeneration* 18: 249-55.

Cintra, V.P., L.C. Bonadia, H.M.T. Andrade et al. (2018). The frequency of the C9orf72 expansion in a Brazilian population. *Neurobiology of Aging* 66: 179. e1–179.e4.

Coatti, G.C., M. Frangini, M.C. Valadares et al. (2017). Pericytes extend survival of ALS SOD1 mice and induce the expression of antioxidant enzymes in the murine model and in IPSCs derived neuronal cells from an ALS patient. *Stem Cell Reviews and Reports* 13 (5): 686-98.

Conselho Federal de Medicina. (2006). Resolution CFM n° 1.805/2006. Retrieved from http://www.portalmedico.org.br/resolucoes/cfm/2006/1805_2006.htm.

de Castro-Costa, C.M., R.B. Oriá, J.A. Machado-Filho et al. (1999). Amyotrophic lateral sclerosis. Clinical analysis of 78 cases from Fortaleza (northeastern Brazil). *Arq Neuropsiquiatr.* 57 (3B): 761-774. https://doi.org/10.1590/s0004-282x1999000500006

Instituto Brasileiro de Geografia e Estatística (IBGE). (2014). Censo Demográfico. Retrieved from http://www.ibge.gov.br/estadosat/perfil.php?sigla¼DF.

Instituto Brasileiro de Geografia e Estatística (IBGE). (2019) Projeção da população do Brasil e das Unidades da Federação. Retrieved from https://www.ibge.gov.br/apps/populacao/projecao/index.html.

Linden-Junior, E., J. Becker, P. Schestatsky et al. (2013). Prevalence of amyotrophic lateral sclerosis in the city of Porto Alegre, in Southern Brazil. *Arq Neuropsiquiatr* 71: 959-62.

Lopes, L.C.G., R. Galhardoni, V. Silva et al. (2017). Beyond weakness: Characterization of pain, sensory profile and conditioned pain modulation in patients with motor neuron disease: A controlled study. *European Journal of Pain* 22 (1): 72-83.

Loureiro, M.P., C.H. Gress, L.C. Thuler et al. (2012). Clinical aspects of amyotrophic lateral sclerosis in Rio de Janeiro/Brazil. *Journal of Neurological Science* 316: 61-66.

Marques, V.D., A.A. Barreira, M.B. Davis et al. (2006). Expanding the phenotypes of the Pro56Ser VAPB mutation: Proximal SMA with dysautonomia. *Muscle Nerve* 34 (6): 731-39.

Matos, S.E., M.T. Conde, F.M. Fávero, et al. (2011). Mortality rates due to amyotrophic lateral sclerosis in São Paulo City from 2002 to 2006. *Arq Neuropsiquiatr* 69: 861-56.

Ministry of Health (2008) PORTARIA N° 1.370, DE 3 DE JULHO DE 2008. Institui o Programa de Assistência Ventilatória Não Invasiva aos Portadores de Doenças Neuromusculares. Retrieved from http://bvsms.saude.gov.br/bvs/saudelegis/gm/2008/prt1370_03_07_2008.html.

Moura, M.C., L.A. Casulari and M.R.C.G. Novaes (2016). Ethnic and demographic incidence of amyotrophic lateral sclerosis (ALS) in Brazil: A population-based study. *Amyotrophic Lateral Sclerosis and Frontotemporal Degeneration* 17: 275-81.

Moura, M.C., L.A. Casulari and M.R.C.G. Novaes (2017). Multidisciplinary care improves survival of patients with Amyotrophic Lateral Sclerosis in the unique health system (SUS) in Brazil. *Journal of Neurological Disorders* 5: 327.

Nishimura, A.L., M. Mitne-Neto, H.C. Silva et al. (2004). A mutation in the vesicle-trafficking protein VAPB causes late-onset spinal muscular atrophy and amyotrophic lateral sclerosis. *Am J Hum Genet.* 75 (5): 822-831. https://doi.org/10.1086/425287

Nzwalo, H., D. de Abreu, M. Swash, S. Pinto, M. de Carvalho (2014). Delayed diagnosis in ALS: The problem continues. *Journal of Neurological Science* 15;343 (1-2): 173–75.

Pena, S.D., L. Bastos-Rodrigues, J.R. Pimenta and S.P. Bydlowski (2009). DNA tests probe the genomic ancestry of Brazilians. *Braz J Med Biol Res* 42 (10): 870-76.

Renton, A.E., A. Chiò and B.J. Traynor (2014). State of play in amyotrophic lateral sclerosis genetics. *Nature Neuroscience* 17 (1): 17-23.

Tavares de Andrade, H.M., V.P. Cintra, M. de Albuquerque et al. (2018). Intermediate-length CAG repeat in ATXN2 is associated with increased risk for amyotrophic lateral sclerosis in Brazilian patients. *Neurobiology of Aging* 69:292.e15–292.e18.

Tavares de Carvalho, R. and H.A. Parsons (2012). Manual de Cuidados Paliativos ANCP 2ª edição. Retrieved from https://paliativo.org.br/download/manual-de-cuidados-paliativos-ancp/.

Vicente dos Anjos, L.G. and M.C. França, Jr. (2013). Epidemiological study of Amyotrophic Lateral Sclerosis in the city of Campinas between January 2012 to April 2013. XXI Scientific Congress of the University of Campinas. B0206.

Zou, Z.Y., Z.R. Zhou, C.H. Che et al. (2017). Genetic epidemiology of amyotrophic lateral sclerosis: A systematic review and metanalysis. *Journal of Neurology, Neurosurgery, and Psychiatry* 88: 540-49.

CHAPTER 5

Public Policy of ALS in Canada

Wendy S. Johnston and Westerly Luth

Abstract The division of responsibilities between federal and provincial governments shapes the care of people with ALS in Canada. Federal policies affect people with ALS through approval of new therapies, research funding, caregiver benefits and legislation including the unsuccessful "right-to-try" bill and the successfully passed Medical Assistance in Dying (MAiD) law. Provinces, responsible for healthcare delivery, approve different services and therapies in their formularies; access to treatments and services therefore vary. ALS-specific care is primarily provided by multidisciplinary clinics in urban tertiary care hospitals. Primary care providers support ALS patients throughout their course including end-of-life care. Palliative care is also available. Since 2016, MAiD has been determined to be a part of healthcare. People with ALS are prominent in media coverage of MAiD. Across Canada, ALS Canada and its federated provincial partners play an important role in advocacy, research funding and engagement with the Canadian public.

W. S. Johnston (✉)
University of Alberta, Edmonton, Canada
e-mail: wendyj@ualberta.ca

W. Luth
School of Public Health, University of Alberta, Edmonton, Canada
e-mail: wluth@ualberta.ca

© The Author(s) 2021
R. H. Blank et al. (eds.), *Public Policy in ALS/MND Care*,
https://doi.org/10.1007/978-981-15-5840-5_5

Keywords Amyotrophic lateral sclerosis • Policy • Federal government • Provincial government • Healthcare • Medical aid in dying • ALS Society

Introduction

Policy impacting the lives of people with amyotrophic lateral sclerosis (ALS) in Canada is shaped by its history and geography. Canada is a federation of ten provinces and three territories. In 1982 the Constitution Act and the Charter of Rights and Freedoms ("The Constitution Act, Schedule B to the Canada Act," 1982) proclaimed that the Constitution is the supreme law of Canada and the Charter is part of the Constitution. The legal authority of provinces to enact laws in their jurisdiction is constitutionally enshrined, whereas territories are delegated legislative authority by the federal government. Quebec follows a civil legal system, while the other provinces and territories follow common law, reflecting their colonial roots in France and Britain, respectively. Therefore, the intersection of healthcare and the law differs from province to province, evidenced in abundance by the decriminalization of medical assistance in dying.

The Canadian federal government makes laws that govern international and national matters and sets national standards for equity between provinces, particularly with respect to healthcare. The Canada Health Act (1984) determines the framework for funding of healthcare. Since Canada is a vast country with a small and dispersed population, with the majority of Canadians living in populous urban areas, there are significant challenges to the delivery of services to people with ALS and their families.

The funding of healthcare is under federal mandate, but the delivery of healthcare and the regulation of healthcare professionals are the responsibilities of the provinces and territories.

Approval of medically therapeutic products is also a federal responsibility (Government of Canada 2019), but again the delivery and reimbursement of those products is the jurisdiction of the provinces. The federal government is a major source of funds for health research. These are distributed through entities like the Canadian Institutes of Health Research and National Research Council, among others.

Public Face of ALS

There is no comprehensive national ALS reporting in Canada. Research suggests the incidence of ALS in Canada is between 2–3 per 100,000 per year (Chiò et al. 2013; Wolfson et al. 2009). A point prevalence of 8.1 per 100,000 in 2016 is supported by ALS Societies across Canada based on approximately 3000 people living with ALS across eight provinces. Using international prevalence data with the Canadian population, the Canadian Neuromuscular Disease Registry (CNDR) estimates that approximately 2800 Canadians live with ALS (Hodgkinson et al. 2018). Mirroring global data, Canadian data suggest a rise in the incidence of ALS diagnoses over time.

Public and Media Perceptions of ALS

The Ice Bucket Challenge can be directly linked to an increase in public awareness in Canada. Additional donations in Canada of $17.2 million between August 1 and December 31, 2014 are attributed to the Ice Bucket Challenge. This initiative helped to raise the profile and awareness of ALS but did not lead to sustained increases in donations beyond 2014 (ALS Canada 2020).

The legal saga that led to the legalization of medical assistance in dying (MAiD) is a uniquely Canadian media depiction of ALS. People with ALS (Sue Rodriguez and Gloria Taylor) were plaintiffs in Canadian court challenges (*Rodriguez v. British Columbia* in 1993 and *Carter v Canada* in 2015) that ultimately led to the decriminalizing of MAiD. They, and others affected by ALS, were prominently featured in media coverage of MAiD, and people with ALS were some of the first to seek MAiD after decriminalization. In some ways, this coverage cast ALS as an archetype/shorthand for the "grievous and irremediable suffering" that would justify MAiD. There was also significant Canadian media coverage of federal politician Mauril Bélanger's diagnosis of ALS, and his death in 2016 brought significant attention to ALS in Canada.

Despite the recent surge in media coverage, the ALS community continues to feel that broad public awareness of ALS still does not exist in Canada, and most people affected by ALS know little about the disease prior to their diagnosis. After their diagnoses, 88 percent of people with ALS will seek information from print media, the Internet, patient organizations and interpersonal contacts (Abdulla et al. 2014; Chiò et al. 2008;

Moir 2019). While much of that information may be helpful and relevant, alternative information sources may also be misleading and subject to partisan framing (Benjaminy and Bubela 2014; Bubela et al. 2012;. Bubela and Caulfield 2004). For example, external sources may encourage persons living with ALS to access unproven interventions (e.g. stem cell therapies) or may focus on MAiD without contextualizing other palliative care options.

Patient organizations engage in online advocacy, including supporting practices that may affect care pathways like "right to try" experimental interventions (Eysenbach et al. 2004). The proliferation and use of non-healthcare sources of information by people with ALS and their caregivers raises concerns amongst healthcare providers (Murray et al. 2003; Oliveira 2014; Potts and Wyatt 2002) who highlight the need for clinical training and up-to-date centers of support and information to which patients with complicated health issues may be referred (Tonsaker et al. 2014).

Active Government and Private ALS Organizations

The ALS Societies in Canada are the primary source of support, information and advocacy for people with ALS. The Federation of ALS Societies across Canada, consisting of ALS Canada and its provincial counterparts, is the largest cohesive advocacy and support group. ALS Canada also has a national research and federal advocacy mandates. Provinces may also provide local research funding.

Canadian ALS societies play a primary role in supporting people to navigate their journey with ALS. Knowledge sharing on how to access local, provincial and federal resources, educational initiatives and support groups helps ensure people have the information necessary to make informed decisions and have access to peer-to-peer support. The societies also fill gaps by providing loaned equipment or funding for assistive devices, equipment and other perceived needs when provincial health and private insurance plans fall short.

ALS Canada, founded in 1977 as the ALS Society of Canada, in its advocacy role and research leadership and funding, has played the major role in raising the profile of ALS research and care needs nationally, as well representing Canada internationally. The annual ALS Research Forum, funded and organized by ALS Canada, brings clinicians and clinical and basic science researchers together to share research findings and forge relationships critical for collaboration and the development of sustainable research networks. The direct support to the Canadian ALS Research Network (CALS) has been critical in the development of robust clinical research. ALS Canada also provides leadership in promoting the best clinical care for patients with ALS, most recently by supporting a group of CALS clinicians to develop the Canadian Best Practice Guidelines for the care of ALS patients (Shoesmith et al. 2020).

There are smaller non-profit organizations and foundations in Canada, often individual patient/family-driven initiatives, that support specific researchers or clinics. People with ALS and their family/friends also fundraise to offset their out-of-pocket costs.

Governmental Action on ALS

Federal advocacy, led by ALS Canada, has yielded positive results. In 2010, following advocacy by ALS societies, veterans with ALS became eligible for, and fast-tracked to, access to disability benefits, medical resources, adapted wheelchairs and home care support (CTV.ca News 2010; Veterans Affairs Canada 2013). Following five years of advocacy initiatives, in 2015, Compassionate Care Leave benefits for people taking unpaid leave to provide care and support to a family member with a serious medical condition with significant risk of death were extended from 6 to 28 weeks (ALS Canada 2015).

The Honorable Mauril Bélanger was diagnosed with bulbar ALS following his election campaign in 2015 (CBC 2016), and he shared his public battle with ALS before his death in 2016. In his memory, an all-party ALS Caucus was established in 2017, to drive greater ALS awareness and support in the federal government. As well, the Honorable Judy A. Sgro put forward a private members' motion, M-105, "That, in light of the death of over 1000 Canadians each year, including the tragic loss of the Honourable Mauril Bélanger, … as a consequence of Amyotrophic Lateral Sclerosis (ALS), the House: (*a*) reiterate its desire and commitment to, in collaboration with provincial and territorial stakeholders, combat ALS via research and awareness; and (*b*) call upon the government to increase funding for ALS research, and to substantially increase national efforts to develop and launch a comprehensive strategy to assist with the eradication of ALS at the earliest opportunity" (House of Commons Canada 2017).

The ALS Caucus "provides an ongoing forum for discussion with the federal government with the goal of raising awareness and securing adequate and stable funding for ALS research to maintain the positive momentum created by the Ice Bucket Challenge. Its members have supported a call to the federal government for $25 million in ALS research funding over a five-year period and a one-time commitment of $10 million in support of Project MinE, an international research partnership that will map the full DNA profiles of 15,000 people with ALS" (ALS Canada 2017).

APPROVAL AND ACCESS TO NEW ALS THERAPIES IN CANADA

Health Canada, a federal agency, approves new therapeutic products and will assess submissions in tandem with the Federal Drug Administration in the United States, upon request. Drug approvals in Canada can take a long time (Salek et al. 2019), and often new therapeutic products are approved and available in other jurisdictions before they are available in Canada (Shajarizadeh and Hollis 2015).

After initial approval, the manufacturer submits a Common Drug Review to the Canadian Agency for Drug and Technologies in Health (CADTH) and Institut national d'excellence en santé et en services sociaux (INESSS) (in Quebec). These quasi-governmental bodies evaluate the clinical effectiveness and cost-effectiveness of the product and make recommendations to reimburse the product to federal, provincial and territorial drug plans. Subsequently the Patent Medicine Prices Review Board (PMPRB) sets a Maximum Average Potential Price for new products (Patent Medicine Prices Review Board 2020) based on drug prices charged in other countries. Canada has the second highest drug expenditures for primary care medicines (second to the US) (Morgan et al. 2017).

Despite having universal public health insurance, Canada does not have universal prescription drug coverage (Morgan and Boothe 2016). Thus, each provincial and territorial health system negotiates the reimbursement price for a new therapeutic product with the developer, although they can negotiate collectively through the pan-Canadian Pharmaceutical Alliance (pCPA). Each will also independently decide whether a new therapeutic product will be added to their formulary and reimbursed by their public drug plan. This can lead to disparities in access between the provinces, which can be felt particularly acutely by patients waiting for novel products to treat conditions with extremely limited, or no other, therapeutic options (Hodgkinson et al. 2018).

Canada has no "right to try" legislation. Advocacy by the ALS community has been recognized by governments federally and provincially, but there are no concrete plans to make "right to try" a reality in Canada. Currently, terminally ill patients can receive investigational treatments outside of clinical trials through the expanded/special access program in Canada (Health Canada 2013; Leever 2011). However, these programs face issues including inequitable access to experimental interventions and patient expectations for a cure (Gleason et al. 2009).

Policy and the Lived Experience of ALS

Medical care, while legislated under the Canada Health Act, publicly funded and universal, is primarily delivered by medical practitioners in private practice, supported by both private and public facilities. Primary care is largely provided in private offices or free-standing clinics. Many specialists maintain private offices as well as hospital practices, and these fee-for-service physicians bill the provincial health system for services covered under the Canada Health Act (1984). All general hospitals are public and financed directly by the provincial health systems. ALS-specific clinical care is primarily provided by multidisciplinary ALS clinics based in tertiary care hospitals, or their ambulatory departments, connected with large academic medical schools. Access to the multidisciplinary clinics is by referral from primary care practitioners or community-based specialists who typically pursue the initial diagnostic assessments and arrive at a diagnosis prior to confirmation at the tertiary ALS clinic.

All ten provinces have at least one multidisciplinary clinic. The multidisciplinary clinics are in large population centers, which can make access for patients living in rural areas and Northern Canada difficult (Fig. 5.1). Many people find attending specialist ALS clinics more difficult as ALS progresses, especially rural patients. Telemedicine is available in many provinces, but care in advanced ALS is undertaken by primary care providers whether in the home or in an institutional setting. Palliative care, both primary and specialist, is available, but admission to hospice at end of life is rare (personal communication from ALS Canada).

The multidisciplinary clinics are all members of the Canadian ALS Research Network (CALS) with the goal of providing all ALS patients in Canada access to research and expert clinical care. CALS, founded in 2007, seeks to include all sites in clinical research, particularly clinical trials. Since its inception, the clinics have become more uniform in their

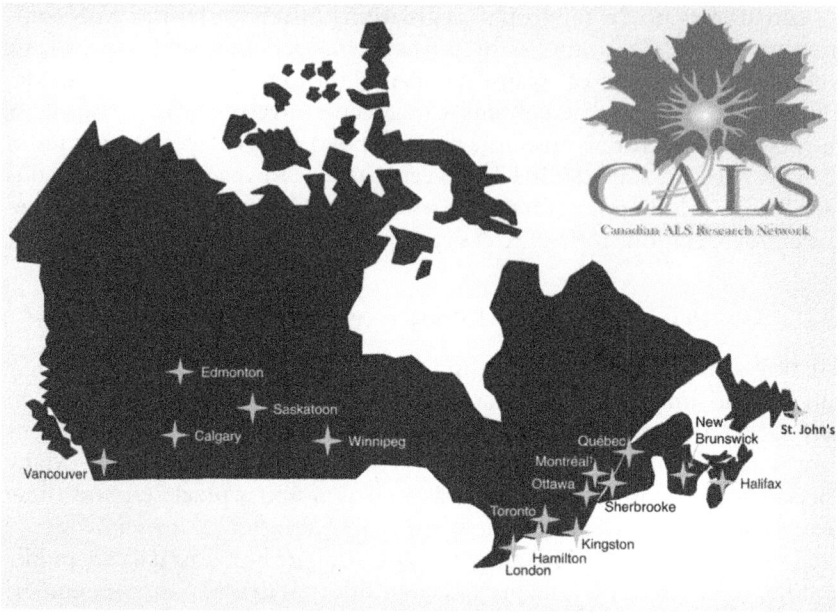

Fig. 5.1 CALS sites. (Adapted from Zinman et al. 2013)

multidisciplinary composition and more centers have been able to participate in clinical trials (Zinman et al. 2013, personal communications CALS
clinic directors). The CALS infrastructure has been supported by ALS
Canada since 2015 with administrative support; this has been critical to
the strengthening of the network and addition of new sites for clinical
research. The Canadian Best Practice Recommendations for care of ALS
patients (Shoesmith et al. 2020), a practice guideline written by CALS
clinicians and supported by ALS Canada, seeks to set the standard for ALS
care across all regions and will promote benchmarking of clinical practice.

DIAGNOSTIC SERVICES INCLUDING GENETIC TESTING

Key diagnostic services to confirm the diagnosis of ALS are available in the
publicly funded system. Access to imaging, such as magnetic resonance
imaging, is hampered by wait-times that vary across provinces (Canadian
Institute for Health Information 2017). Private independent imaging
facilities are available on a fee-for-service basis in parts of Canada but are
not reimbursed by provincial health systems.

Genetic testing is available through provincially funded labs or commercial companies. Most provinces will cover the cost of at least some testing with restrictions based on age and family history, often requiring specific applications to be completed prior to testing (CALS members, personal communication). Routine genetic testing of all consenting ALS patients is not widely practiced; only clinics in Alberta and Quebec offer genetic testing to all patients, 'and not for all genes (Genge, Dupre, personal communication).

The disclosure of genetic test results to a patient's relatives is not fully resolved. There can be tension between different ethical principles that may guide a Canadian physician's decision to disclose genetic test results to relatives of a patient including the relative's right not to know, a duty to prevent harm to relatives and the patient's right to privacy and autonomy (Godard et al. 2006). The CMA Code of Ethics and professionalism states: "sharing information only to benefit the patient and within the patient's circle of care" unless "the informed consent of the patient has been obtained for disclosure or as provided by law" (Canadian Medical Association 2018). The Genetic Non-Discrimination Act (2017) protects genetic test information from individuals or service providers entering into a contract (Bombard and Heim-Myers 2018). However, regulatory bodies in different provinces may have additional guidance for their members.

CARE AND SUPPORT THROUGHOUT THE COURSE OF ALS

The location and provision of care is not systematically reported, nor has it been prospectively studied for ALS in Canada and there is no population-based data available. There is indirect evidence that many Canadians prioritize living at home for as long as possible. Currently available data suggest the mean annual cost per patient with ALS was $32,337. About two-thirds of costs are paid out of pocket by patients: 90 percent of patients report home renovations, and 80 percent of the $12,585 mean annual home renovation cost were out of pocket (Gladman et al. 2014). A recent benchmarking report from ALS Canada, on behalf of the Federation partners, indicates the majority of people with ALS live and die in the home (personal communication from ALS Canada). The number of people with ALS in long-term care rises as the disease progresses, and it is variable across provinces. Informal caregivers predominate; the availability of funding for paid caregivers for home-based patients can be highly variable even within the same province (personal communication from ALS Canada).

Provincial health plans are more likely to provide and fund respiratory and nutritional interventions than other assistive devices, such as mobility aids (walkers, braces, wheelchairs) or augmentative communication devices. Private insurance plans cover costs for some devices at least in part, and the ALS Societies attempt to fill in the gaps. However, people with ALS and their families are left with a significant financial burden.

GOVERNMENTAL AID FOR FAMILY CAREGIVERS

Compassionate Care Leave ("Canada Labour Code" 1985) and leave related to critical illness ("Canada Labour Code" 1985) permit unpaid leave of up to 28 weeks (Compassionate Care Leave) or 17 weeks (leave related to a critical illness) in a 52-week period to care and support a family member with a serious medical condition with a significant risk of death. Both require a medical certificate from a medical provider. A person cannot take both leaves at the same time.

Additionally, employees may be entitled to benefits under employment insurance (EI), which are available regardless of the employee's length of service with their employer (Government of Canada 2020). This provides financial assistance up to 55 percent of earnings (maximum $573 per week) for up to 26 weeks payable during a 52-week period following the date the person is certified by a medical doctor or nurse practitioner to be critically ill/injured/in need of end-of-life care. This benefit can be used by numerous caregivers and can be requested by anyone close to the patient, not just immediate family.

Publicly funded in-home care is available to a greater or lesser extent in the provincially funded health systems, as is respite care whether in-home or in a care facility or hospital. However, the availability and funding of respite care is highly variable even within the same provincial health system (ALS Canada 2015).

PALLIATIVE CARE

Variations between and within provincial and territorial policies and funding models affect the delivery, organization and accessibility of palliative care across Canada (Canadian Institute for Health Information 2018).

There are also information gaps on access to palliative care. Canadians would prefer to die at home if they could receive the support they need (Canadian Institute for Health Information 2018). Receiving palliative care at home the year prior to death increases the chance a person will die at home by 2.5 times (Canadian Institute for Health Information 2018). Most people who had palliative care in 2016 received it only in the last month of life, despite reports that people receiving palliative care earlier were less likely to use emergency departments or intensive care units (Zwicker et al. 2019; Russell and Dorsey 2019).

Palliative care in Canada is largely provided by primary care practitioners with special training in palliative care, rather than by specialist palliative care providers or service. Data from the Federation of ALS Societies suggest less than 10 percent are admitted to inpatient hospice, but utilization of palliative care services on a consultative basis is not reported.

People with ALS are encouraged to have advance directives and to engage in end-of-life planning, with formal goals of care instruments or physician orders for life-sustaining therapies available in some provinces. Advance care planning tools are available in most provinces but vary in their ease of use (Richard et al. 2018) and in the terminology and specific documentation required (Hanvey 2020). Withholding or withdrawing mechanical ventilation and other life-extending interventions is recognized as both legal and ethical in Canada ("Nancy B V Hotel-Dieu de Quebe," 1992), and palliative sedation is offered when indicated as part of medical care (Government of Canada 2017).

MEDICAL ASSISTANCE IN DYING

Suicide was removed from the Criminal Code in 1972, but the cases of Rodriguez (1993) and Carter (2015) brought to light that assisting someone seeking to commit suicide but physically incapable of doing so was still illegal. In Quebec, the Act Respecting End-of-Life Care (2014) was approved by the provincial government and came into force on December 10, 2015. It established rights with respect to end-of-life care, specifically a person's right to obtain the end-of-life care required by their state of health, including medical aid in dying (MedAID). It framed the legislation as extending medical care at end of life, a provincial responsibility, and set out rules for the regulation and organization of end-of-life care in the health and social services network, including specific requirements for continuous palliative sedation and medical aid in dying. MedAID was available in Quebec before Bill C-14 (Medical Assistance in Dying 2016) legalized Medical Assistance in Dying (MAiD) across Canada.

The federal government passed Bill C-14 ("Medical Assistance in Dying," 2016), changing the Canadian Criminal Code so that physicians and nurse practitioners could assist eligible adults (see Box 5.1) in dying at the time of their choosing in accordance with proper procedure without fear of prosecution. At the same time, with MAiD decriminalized, provinces had to establish policies and procedures to make MAiD accessible to their residents once the MAiD Act came into effect. Consultation with multiple groups determined that MAiD would be viewed as a medical act, with mandatory reporting and adherence to standard protocols.

Physicians and nurse practitioners are regulated by separate professional colleges, also on provincial and territorial levels. Across provinces it is agreed that two physicians or nurse practitioners must undertake independent assessments of the person seeking MAiD, followed by a ten-day "contemplation" period, and that patients must maintain legal decision-making capacity until the completion of MAiD. Most provinces require drug procurement and attendance by the provider throughout. Each province established different procedures: for example, Alberta has central MAiD coordinators, while Ontario mandates direct referrals to MAiD specialists. Provinces also differ in how conscientious objections were handled: some provinces require physicians to refer directly to a MAiD provider regardless of their objections, while in others there is a neutral third party to whom physicians can refer people interested in MAiD.

Since December 15, 2015 (when MedAiD was available in Quebec), there have been 6749 assisted deaths in Canada (Health Canada 2019b). A by-product of the requirement for practitioner attendance and drug procurement meant that the majority of these were by lethal injection, not lethal prescription. By comparison, in Oregon, there were 1179 assisted deaths over 20 years (Hedberg and New 2017), and in the Netherlands, there were 49,287 assisted deaths over 15 years (Preston 2018). Medical assistance in dying, then, is legal in Canada, but it is not a "right" under the Charter of Rights and Freedoms. However, the right to access MAiD is under the Canada Health Act as part of medical care.

Box 5.1 Eligibility Criteria for People Seeking MAiD ("Medical Assistance in Dying," 2016)
Basics of eligibility criteria under law for Medical Assistance in Dying

Medical Assistance in Dying is available to competent adult with a grievous and irremediable medical condition who is suffering intolerably and where death is reasonably foreseeable.

The patient must:

- Have a serious illness, disease or disability.
- Be in an advanced state of decline that cannot be reversed.
- Be suffering unbearably from an illness, disease, disability or state of decline.
- Be at a point where natural death has become reasonably foreseeable, which takes into account all of medical circumstances ("A.B. v. Canada (Attorney General)," 2017).
- But does not need to have a fatal or terminal condition to be eligible for medical assistance in dying.
- Must voluntarily request and provide consent, with ten clear days between formal request and provision (interval can be shortened).
- Eligible for funded health services delivered by a Canadian jurisdiction.

RESEARCH IN ALS

Government prioritization of support for ALS research started in 2000 when the Canadian Institutes of Health Research (CIHR) formed a partnership with the ALS Society of Canada and Muscular Dystrophy Canada. Three institutes—the Institute of Neurosciences, Mental Health and Addiction (INMHA), the Institute of Musculoskeletal Health and Arthritis (IMHA) and the Institute of Genetics (IG)—contributed matching funds with the health charities to form the Neuromuscular Research Partnership (NRP). The NRP created a pool of funds to provide full, multi-year support to the top relevant grant applications that scored closest to the overall funding threshold for the CIHR biannual Open Operating Grant competition.

The NRP was an important mechanism to build a dedicated ALS research community in Canada. It was ended in 2012 when CIHR programs were reformed. For a time, CIHR also provided matched funds to PhD studentships and postdoctoral fellowships, delivered through partnership with ALS Canada.

In 2011, Health Canada designated a $100 million Canada Brain Research Fund to be delivered as a set of matching programs stewarded through Brain Canada. Following the windfall of the Ice Bucket Challenge ($17.2 million in Canada), ALS Canada utilized $10 million to create a $20 million partnership with Brain Canada. Between 2014 and 2017, the partnership funded numerous programs, including numerous small Discovery Grants, Career Transition Awards, studentships and postdoctoral fellowships and large multi-institutional team grants. This represented an opportunity for further expansion of the Canadian ALS research community. Following the full allocation of the original Canada Brain Research Fund, the federal government dedicated an additional $40 million through Brain Canada in the 2019 Budget. ALS Canada leveraged a $2 million partnership ($1 million matched) to deliver an increased size and number of grants in 2020.

The ALS Society of Canada remains the largest dedicated funder of ALS research in the country, with an annual allocation of approximately $2 million, spread across several grant and award competitions, support for conference travel, sponsorship of Canadian ALS meetings and directed funding to projects of national and international importance. In addition, the ALS Canada Research Program is a collaborative pool of funds raised through the national Walk to End ALS across the Federation of ALS Societies. These funds represent approximately 10 to 15 percent of the total funds raised in Canada. Private foundations and philanthropy, particularly research institutes and medical schools, are also significant partners in ALS research, and small regional, usually temporary, fundraising efforts surrounding a specific individual, family or group of individuals with ALS provide directed support of local clinics or researchers.

As a result of government support that does not match the need or sustainability of Canadian ALS research, ALS Canada advocates continuously for a dedicated source of ALS funding in the federal budget. Most other dedicated government funding with neurological or rare disease focus provides an opportunity for ALS funding, but has not yielded strong impact. For example, in partnership with Neurological Health Charities Canada, the federal government invested $15 million into a National Population Health Study of Neurological Conditions. ALS was one of fourteen neurological conditions studied with the long-term goal of reducing the burden of neurological conditions in Canada through an increase in understanding of these conditions in a Canadian context (Health Canada 2014). Unfortunately, almost every measure in the report has unreportable data for ALS due to small sample size or high variability, indicating a lack of prioritization compared with more prevalent conditions.

FACTORS UNIQUE TO CANADA

Canada is a secular country whose federated model of government is reflected in the organization of the main ALS-focused health charities. The national or federal arm brings together the regional partners for common purpose while respecting autonomous management of provincial clinical and fundraising endeavors. This is a strength, since centralized decision-making is not sensitive to regional or local priorities, but also a vulnerability as maintaining a well-functioning federation can be challenging when regional interests pull a partner away from the federation. Moreover, the relatively sparse and geographically dispersed population has implications for delivery of equitable clinical care and effective clinical research collaboration.

The national ALS-focused health charity, ALS Canada, has promoted clinical and research collaboration and has leveraged this relatively small community to a leadership role at the national level, raising the profile of ALS and the needs of the community to the federal government while supporting the creation of clinical guidelines and research networks that draw on regional supports for delivery of evidence-based clinical care.

Universal health care insurance ensures basic health needs of ALS patients are not financially prohibitive; however, regional variations in advanced care still occur. The stability of funding of medical care ensures that people with ALS can participate in research, knowing clinical supports are constant.

Recommended Policy Changes to Improve Care of ALS/MND Patients

- The infrastructure for medical therapeutics development and approval is complex and insufficiently responsive to the pace required for identification of new therapeutics and access to life-altering therapies for ALS patients.
- Access to approved therapies requires a national strategy for managing the cost and delivery of treatments in a fair and equitable manner given the dispersed population with rural and northern Canadians being disadvantaged.
- Both corporate and philanthropic engagement in ALS interests needs to be a priority; these strategies are underdeveloped in Canada.

Acknowledgments The authors would like to thank the following individuals who contributed to the chapter: ALS Canada: Tammy Moore, David Taylor, Lisa Droppo and Federated ALS Society partners, Wendy Toyer (BC), Diana Rasmussen (MN); CALS: Hannah Briemberg, Angela Genge, Ian Grant, Charles Krieger, Kerri Schellenberg, Christen Shoesmith.

References

A.B. v. Canada (Attorney General), 3759. (2017).

Abdulla, S., S. Vielhaber, J. Machts, H.J. Heinze, R. Dengler and S. Petri (2014). Information needs and information-seeking preferences of ALS patients and their carers. *Amyotrophic Lateral Sclerosis Frontotemporal Degeneration* 15 (7–8): 505-12. https://doi.org/10.3109/21678421.2014.932385

Act Respecting End-of-Life Care, S-32.0001, LégisQuébec (2014).

ALS Canada. (2015). ALS Canada Supports the Government of Canada's Decision to Extend the Compassionate Care Benefit to 26 weeks. Retrieved from https://www.als.ca/media-room/als-canada-supports-government-canadas-decision-extend-compassionate-care-benefit-26-weeks/

ALS Canada. (2017). MPs give ALS a voice in Parliament. Retrieved from https://www.als.ca/blogs/mps-give-als-voice-parliament/

ALS Canada. (2020). Research Funding to Create a Future Without ALS. Retrieved from https://www.als.ca/advocacy/research-funding-to-create-a-future-without-als/

Benjaminy, S. and T. Bubela (2014). Ocular gene transfer in the spotlight: Implications of newspaper content for clinical communications. *BMC Medical Ethics* 15: 58-68. https://doi.org/10.1186/1472-6939-15-58

Bombard, Y. and B. Heim-Myers (2018). The Genetic Non-Discrimination Act: Critical for promoting health and science in Canada. *CMAJ: Canadian Medical Association Journal = journal de l'Association medicale canadienne 190* (19): E579-E580. https://doi.org/10.1503/cmaj.180298

Bubela, T.M. and T.A. Caulfield (2004). Do the print media "hype" genetic research? A comparison of newspaper stories and peer-reviewed research papers. *Canadian Medical Association Journal* 170 (9): 1399-1407. https://doi.org/10.1503/cmaj.1030762

Bubela, T., M.D. Li, M. Hafez, M. Bieber and H. Atkins (2012). Is belief larger than fact: Expectations, optimism and reality for translational stem cell research. *BMC Medicine* 10: 133-33. https://doi.org/10.1186/1741-7015-10-133

Health Canada. (2019a). *Fourth Interim Report on Medical Assistance in Dying in Canada* (80947). Ottawa, ON: Government of Canada

Canada Health Act, 6, 3 Stat. (1984).

Canada Labour Code, c. L-2 § Compassionate Care Leave, 206.3 Stat. (1985).

Canadian Institute for Health Information (2017). *Wait Times for Priority Procedures in Canada, 2017.* Retrieved from Ottawa, ON: https://www.cihi.ca/sites/default/files/document/wait-times-report-2017_en.pdf

Canadian Institute for Health Information. (2018). *Access to Palliative Care in Canada*. Retrieved from Ottawa, ON: https://www.cihi.ca/en/access-data-and-reports/access-to-palliative-care-in-canada

Canadian Medical Association (2018). *CMA Code of Ethics and Professionalism*. CMA Board of Directors. Retrieved from https://www.cma.ca/cma-code-ethics-and-professionalism

Carter v. Canada (Attorney General), No. 331, 1 (Supreme Court of Canada 2015).

CBC. (2016, August 16). Mauril Bélanger, longtime Ottawa-Vanier MP, dies of ALS at 61. *CBC News.* Retrieved from https://www.cbc.ca/news/canada/ottawa/mauril-belanger-obituary-als-1.3555135

Chiò, A., A. Montuschi, S. Cammarosano, S. De Mercanti et al. (2008). ALS patients and caregivers communication preferences and information seeking behaviour. *European Journal of Neurology* 15 (1): 55-60. https://doi.org/10.1111/j.1468-1331.2007.02000.x

Chiò, A., G. Logroscino, B.J. Traynor, J. Collins et al. (2013). Global epidemiology of amyotrophic lateral sclerosis: A systematic review of the published literature. *Neuroepidemiology* 41 (2): 118-30. https://doi.org/10.1159/000351153

CTV.ca News. (2010). Veterans with Lou Gehrig's to get benefits. *CTV.* Retrieved from https://www.ctvnews.ca/veterans-with-lou-gehrig-s-to-get-benefits-1.563687

Eysenbach, G., J. Powell, M. Englesakis, C. Rizo and A. Stern (2004). Health related virtual communities and electronic support groups: Systematic review of the effects of online peer to peer interactions. *BMJ (Clinical research ed.)* 328 (7449): 1166. https://doi.org/10.1136/bmj.328.7449.1166

Genetic Non-Discrimination Act, C-3 (2017).

Gladman, M., C. Dharamshi and L. Zinman (2014). Economic burden of amyotrophic lateral sclerosis: A Canadian study of out-of-pocket expenses. *Amyotrophic Lateral Sclerosis and Frontotemporal Degeneration* 15 (5–6): 426-32. https://doi.org/10.3109/21678421.2014.932382

Gleason, M.E.J., F.W.K. Harper, S. Eggly, J.C. Ruckdeschel and T.L. Albrecht (2009). The influence of patient expectations regarding cure on treatment decisions. *Patient Education and Counseling* 75 (2): 263-69. https://doi.org/10.1016/j.pec.2008.10.015

Godard, B., T. Hurlimann, M. Letendre and N. Egalite (2006). Guidelines for disclosing genetic information to family members: From development to use. *Family Cancer* 5 (1): 103-16. https://doi.org/10.1007/s10689-005-2581-5

Government of Canada (2017). *Options and decision-making at end of life.* Retrieved from https://www.canada.ca/en/health-canada/services/options-decision-making-end-life.html

Government of Canada (2019). *Canada's Health Care System.* Ottawa, ON: Government of Canada Retrieved from https://www.canada.ca/en/health-canada/services/health-care-system/reports-publications/health-care-system/canada.html

Government of Canada (2020). *EI Caregiving benefits and leave: What caregiving benefits offer.* Retrieved from https://www.canada.ca/en/services/benefits/ei/caregiving.html

Hanvey, L. (2020). You say proxy, I say power of attorney. Retrieved from https://www.advancecareplanning.ca/across-canada/you-say-proxy-i-say-power-of-attorney/

Health Canada (2013). *Guidance Document for Industry and Practitioners: Special Access Programme for drugs* Minister of Heatlh, Retrieved from https://www.canada.ca/en/health-canada/services/drugs-health-products/special-access/drugs/guidance-industry-practitioners-special-access-programme-drugs-health-canada-2008.html

Health Canada (2014). *Mapping Connections: An understanding of neurological conditions in Canada* (140100). Government of Canada Retrieved from https://www.canada.ca/en/public-health/services/reports-publications/mapping-connections-understanding-neurological-conditions.html

Health Canada (2019b). *Guidance Document: Management of Drug Submissions and Applications* (190059). Government of Canada Retrieved from https://www.canada.ca/en/health-canada/services/drugs-health-products/drug-products/applications-submissions/guidance-documents/management-drug-submissions/industry.html

Hedberg, K. and C. New (2017). Oregon's Death with Dignity Act: 20 Years of experience to inform the debate. *Annals of Internal Medicine* 167 (8): 579-83. https://doi.org/10.7326/m17-2300

Hodgkinson, V.L., J. Lounsberry, A. Mirian, A. Genge et al. (2018). Provincial differences in the diagnosis and care of amyotrophic lateral sclerosis. *Canadian Journal of Neurological Sciences* 45 (6): 652-59. https://doi.org/10.1017/cjn.2018.311

House of Commons Canada (2017). *42nd Parliament, 1st Session* Ottawa: Government of Canada Retrieved from https://www.ourcommons.ca/Members/en/judy-a-sgro(1787)/motions/8659380

Leever, M.G. (2011). Cultural competence: Reflections on patient autonomy and patient good. *Nursing Ethics* 18 (4): 560-70. https://doi.org/10.1177/0969733011405936

Medical Assistance in Dying. (2016). An Act to amend the Criminal Code and to make related amendments to other Acts (medical assistance in dying) 3, Annual Statutes.

Moir, M. (2019). Communication, information gathering and use among ALS stakeholders: Diagnosis and care. (Master of Science). University of Alberta.

Morgan, S.G. and K. Boothe (2016). Universal prescription drug coverage in Canada: Long-promised yet undelivered. *Healthcare Management Forum* 29 (6): 247-54. https://doi.org/10.1177/0840470416658907

Morgan, S.G., C. Leopold and A.K. Wagner (2017). Drivers of expenditure on primary care prescription drugs in 10 high-income countries with universal health coverage. *Canadian Medical Association Journal* 189 (23): e794-e799. https://doi.org/10.1503/cmaj.161481

Murray, E., B. Lo, L. Pollack, K. Donelan et al. (2003). The impact of health information on the Internet on health care and the physician-patient relationship: National U.S. survey among 1.050 U.S. physicians. *Journal of Medical Internet Research* 5 (3): e17. https://doi.org/10.2196/jmir.5.3.e17

Nancy B V Hotel-Dieu de Quebe, No. (1992) 86 DLR (4th) 385, [1992] RJQ 361 385 (RJQ 1992).

Oliveira, J.F.D. (2014). The effect of the internet on the patient-doctor relationship in a hospital in the city of São Paulo. *JISTEM—Journal of Information Systems and Technology Management* 11: 327-44. Retrieved from http://www.scielo.br/scielo.php?script=sci_arttext&pid=S1807-17752014000200327&nrm=iso

Patent Medicine Prices Review Board (2020). Patented Medicine Prices Review Board. Retrieved from https://www.canada.ca/en/patented-medicine-prices-review.html

Potts, H.W. and J.C. Wyatt (2002). Survey of doctors' experience of patients using the Internet. *Journal of Medical Internet Research* 4 (1): e5. https://doi.org/10.2196/jmir.4.1.e5

Preston, R. (2018). Death on demand? An analysis of physician-administered euthanasia in The Netherlands. *British Medical Bulletin* 125: 145-55.

Richard, A., J. Richard, W. Johnston and J. Miyasaki (2018). Readability of advance directive documentation in Canada: A cross-sectional study. *CMAJ Open* 6: e406-e411. https://doi.org/10.9778/cmajo.20180037

Rodriguez v. British Columbia (Attorney General), No. 519, 3 (Supreme Court of Canada 1993).

Russell, J.A. and E.R. Dorsey (2019). Cost vs care. *Neurology* 93: 985-86.

Salek, S., S. Lussier Hoskyn, J.R. Johns, N. Allen and C. Sehgal (2019). Factors influencing delays in patient access to new medicines in Canada: A retrospective study of reimbursement processes in public drug plans. *Frontiers in Pharmacology* 10: 196. https://doi.org/10.3389/fphar.2019.00196

Shajarizadeh, A. and A. Hollis (2015). Delays in the submission of new drugs in Canada. *Canadian Medical Association Journal* 187 (1): E47–E51. https://doi.org/10.1503/cmaj.130814

Shoesmith, C., T. Bensted, M. Chum, N. Dupre et al. (2020). Canadian Medical Association Journal (in press).

The Constitution Act, Schedule B to the Canada Act, C. 11 (1982).

Tonsaker, T., G. Bartlett and C. Trpkov (2014). Health information on the Internet: Gold mine or minefield? *Canadian Family Physician Medecin de famille canadien* 60 (5): 407–08. Retrieved from https://www.ncbi.nlm.nih.gov/pubmed/24828994

Veterans Affairs Canada (2013). *Amyotrophic Lateral Sclerosis (ALS)*. Government of Canada Retrieved from https://www.veterans.gc.ca/eng/about-vac/legis-lation-policies/policies/document/1177

Wolfson, C., S. Kilborn, M. Oskoui and A. Genge, (2009). Incidence and prevalence of amyotrophic lateral sclerosis in Canada: A systematic review of the literature. *Neuroepidemiology* 33: 79-88. https://doi.org/10.1159/000222089

Zinman, L., A. Genge and D.A. Figlewicz (2013). Developing a consortium for ALS clinical research: The Canadian ALS Research Network. *Clinical Investigation* 3 (12): 1113-17.

Zwicker, J., D. Qureshi, R. Talarico, P. Bourque et al. (2019). Dying of amyotrophic lateral sclerosis: Health care use and cost in the last year of life. *Neurology* 93: e2083-e2093.

CHAPTER 6

Public Policy for Amyotrophic Lateral Sclerosis in China

Lu Chen and Dongsheng Fan

Abstract The prevalence and incidence of amyotrophic lateral sclerosis (ALS) in mainland China in 2016 were 2.97 and 1.62 per 100,000 person-years, respectively. However, the mortality of ALS is still unclear. The government and the public are very concerned. Although, the precise incidence, prevalence and mortality of amyotrophic lateral sclerosis (ALS) in mainland China are still unclear; however, the government and the public are very concerned. Although funding from the government, society and other organizations to support ALS-related research, care, rehabilitation and caregiver assistance is growing continuously, it still lags behind developed countries and needs to be further increased. Due to traditional Chinese beliefs, ALS patients and their families generally have low acceptance rates for invasive treatments, thus highlighting the importance of increasing the relevant knowledge regarding this disease.

L. Chen • D. Fan (✉)
Department of Neurology, Peking University Third Hospital,
Beijing, China
e-mail: chenlu88@bjmu.edu.cn; dsfan2010@aliyun.com

© The Author(s) 2021
R. H. Blank et al. (eds.), *Public Policy in ALS/MND Care*,
https://doi.org/10.1007/978-981-15-5840-5_6

Keywords Amyotrophic lateral sclerosis • Oriental Rain ALS Care • Chinese Medical Doctor Association • China Disabled Person's Federation • ALS Collaboration Group of the Chinese Medical Association Neurology Branch

Incidence, Prevalence and Deaths of ALS in China

Recently published population-based research reported that the estimated age-adjusted ALS prevalence in mainland China was 2.97 per 100,000 person-years, and the incidence was 1.62 per 100,000 person-years in 2016 (Xu et al. 2020). There has been no population-based research on mortality of ALS in mainland China. Besides, previous studies reported that the incidence of ALS in Hong Kong and Taiwan are 0.60/100,000 per year and 0.51/100,000 per year, respectively (Fong et al. 2005; Tsai et al. 2015). Recent capture-recapture studies based on hospitals concluded that the incidence of ALS in Beijing is 0.8/100,000 per year (Zhou et al. 2018a, b). Data analysis from Peking University Third Hospital and Oriental Rain ALS Care estimated that the incidence of ALS in the Beijing area is approximately 1.23/100,000 per year.

Governmental and Private Action on ALS

There has been much activity surrounding ALS over the last decade in China. In December 2004, the ALS Collaboration Group of the Chinese Medical Association Neurology Branch (2019) was established by neurologists working at ALS clinical centers in five hospitals. The aim was to promote ALS clinical research and improve care for patients. After fifteen years of development, it has expanded into a collaborative academic group of dozens of hospitals and more than 100 doctors. On June 26, 2016, it became an official organization of the Chinese Medical Association Neurology Branch.

Similarly, in 2005 the Chinese Medical Doctor Association (2019), together with 70 tertiary hospitals and more than 100 neurologists, launched the social welfare program "Melting the Freezing Heart". The program focuses on improving the therapy and survival of ALS patients in poor economic conditions by providing free medications. Events planned by the program have garnered the attention of the whole society and provided support and help for ALS patients.

The National People's Congress representatives and the Chinese People's Political Consultative Conference members have worked to speed up legislation pertaining to rare diseases, including ALS (http://www.npc.gov.cn/; http://www.cppcc.gov.cn/). Since 2010, the representatives from the medical and health sector have made a series of proposals to the National People's Congress of the People's Republic of China and the Chinese People's Political Consultative Conference with regard to the prevention and treatment of rare diseases and the inclusion of rare diseases in medical insurance. This included the passage of the National Rare Disease Prevention and Control Act, which includes ALS, to accomplish as soon as possible the inclusion of rare diseases in medical insurance, reimbursement for important therapeutic medications and the selection of a number of pharmaceutical factories to produce essential drugs for rare diseases with a state subsidy. Under the Chinese government's national health goal of "Healthy China 2020," the social security system for patients with rare diseases, including ALS, has developed and improved rapidly.

Patients with ALS can apply for disability identification and disability certificates and receive a monthly subsidy according to national regulations. Under the deployment of the State Council of China's "establishment of living allowances for disabled persons and care subsidies for severely disabled persons," provinces have successively introduced social security systems for disabled people. With the support and guidance of the China Disabled Persons' Federation (2019), an ALS Expert Committee was established and completed the first Chinese ALS Rehabilitation and Care Guidelines in 2018. These guidelines have been published recently and will be used as the textbook for training.

Meanwhile, the China Social Welfare Foundation (2019) has also been active in setting up civil ALS patient associations. The first Chinese ALS patient association, Oriental Rain ALS Care Center (also known as Oriental Rain ALS Patient Association), was established in November 2013 and is subordinate to China Social Welfare Foundation. It joined the International Alliance of ALS/MND Association in 2015, established the Home of ALS China in 2017 and has been open to patients from all over the country ever since. The ALS Million Respiratory Project (http://www.jiandongren.org/) was the first project Oriental Rain ALS Care Center launched after it was established. The project aims to support breathing management for economically poor ALS patients to improve their quality of life (QoL). Since the launch in November 2014, the project has raised more than 5 million RMB (700,000 USD), provided free medical equipment (i.e., breathing apparatus, airway clearance devices and oxygen generators) to nearly 2000 ALS patients and organized nearly 100 training sessions for ALS breathing management and care, which has greatly improved the QoL of ALS patients.

Another active public organization is the Rehabilitation Division of China Disabled Persons' Federation (2019) that focuses on the care and rehabilitation of disabled persons, assisting in the establishment of ALS patient care centers and providing nursing care guidance. Funded by the Federation, the guidelines for ALS rehabilitation and care have been completed by Oriental Rain ALS Care and have been published recently. Moreover, for three consecutive years, the Beijing Disabled Persons' Federation (2019) has cooperated with Oriental Rain ALS Care to hold ALS rehabilitation and care training sessions at the Rehabilitative Service Center of Beijing Disabled Persons' Federation. Finally, on August 20, 2014, inspired by the Ice Bucket Challenge that swept the world that year, China Social Welfare Foundation set up an ALS fund to help improve the care of ALS patients.

Similarly, the Shaanxi ALS Association (SNALSA) is a non-profit volunteer social organization that was created by healthcare workers, ALS patients and their family members and medical institutes of Shaanxi Province. Its establishment was formally approved by the Bureau of Civil Affairs, Shaanxi, in January 2014 and was admitted as a member of the International Alliance of ALS/MND Association in 2015. In addition, BingYuGe WeChat Official Platform is a public platform created by Ms. Min Ge and other ALS patients in early 2018. It draws together ALS patients from all over the country, through which they communicate and comfort each other and seek peace of mind. Behind each article is a moving story of persistence.

Public Funding for Research and Care

National Natural Science Foundation of China (2019) recently has increased overall research funding, prioritized rare diseases (including ALS) in research grant approvals and involved rare diseases in key projects. In addition, the Key Project of Precise Medicine Research, Ministry of Science and Technology of China (http://www.most.gov.cn/) focuses both on prevalent diseases that are threatening public health and rare diseases with a relatively high incidence. It aims to establish a research cohort for each specific disease; an experimental and analytic system for disease risk, diagnosis and therapeutic outcomes; the precise criteria for disease prevention, diagnosis and treatment; a clinical decision-making system and a structure to demonstrate, apply and promote effective clinical programs to address diseases among the Chinese population.

The ALS Clinical Center of Peking University Third Hospital closely collaborates with top foreign research institutes and laboratories. In recent years, it has established several international cooperative fund projects with scientific teams from Germany, the United States and Australia in order to advance ALS research.

Incomplete statistics show that the overall funding from the Ministry of Civil Affairs, China Disabled Persons' Federation and other governmental and civil organizations has exceeded 10 million RMB ($1.4 million US), which is used to purchase breathing apparatus, write textbooks, train professionals, help economically poor families, provide assistive devices for patients with limb dysfunctions, partially fund the Home of ALS China and the Taikang Nursing Centre and provide subsidies for volunteers. Public funds for ALS research and care are gradually growing but are much lower than that of Western countries, indicating a need to be increased further.

PUBLIC AND MEDIA PERCEPTIONS OF ALS

Since the 2014 Ice Bucket Challenge, public awareness of ALS has increased dramatically through the media. The rapid development of new media (Weibo, WeChat) has further elevated the public understanding of ALS. Some celebrities, through their own promotion and influence, inspire fans to participate in social welfare events and volunteer help for ALS patients. At present, most ALS-related activities are initiated by the public, with very little commercial contribution. However, increasingly more companies are willing to be sponsors. ALS-related companies are willing to donate free equipment supplies, while unrelated companies usually donate funds for public ALS welfare programs.

CARE OF ALS PATIENTS IN CHINA

Long-term follow-up data from Peking University Third Hospital show that most ALS patients are cared for by family members at home, some patients live in care centers and a very small number of patients stay in a hospital long term. The location of patient care selected by the family members is closely related to the family structure as well as economic status.

Those who care for ALS patients are mainly family members and personal support workers (full-time, nonprofessional, paid). Most caregivers are nonprofessional. Because it is costly to hire professional nurses, only a few wealthy families can afford it. However, care for ALS patients is becoming increasingly more professional and refined despite a continuing shortage of trained professionals. Therefore, more dedicated training in ALS care is required to improve professionalism. Most importantly, more people are needed to join caregiver teams.

Governmental Aid for Family Caregivers

Initiated three years ago, severely disabled individuals are granted a monthly allowance of 300 RMB ($43 US). Also, through the China Disabled Persons' Federation, family caregivers of ALS patients are provided training and re-employment opportunities. Furthermore, respite care services for the disabled are currently being developed and will provide family caregivers opportunities to rest.

The Beijing Disabled People's Federation provides rehabilitation homecare services to home-bound disabled individuals. It has also set up a service platform to provide assistive supplies under which most of the expenses are waived if patients provide a disability certificate and state their needs for the assistive supplies. Presently, the organization is seeking a list of special supplies for ALS patients, thereby increasing assistance to them. Additionally, the China Social Welfare Foundation provides support to ALS patients from economically poor families by providing them with breathing apparatus. The ALS medication, riluzole, is covered by medical insurance, which greatly reduces the financial burden on patients and their families.

Access to Assistive Technologies and Drugs

If patients can afford it, a variety of electronic communication devices are currently available, including eye-tracking systems and brain-computer interfaces to help patients communicate with others. Artificial intelligence equipment is also being developed. However, electronic communication devices are still very expensive for average income families, which restricts their application. Therefore, accessibility needs to be further improved.

There are no relevant laws regarding right to try unapproved drugs in China at present. In fact, the government does not permit the use of unapproved drugs, although it is possible that patients may obtain such drugs privately.

Status of Multidisciplinary Team Care and Clinics

Currently, some major Chinese cities have a comprehensive, multidisciplinary, multicenter medical teams. Peking University Third Hospital is an example. Every week, ALS patients can visit the multidisciplinary team (MDT) Joint Consultation Center, where multidisciplinary experts can make diagnoses and develop treatment plans for them. To help patients living in remote areas, Peking University Third Hospital developed an online teleconsultation system to resolve patients' problems and concerns in a timely fashion.

GENETIC TESTING FOR ALS

Genetic testing is performed for familial ALS patients, young ALS patients or patients with specific clinical manifestations. With fully informed consent, second-generation sequencing, whole-exome sequencing and whole-genome sequencing can be selected. If their finances permit, patients are charged for the cost of the test. If patients are financially unable to pay and genetic testing will add substantial data for patient care, the hospital or a foundation can sponsor the test. The test results, in the form of a formal written report, are given only to the patient or his or her authorized family member.

PALLIATIVE AND HOSPICE CARE FOR ALS PATIENTS

Due to the shortage of medical resources as well as the prevalence of the traditional Chinese concept of family, only a small number of patients receive palliative treatment and hospice care. From the hospitals' perspective, more social workers and volunteers are needed. Due to inconvenience to patients, patients and their family members want to receive home care services from physicians and personal support workers to improve QoL at the end-stage. This situation has already drawn government attention and has gradually improved, but there is still great room for further improvement.

According to Chinese policy, a death certificate issued by a hospital is required after death; thus, most of patients die in a hospital even though only a minority of them are hospitalized patients. A small number of patients die at home or in care centers.

END-OF-LIFE DECISION-MAKING

Currently, in China, patients and family members can choose not to use mechanical ventilation or ventilators, but it is illegal to withdraw mechanical ventilation and other life-prolonging measures and mechanical support once they are started. Overall, Chinese ALS patients have low acceptance rates for invasive treatments due to the following reasons:

1. Cultural reasons: Because of fear and resistance, Chinese patients generally have low acceptance rates for invasive interventional treatments, leading to an extremely low rate of endotracheal intubation and tracheotomy. Some patients deliberately conceal the severity of their condition to their doctor to postpone using noninvasive breathing apparatus as long as possible. As a result, treatment initiation is often very late, and the overall number of patients using noninvasive breathing apparatus is low. Through persistent patient education, patients' traditional beliefs have somewhat changed, and the application of invasive and noninvasive breathing apparatus is gradually increasing.

2. Economic reasons: The use of an invasive ventilator and the resulting management costs are an unbearable financial burden to most Chinese families. The high prices of in-home invasive and noninvasive breathing apparatus restrict their application and promotion. In the end, however, the decision of patients and their families to use ventilation and other mechanical support is totally respected in China.

For end-stage patients suffering from pain, sleep disorders or other physical discomforts, palliative pain relief, soothing treatment and other methods can be used to alleviate suffering. However, euthanasia and physician-assisted suicide are illegal in China. Suicide is difficult to implement because of the difficulty of movement in end-stage patients; therefore, it is extremely rare. Moreover, in Chinese culture, suicide and euthanasia are contrary to ethical and moral behavior because of the strong family concept and integrity; thus, few people attempt suicide or would accept euthanasia. In addition, Chinese culture is lacking death education. Patients and their families usually avoid talking about death, as they are unable to accept or face death. Patients with very traditional thoughts do not accept invasive treatments such as ventilators and gastrostomy. Most Chinese families are small and without religious beliefs, and there is very little support from outside the family.

SUGGESTED POLICY CHANGES TO IMPROVE THE CARE OF ALS PATIENTS

There is a need for increased funding for scientific research and clinical care. In addition, more nurses with professional skills should be trained to provide quality care to improve the QoL of patients, and additional professional training and psychological and economic support should be provided to caregivers. We also recommend conducting more international clinical trials in China because of the vast population and the large number of patients. Finally, both caregivers and patients require whole-person care and increased efforts by all sectors of society.

REFERENCES

Beijing Disabled Persons' Federation (2019). http://www.bdpf.org.cn/.

China Disabled Persons' Federation (2019). http://www.cdpf.org.cn/.

Chinese Medical Association Neurology Branch (2019). http://www.cmancn.org.cn/.

Chinese Medical Doctor Association Melting the Freezing Heart Program (2019). http://www.cmda.net/hydt11/10333.jhtml.

Fong, G.C., T.S. Cheng, K. Lam et al. (2005). An epidemiological study of motor neuron disease in Hong Kong. *Amyotrophic Lateral Sclerosis and Other Motor Neuron Disorders* 6 (3): 164–68.

National Natural Science Foundation of China (2019). http://www.nsfc.gov.cn/.

The China Social Welfare Foundation (2019). http://www.cdpf.org.cn/.

The Rehabilitation Division of China Disabled Persons' Federation (2019). http://www.cdpf.org.cn/ywzz/kf_211/.

Tsai, C-P, K-C. Wang, C-S. Hwang, I.T. Lee and C.T. Lee (2015). Incidence, prevalence, and medical expenditures of classical amyotrophic lateral sclerosis in Taiwan, 1999–2008. *Journal of the Formosan Medical Association* 114: 612–19.

Xu L., L. Chen, S. Wang, J. Feng et al. (2020). Incidence and prevalence of amyotrophic lateral sclerosis in urban China: a national population-based study. *Journal of Neurology, Neurosurgery and Psychiatry* 91 (5): 520–525.

Zhou, S., S. Qian, X. Li, L. Zheng, W. Chang and L. Wang (2018a). Using the capture-recapture method to estimate the incidence of amyotrophic lateral sclerosis in Beijing, China. *Neuroepidemiology* 50: 29–34.

Zhou, S., Y. Zhou, S. Qian, W. Chang, L. Wang and D. Fan (2018b). Amyotrophic lateral sclerosis in Beijing: Epidemiologic features and prognosis from 2010 to 2015. *Brain and Behavior* 8:e01131.

CHAPTER 7

German Perspective on ALS/MND Policy

Maike F. Dohrn and Roman Rolke

Abstract Guideline development on motor neuron disease (MND) in Germany is driven mainly by the German Neurological Society and German Association for Muscle Diseases. Greater research funding, a national strategy, and programs on MND are still lacking. General and specialized palliative care home services, palliative care units, or hospice care are accessible for all MND patients in Germany. Assistive technologies can be ordered by treating physicians in experienced centers. In symptomatic patients, qualified neurologists can request genetic testing of about five to ten genes per year. Withholding or withdrawing mechanical ventilation in end-of-life situations of MND can be described as "passive help in dying," and the German Ethics Council recommends use of the term "letting die." Palliative sedation therapy is allowed in Germany, euthanasia is prohibited.

Keywords MND • ALS • German Ethics Council • Deutscher Ethikrat • Genetic counseling • Passive euthanasia • Letting die • End-of-life

M. F. Dohrn • R. Rolke (✉)
RWTH Aachen University Hospital, Aachen, Germany
e-mail: mdohrn@ukaachen.de; rrolke@ukaachen.de

© The Author(s) 2021
R. H. Blank et al. (eds.), *Public Policy in ALS/MND Care*,
https://doi.org/10.1007/978-981-15-5840-5_7

Incidence and Prevalence of ALS/MND in Germany

With an estimated prevalence of 6–8/100,000 inhabitants, amyotrophic lateral sclerosis (ALS) is considered a rare disease in Germany. It affects approximately 4800 to 6500 individuals. The German Federal Statistical Office (Statistisches Bundesamt, https://www-genesis.destatis.de) registered 9345 patients released from hospital with the diagnosis of motor neuron disease (MND) in 2017, although multiple entering of an individual is possible. Assuming a life span of two to four years after diagnosis, the overall incidence is 2/100,000 individuals. This is consistent with the European estimates (Logroscino et al. 2010). However, results from the Swabian ALS register reported an incidence rate of 3.1/1,000,000 individuals for southern Germany (Rosenbohm et al. 2017). There might be regional differences which have not been systematically assessed so far, but there are no known endemic areas for familial or sporadic ALS in Germany. Only 5 percent of all ALS patients report a positive family history.

Government and Private Activity

There have been no governmental actions, reports or committees on ALS/MND to date in Germany. However, the German Society of Neurology (Deutsche Gesellschaft für Neurologie, DGN) in 2003 established a national guideline for the diagnosis and treatment of MND, and especially ALS, which was last updated in 2014/2015. It is dedicated to all professions involved in the diagnosis and care of MND patients including physicians, therapists, social workers and nurses and focuses on both in- and outpatient treatment settings.

A traditional advocacy group for ALS/MND patients is the German Association for Muscle Diseases (Deutsche Gesellschaft für Muskelkranke, DGM). Founded in 1965, this association originated as a parents' initiative, receiving support by physicians and nurses. The principal aims are to promote research and support the affected by means of financial assistance and self-help. It has published online and in printed form many information booklets addressed to ALS patients and/or their relatives that cover important matters like breath assistance and end-of-life considerations in a patient-friendly way. The Association also provides a specialized emergency passport for patients with all types of neuromuscular diseases that summarizes the most important information on the patient's diagnosis, current treatment, private and professional contacts, anesthetic risks and special requirements of ventilation and care. In 2018, the Association founded a diagnosis-related subgroup for ALS patients which collaborates closely with the official Network for Motorneuron Diseases (MND-NET) and other neuromuscular or clinical trial centers. Organized on a national level, there are counterparts in different regions that can provide information and contact for patients and families.

Examples of other self-organized advocacy groups are "ALS—der Wunsch zu leben e.V." (ALS—the desire to live association), "ALS mobil e.V." (ALS mobile association) and "Initiative Therapieforschung ALS e.V." (initiative for ALS treatment research association), which work together with each other and with the German MND-NET as well. When the Federal Ministry of Education and Research (Bundesministerium für Bildung und Forschung, BMBF) announced it would no longer maintain the high level of ALS funding following the Ice Bucket Challenge in 2015, the aforementioned associations started a collaborative initiative called "Stop! ALS" and collected about 20,000 signatures.

Several other self-help groups are organized on the regional level, mostly localized around hospitals or outpatient clinics. An exemplary advocacy group, the association "Alle-Lieben-Schmidt" ("all love Schmidt"), was founded by an ALS patient named Bruno Schmidt and is highly active particularly on a regional level. Its members provide individual counseling and help to affected patients and families and organize fundraising events such as runs or biking tours. With this money, the association supports families in need as well as research projects on ALS. It raises not only money but also public awareness which is needed to create pressure on governmental and research organizations and overcome stigmatization. A documentary on Bruno Schmidt visiting other ALS patients and their families at home during his last biking tour throughout Germany has been shown at various cinematic events and has won national awards.

FUNDING PATIENT CARE AND RESEARCH IN GERMANY

Patient care is organized on a national level, and since 1995, it is obligatory to have insurance which covers care dependency. As a consequence, every citizen has the right to receive regular care services, financial support or payment in kind, from the federal government. The Federal Ministry of Health (Bundesministerium für Gesundheit) is the core governmental agency involved. Since the enactment of two federal laws in 2015 and 2016, the extent of care dependency is now distributed into five instead of three categories with the intent to offer more flexible support to patients and families according to their respective health care needs. However, this needs-oriented approach is not related to any particular diagnosis, and there is no governmental care program specifically for ALS/MND patients.

ALS/MND research is financially supported by both public and private organizations and foundations. Historically, university research policy was largely organized on a state level. However, since 2015, Article 91b of the German constitutional law (Grundgesetz) assures that projects of suprare-gional importance can be subsidized both by federal and state institutions. The Federal Ministry of Education and Research (Bundesministerium für Bildung und Forschung, BMBF) determines general educational and research policy and provides funding for single projects, collaborative groups and institutions. Since 2003, the BMBF has fostered various rare disease initiatives, one being the National Action League for People with Rare Diseases (NAMSE, founded in 2010) which produced a complex action plan with fifty-two proposals to shorten latencies to diagnosis and improve patient care and research. In the past five years, the BMBF has provided funding for ten ALS/MND projects to research groups in Aachen, Bad Nauheim, Berlin, Göttingen, Hannover, Jena, München (twice), Regensburg and Tübingen, with a total sum of about ten million euros.

Another important share of public funding for research and care comes from the German Research Foundation (Deutsche Forschungsgemeinschaft, DFG) which is a self-governed association under private law. Drawing their financial sources from both the states and the federal government, the DFG has supported ten projects on ALS/MND since 2014, six of those by providing material grants, two by supporting a priority program, one by funding a collaborative research center and one by financing a research fellowship. Other sources of funding are provided by centers for interdisciplinary clinical research and university organizations associated with medical faculties. Additionally, patient organizations and self-help groups invest in research, but the amount and focus is based on patients' and collaborators' discretion.

Research on cure and care of such a tragic disease like ALS can hardly be overfunded. Not only do the pathomechanisms need to be further addressed, requiring molecular genetic screening tools, complex cell and animal models, clinical trials and real-life assessments, but also the ethical and practical aspects of patient needs deserve to be further assessed. The overall funding rate of neuroscientific projects, however, is currently relatively high (according to personal information, up to 70 percent of the submitted research proposals are accepted by the DFG to date), so that in a country like Germany that is at the cutting edge of Western medicine, the possibilities to advance in MND research are comparatively good.

PUBLIC AWARENESS AND MEDIA INTEREST

The public and media perception of ALS in Germany has been influenced significantly by prominent athletes. When the Polish national soccer player Krzysztof Nowak was diagnosed with ALS at the age of 25, his own and several other German soccer clubs raised awareness of the—at the time relatively unknown—disease. By setting up the Krzysztof-Nowak Foundation in 2002, his former soccer club VfL Wolfsburg began to actively support ALS patients and also research. Krzysztof Nowak died in 2005 at the age of 29. The German racing cyclist André Greipel successfully participates in many Grand Tours such as the Tour de France. Through his openness about his mother having died from ALS, he became one of the public advocates for ALS patients in Germany. With his "Fight-ALS" bike racing team consisting of professional and hobby bikers, he regularly participates in fundraising and beneficial events to raise awareness and collect money.

WHERE ALS PATIENTS LIVE AND DIE

There are no standardized data on the proportion of German ALS patients living at home and of those living in a care home, so a statistical percentage cannot be provided. Based on personal experience, most patients appear to live at home until the very last stage of the disease and then prefer to either die at home supported by a palliative home care service or in a hospice. However, this impression could be biased because only those patients who are mobile enough or sufficiently supported by family members come to our center.

In Germany, the place of death is not part of the death certificate. The proportion of ALS/MND patients who die at home, in care facilities, hospitals or hospices can, therefore, only be estimated indirectly on the basis of data from the health insurance companies. Such data are currently not available.

PALLIATIVE CARE AND HOSPICES IN GERMANY

General and specialized palliative care home services are widely available. The reimbursement rate of these professional caregiver services is 100 percent and completely covered by all health insurance companies in Germany. This also applies for professional caregivers in palliative care units and hospices. Professionals such as physicians, nurses, physiotherapists, psychologists, social workers or chaplains act hand in hand with family caregivers. In Germany, the number of ambulatory hospice services involving qualified volunteers is growing. To date, more than 1300 of these hospice services exist for adults.

Although all MND patients in Germany have adequate access to palliative and hospice care, many palliative or hospice caregiver teams are trained and have experience in caring for predominately cancer patients. For many teams, there remains a lack of knowledge, and they perform with less developed neurological skills when caring for MND patients. Table 7.1 demonstrates the wide distribution of these services.

SUPPORT FOR FAMILY CARE AND ASSISTIVE TECHNOLOGIES

All family caregivers—not restricted to MND patients—receive financial aids from the special care insurance (Pflegeversicherung) in Germany. This type of financial aid is aimed at coverage of costs for home care services. The money is paid to families who can then decide how to use it, either for the care they deliver or for a nursing team.

Assistive technologies such as (electronic) wheelchairs or speech computers can be ordered by treating physicians mostly in experienced centers. Patients usually borrow such assistive devices from the manufacturer to test the respective advantages, and then as a second step, the physician prescribes the already tested device. Both the prescription and the patient's report of successful use are submitted for approval to the responsible health insurance. In case of rejection of the claim for reimbursement, the patient can file an objection. Compared to other rare diseases such as muscular dystrophy or hereditary neuropathies, ALS/MND patients tend to experience less rejection when applying for support.

Table 7.1 Overview of palliative care and hospice services across Germany

Germany States	PC counseling services in hospitals	PC units in hospitals	Specialized PC at home services	Hospice volunteer services	Hospice at home
Baden-Württemberg	8	45	36	26	281
Bayern	21	53	45	19	153
Berlin	1	11	10	13	35
Brandenburg	4	10	11	11	25
Bremen	3	2	3	2	8
Hamburg	2	6	8	6	20
Hessen	3	21	27	22	103
Mecklenburg-Vorpommern	1	10	11	8	18
Niedersachsen	3	36	50	26	147
Nordrhein-Westfalen	12	72	34	67	288
Rheinland-Pfalz	4	25	9	12	52
Saarland	1	6	4	3	26
Sachsen	1	19	12	8	54
Sachsen-Anhalt	0	10	8	7	26
Schleswig-Holstein	3	9	16	6	55
Thüringen	1	8	8	7	33
Overall sum	**68**	**343**	**292**	**243**	**1324**

ALS/MND patients are supported by all types of PC units or services in Germany. Numbers are current as of August 6, 2019 (Data source: Wegweiser Hospiz- und Palliativversorgung Deutschland; Guide to Hospice and Palliative Care in Germany, personal communication)

MULTIDISCIPLINARY TEAMS

Multidisciplinary teams are becoming increasingly important in ALS care. In a German outpatient network ("Ambulanzpartner"), there are currently 245 clinics and private practices listed as specialist contact persons for patients. Around twenty university centers are specialized in MND, but are not completely accessible as some centers have separate MND consultants and others integrate these patients into a broader neuromuscular outpatient clinic. To varying degrees, these centers not only provide a high neurological expertise for in- and outpatient care but also offer a fast and easy transfer to a pulmonologist for non-invasive or invasive ventilation and cough-assist machines, to the gastroenterologist for applying a percutaneous endoscopic gastrostomy tube, to a human geneticist if family counseling is required and to a palliative care specialist and/or psychologist to better control other symptoms such as depression and anxiety.

Besides the medical staff, however, there are speech therapists, physiotherapists and ergotherapists to assess a patient's functional status and provide recommendations for nearby family therapists. Assistive devices as well as symptomatic drugs can be prescribed at the specialized centers. With a centralized expertise, it is easier to meet the specific needs of each patient while unburdening neurologists and family physicians. Connecting the centers by networks and registers such as MND NET, patient care can be assessed, compared and harmonized, providing national standards and common goals. The presence of specialized centers can persuade patients and families that even if there is no cure, there are still options open to provide help.

AVAILABILITY OF UNAPPROVED DRUGS

Since 1976, medicinal products can only be prescribed after officially being approved by either the Federal Institute for Drugs and Medical Devices (Bundesinstitut für Arzneimittel und Medizinprodukte, BfArM) or the European Medicines Agency (EMA). Vaccines receive their approval by the Robert Koch Institute.

In Germany, there is no "right to try" defined by law. However, if the treating physician sees a potential benefit of a certain treatment that is off or beyond its approval for the respective patient, there are two options for obtaining access depending on the type of medication. For treatment modalities already approved for diseases other than ALS, the Federal Joint Committee (Gemeinsamer Bundesausschuss, G-BA) has defined criteria for a so-called off-label use. Following these criteria, the disease of interest needs to be severely disabling or life threatening, there must not be any other approved treatment alternative for this patient and there have to be data from the literature suggesting a potential benefit of this particular drug.

In case a prospective treatment is still in the process of approval or in clinical trials and the expected approval might come too late for a certain patient, the current legislation, last modified by the amendment of the German Medicinal Product Act (Arzneimittelgesetz, AMG) in July 2009, stipulates a compassionate use program. Therefore, a marketing authorization is not required if a medicinal product is provided free of charge "for administration to patients with a seriously debilitating disease or whose disease is life-threatening, and who cannot be treated satisfactorily with an authorized medicinal product" (Section 21, sub-section 2, No. 6 of the German Medicinal Product Act). Both off-label and compassionate use have to be requested and justified by the treating physician.

GENETIC TESTING FOR MND

The national guideline for the diagnosis and care for MND patients recommends offering genetic analyses to affected patients with a positive family history (Ludolph 2015). Since young ALS patients have a greater probability of carrying a de novo mutation, they are exempted from this recommendation since family members are not likely to be affected. Genetic counseling and written informed consent are essential requirements for any genetic tests. Psychological support can be offered but is not a routine part of the counseling process. The German Genetic Diagnostics Act (Gendiagnostikgesetz) stipulates that predictive tests and analyses in children can only be performed by human geneticists, who are physicians with a five-year specialization in human genetics. In symptomatic patients, however, the informed consent for genetic testing can also be obtained by a qualified specialist in the field of the respective disease.

Since July 2016, the general health insurances cover 25 kilobases of molecular genetic analysis per year, which allows a panel analysis of about five to ten genes for any individual patient. Since there are currently about 22 genes known to cause MND if mutated (Volk et al. 2018), it is necessary that the requesting physician chooses an appropriate number of the most likely genes. This requires knowledge on genotype-phenotype patterns such as age of onset, predominantly affected systems, associated features and mode of inheritance. Specialists are typically located at MND or neuromuscular centers. In Germany, the most common gene associated with ALS is *C9ORF* affecting 25 percent of patients with a positive family history and up to 10 percent of the sporadic cases. Other commonly identifiable genes are *SOD1, TDP43* and *FUS.*

If the significance of a genetic mutation is unclear, this might cause major confusion to both patients and relatives. It is up to the requesting physician's discretion whether and how a test result should be reported. Another potential problem can be occasional findings that disclose heritable diseases other than the one in question. It is now common in Germany that patients are asked whether they want or do not want to be informed about additional findings prior to the analysis, which is then documented on the consent form. Predictive tests (Benatar et al. 2016) can only be performed if a known pathogenic mutation has already been proven in a first-degree related family member, so that the result will be a clear yes or no constellation. The counseling protocols for individuals at risk resemble those of other fatal diseases such as Huntington's and meet international standards. At least two appointments are recommended including pre-decision, pre-test and post-test counseling. The responsible counselor is supposed to assess psychological readiness and offer psychological support.

ADVANCE DIRECTIVES AND END-OF-LIFE DECISIONS

Based on the third law to change the right for care in Germany, in force since September 2009 (Advance Directive Act), advance directives (ADs) must now be written (not necessarily handwritten). A revocation can be made "informally" (i.e. also verbally) at any time. They are only binding if (1) the patient's will for the specific treatment situation can be clearly and reliably determined, (2) the patient does not visibly change his/her mind and (3) the advance directive has been drawn up in a state of consent (decision-making ability). The validity of such advance directive is not limited in time.

Withholding or withdrawing mechanical ventilation in end-of-life situations of patients with ALS/MND can be described as "passive help in dying." According to the recommendations of the German Ethics Council (Deutscher Ethikrat), the term "passive euthanasia" should not be used to avoid confusion with the term "direct or active euthanasia," a procedure that is forbidden in Germany. Instead, the German Ethics Council recommends use of the term "letting die" which reflects the practical and ethical process including the termination of all types of life-extending procedures and mechanical support if ongoing treatment has become futile.

Palliative sedation is allowed in Germany. A controversial debate has been fought on the German end-of-life regulations, at the center of which fatal diseases such as ALS have often been discussed. In Germany, "direct or active euthanasia" is prohibited by law. Individual cases of physician-assisted suicide (PAS) are not prosecuted by official authorities, but they are not accepted as part of the Medical Association's professional code of conduct. Just as suicide itself cannot be prosecuted in Germany, so assistance to it is also exempt from punishment by law. Killing on request (euthanasia), however, is punishable (§216 Criminal Code) in Germany.

According to the German Medical Association (Bundesärztekammer), collaboration in suicide conflicts with a physician's professional duty to maintain respect for life. The alleviation of suffering, which is indeed one of the physician's responsibilities, should rather be provided by palliative care. The German Ethics Council has passed several opinion papers on end-of-life considerations, for example, in 2006 and 2014 (German Ethics Council Opinion Report on "Self-determination and Care at the End of Life," www.ethikrat.org), that recommended prohibiting systematic assisted suicide but acknowledged the individual moral implications within a doctor–patient relationship that might arise in an exceptional situation.

CULTURAL AND HISTORICAL PARTICULARITIES IN THE GERMAN POSITION ON END-OF-LIFE DECISIONS

Some data suggest that in comparison to neighbor countries such as Belgium and the Netherlands, euthanasia and PAS are less commonly requested by patients and less frequently accepted by physicians in Germany. This information, however, has been extracted from small studies in which the perspectives of patients (Lule et al. 2008), relatives (Kuhnlein et al. 2008) and physicians (Maitra et al. 2005) were assessed by questionnaires or structural interviews. Solid evidence representing the cultural diversity of the entire country is lacking and a selection bias might have occurred in some studies.

In a Bavarian cohort for instance, only 10 percent of related caregivers of an already deceased ALS patient admitted that the affected family member had expressed an interest in PAS, whereas 17 percent temporarily had mentioned suicidal thoughts within the course of the disease (Kuhnlein et al. 2008). In an anonymous questionnaire, more than 90 percent of palliative caregivers expressed their disagreement of the legalization of "killing on request" and about 75 percent did not support PAS (Muller-Busch et al. 2004). Contrarily, 62 percent of general practitioners stated they had already been approached by a patient asking for euthanasia at least once in their career and 73 percent were asked for PAS (Maitra et al. 2005). The German neurologists' attitude toward these end-of-life considerations has so far not been systematically assessed. In a patient cohort with multiple sclerosis, as distinct from ALS/MND, however, 25 percent of the treating neurologists were asked for euthanasia, of whom about 80 percent strictly declined (Kumpfel et al. 2007).

To delineate the differences with neighboring countries, several hypotheses have been presented. Religiosity, shown as believing in life after death, seemed to be one factor to be influential, particularly as patients interested in PAS displayed a lower tendency to be religious (Kuhnlein et al. 2008). The fact that the term "euthanasia" was used by Nazi prosecutors as an euphemism to deflect the systematic homicide of disabled people seems to have a minor effect on the current physicians' attitudes (Muller-Busch et al. 2004). However, the National Ethics Council revealed that the sensitivity about the term "euthanasia" might still influence the German opposition toward active euthanasia in favor of historical responsibility (Schicktanz et al. 2010). Instead of the internationally conventional term "euthanasia" (in German: "Euthanasie"), a vague translation (active or direct "help in dying"/ "aktive/direkte Sterbehilfe") is actually used.

Both withholding and withdrawal of life-prolonging medical interventions such as non-invasive or invasive ventilation, the administration of antibiotics or the implementation of a percutaneous gastrostomy tube are considered "passive euthanasia" in Germany, which is legal when following the patient's wish. The national guidelines for the diagnosis and treatment of MND, therefore, recommend addressing the affected individual's attitudes and preoccupations toward death and the process of dying as early in the clinical course as possible. ADs were first brought into consideration when the German Medical Association published an article on new principles for medical care of the terminally ill in 1998 (Bundesärztekammer 1998). A 2009 law on living wills (German Civil Code §1901a) strengthened the binding character of the patient's wish without the requirement of a notarial act. Several examples and formulation patterns are provided for patients by lawyers, physicians and churches. If clearly written, an AD can assist both caregivers and medical support teams in the final stage of ALS. If a patient's wish remains doubtful, however, the National Ethics Council recommends deciding in favor of life and continuing sustaining treatment.

CONCLUSIONS

With an estimated incidence of 2/100,000 inhabitants per year, the number of annually diagnosed ALS cases ranges in the same level as new HIV infections in Germany, but is more frequent than infectious diseases such as meningococcal meningitis. ALS/MND remains underrepresented in the public awareness, but this has recently begun to change with the increasing activities of self-help groups and patient organizations, public advocates, networks and specialized outpatient centers. With a heightened emphasis on both care and eventual cure, many milestones still have to be reached to better meet the needs of patients and their families. Besides pathomechanistic and therapy-oriented research, important subjects such as home and hospice care, family counseling and end-of-life considerations merit further investigation to face the complexity of this terrible disease.

References

Benatar, M., C. Stanislaw, E. Reyes, S. Hussain et al. (2016). Presymptomatic ALS genetic counseling and testing: Experience and recommendations. *Neurology* 86 (24): 2295–2302.

Kuhnlein, P., A. Kubler, S. Raubold, M. Worrell et al. (2008). Palliative care and circumstances of dying in German ALS patients using non-invasive ventilation. *Amyotrophic Lateral Sclerosis 9* (2): 91–98.

Kumpfel, T., L.A. Hoffmann, W. Pollmann, P. Rieckmann et al. (2007). Palliative care in patients with severe multiple sclerosis: Two case reports and a survey among German MS neurologists. *Palliative Medicine* 21 (2): 109–14.

Logroscino, G., B.J. Traynor, O. Hardiman, A. Chio et al. (2010). Incidence of amyotrophic lateral sclerosis in Europe. *Journal of Neurology, Neurosurgery and Psychiatry* 81 (4): 385–90.

Ludolph, A. (2015). ALS (motor neuron disease) guideline Retrieved from https://www.dgn.org/images/red_leitlinien/LL_2014/PDFs_Download/030001_DGN_LL_ALS.pdf

Lule, D., S. Hacker, A. Ludolph, N. Birbaumer and A. Kubler (2008). Depression and quality of life in patients with amyotrophic lateral sclerosis. *Dtsch Arztebl Int* 105 (23), 397–403. https://doi.org/10.3238/arztebl.2008.0397

Maitra, R.T., A. Harfst, L.M. Bjerre, M.M. Kochen and A. Becker (2005). Do German general practitioners support euthanasia? Results of a nation-wide questionnaire survey. *European Journal of General Practice* 11 (3–4): 94–100.

Muller-Busch, H.C., F.S. Oduncu, S. Woskanjan and E. Klaschik (2004). Attitudes on euthanasia, physician-assisted suicide and terminal sedation--a survey of the members of the German Association for Palliative Medicine. *Med Health Care Philosophy* 7 (3): 333–39.

Rosenbohm, A., R.S. Peter, S. Erhardt, D. Lule et al. (2017). Epidemiology of amyotrophic lateral sclerosis in Southern Germany. *Journal of Neurology* 264 (4): 749–57.

Schicktanz, S., A. Raz and C. Shalev (2010). The cultural context of end-of-life ethics: A comparison of Germany and Israel. *Cambridge Quarterly of Healthcare Ethics* 19 (3): 381–94.

Volk, A.E., J.H. Weishaupt, P.M. Andersen, A.C. Ludolph and C. Kubisch (2018). Current knowledge and recent insights into the genetic basis of amyotrophic lateral sclerosis. *Medical Genetics* 30 (2): 252–58.

OTHER RESOURCES

Guideline of the German Neurological Association (DGN) on ALS (motor neuron disease) (2015). https://www.dgn.org/images/red_leitlinien/LL_2014/PDFs_Download/030001_DGN_LL_ALS.pdf

Recommendations of the German Ethics Council (Deutscher Ethikrat) (2014). https://www.ethikrat.org/fileadmin/Publikationen/Ad-hoc-Empfehlungen/deutsch/empfehlung-suizidbeihilfe.pdf

Statement of the German Medical Association (Bundesärztekammer) (1998). 'Grundsätze der Bundesärztekammer zur ärztlichen Sterbebegleitung' Deutsches Ärzteblatt 95, A2365–2366.

CHAPTER 8

Living and Dying with ALS/MND in India: Public Policy and Private Realities

Roop Gursahani and Satish Khadilkar

Abstract Amyotrophic lateral sclerosis/motor neuron disease (MND/ALS) is an uncommon disease in India with a prevalence of about 4/100,000. Available care is shared with other chronic diseases and is largely pay-as-you-go. There are no dedicated multidisciplinary clinics or services for management. Almost all patients are cared for at home by family or by paid caregivers. Palliative and rehabilitative care are particularly underdeveloped in India. The major barrier is a taboo on the discussion of death and dying; truth-telling is the exception and collusion is the rule. The legal system has only just begun to recognize advance directives, and medical aid in dying may not be considered for at least two decades. The way ahead consists of neurologist training in the basics of palliative care, advocacy for appropriate end-of-life legislation and public awareness and

R. Gursahani (✉)
P.D. Hinduja National Hospital, Mumbai, India
e-mail: roop_gursahani@hotmail.com

S. Khadilkar
Bombay Hospital Institute of Medical Sciences, Mumbai, India
e-mail: khadilkarsatish@gmail.com

R. H. Blank et al. (eds.), *Public Policy in ALS/MND Care*,
https://doi.org/10.1007/978-981-15-5840-5_8

support for palliative care. The emergence of a patient-run support group for MND is a major positive.

Keywords Amyotrophic lateral sclerosis • Motor neuron disease • Palliative care • End-of-life care • Support groups • Health care in India

Introduction: ALS/MND in India

There is limited published data available on the incidence and prevalence of amyotrophic lateral sclerosis (ALS) in India. One study conducted in 1987 estimated the prevalence of ALS to be 4/100,000 (Gourie-Devi et al. 1987). The clinical features have been documented in a large series of 1153 patients (Nalini et al. 2008). In this study, the male-to-female ratio was 3:1. The clinical manifestations were similar to findings from other developing countries with regards to age of onset, sex ratio and survival. When compared to studies among Caucasians, the age of onset was one to two decades earlier. The survival pattern followed that documented from Africa and was much longer than the studies of Caucasian populations. Indians appear to have a relatively younger age of onset and prolonged survival. While no systematic studies exist, the bulk of ALS in India is formed by sporadic cases. The recent availability of genetic studies in India has identified only a few cases where genetic mutations have been associated with ALS.

Case Studies

The three patients discussed in the chapter exemplify the challenges and the opportunities available for the palliative care of motor neuron disease (MND) patients in India today. All three come from the practice of one of the authors. Cases 2 and 3 were personally examined, while only the case papers of the first patient were available for review together with the family's account. All three patients resided in Maharashtra, a state ranked high on socioeconomic indicators among Indian states (World Bank Group 2017). Maharashtra is one of the larger Indian states, and its capital Mumbai exemplifies the high degree of socioeconomic inequality that pervades India.

Case 1: KN, male, born 1971, usually resident in Hanwatkhed village, Buldana district, Maharashtra state. He was educated till 8th standard, married with 3 children (M 16, M 14, F 11) and working as construction laborer in Mumbai and on a family farm (seasonal migration). He developed right foot drop in Dec 2014 and was examined and diagnosed MND in public hospitals in Aurangabad and subsequently Mumbai. He was started on riluzole and then was discharged and his brothers were told that 'Nothing more can be done' but there was no discussion with the patient. He returned to the family farm and continued to work with diminishing capacity over the next year and began developing bulbar symptoms and breathing difficulty in June 2016. He was finally admitted in crisis in Oct 2016 to a small private hospital in Buldana, intubated and ventilated, with a tracheostomy 10 days later. His family (brothers and wife) ran out of funds and asked for transfer to a local public hospital where he was ventilated but developed ventilator associated pneumonia and septicemia. At the request of his family he was disconnected from the ventilator and unconscious, febrile and tachypneic put in an ambulance for transfer to his village home but died halfway home in early Nov 2016.

Case 2: SM, female, born 1948, resident in Mumbai. She was educated, postgraduate in Hindi literature, married 1968, one son and daughter by 1971 and widowed in 1976. She started working as a college lecturer until retirement at age 58. She began developing bilateral hand weakness in mid-2015 and was diagnosed MND, separately by two senior colleagues and started on riluzole. She was seen by one of us in September 2018 accompanied by son (primary carer) and daughter, both in their late 40s and by this point had limited mobility and came in a wheelchair. She was dysarthric and had lost a 'few kilos' in two months. After the examination, she wanted to know what was wrong with her, but her son intervened and wheeled her out. The son and daughter were counselled about collusion and its consequences, but they asked for time to reconsider since their wider family did not think it appropriate to inform the patient. In the son's words "My eldest uncle said that we should not trouble her with the knowledge of her illness". Three weeks later the son reported that his mother had voluntarily stopped eating and drinking and had died at home.

Case 3. DT, male, born 1961, resident of Kalyan, near Mumbai. He was educated until 12th standard and worked in a public sector firm and was living in an extended family with wife and married son and his family. The patient's married daughter stayed in the vicinity and was available to help. He developed left hand weakness in January 2015 and was examined and diagnosed over the next three months in Mumbai as MND and was started on riluzole with apparent arrest of progression for about one year. He began to deteriorate again in mid-2016, was given three cycles of edaravone without benefit and was almost wheelchair bound by end 2017. His family had begun planning stem cell therapy and decided to get a second opinion. The patient himself had no knowledge of his illness. With his family's consent, one of us explained the diagnosis and prognosis appropriately to patient and family and advised against the stem cell program. A palliative care referral was made, and the family enrolled in a support group. Bulbar symptoms appeared in mid-2018 and respiratory function began to deteriorate. The patient was counselled about, but refused PEG, and was started on oral morphine by palliative care. By early December 2018, NIV was begun with the acceptance of the patient and he was apparently comfortable when he passed away at home two weeks later. In the last six weeks, the local GP managed issues with weekly home visits and phone support from the palliative care team. A bereavement interview by the PC physician with the family documented fairly-high satisfaction with his care at the end of life.

HEALTH CARE SETTING

Much of what is reported here is based on our experience in Mumbai and Maharashtra, but the care that is accessible to MND patients is no different from that available for other chronic diseases. It has been estimated that the private sector supplies almost 80 percent of health services, while publicly funded health care serves about 20 percent and is probably utilized only by the bottom of the pyramid (Wikipedia 2019). There is almost no overlap or coordination between public and private health care. Public health facilities are largely funded by the state (provincial) government and vary substantially in quality and scope. Even within Maharashtra, health facilities depend mainly on location.

In general, publicly funded tertiary health care in the large cities is much better than primary or secondary level care, although efforts are being made to increase investment in rural areas. At all levels, this care is almost completely free at the point of contact and delivery. Most public facilities do not have a system of appointments, and waiting periods tend to be short. Patients and families coming from rural areas are known to camp in the vicinity of the hospital until attended to. There are no dedicated facilities for MND or even for neuromuscular diseases. However, since neurologists and neurological investigations are available in most referral hospitals, it is probable that no patient needs to travel more than about 300 km for a diagnosis or wait for longer than a week.

Private health care is patchy with poor standardization, but it is available everywhere, almost always pay-as-you-go basis. It ranges in quality from world class to outright quackery largely because of regulatory weakness, but it thrives because the public generally has a very low opinion of overcrowded government hospitals. Top-of-the-line care costs are much lower than elsewhere. Only admissions are generally covered by insurance, and most people utilize it for serious illnesses only. Given income levels in India, health care costs in the private sector are prohibitive for lower-income families, and thus private insurance covers less than 10 percent of the population. The government has just begun a national plan for poorer families for admissions and surgery only, mainly because serious illness-related health expenditure can be financially catastrophic.

NEUROLOGY AND ALS/MND CARE IN INDIA

The Indian Academy of Neurology currently has close to 2000 full members with approximately another 1000 neurologists practicing independently. There are approximately 400 neurologists currently qualifying annually, but with the Indian population at 1.2 billion and growing, India will have a shortage of neurology work force for some decades. As a result, most of the patients with ALS are seen by the internists and general practitioners at least initially and often throughout the course of the illness. Hence, a diagnosis may take a long time to be made and confirmed by a neurologist.

Most neurologists are based in the large cities, although many monthly or weekly extension clinics are run in smaller towns. Neurology consultation charges in the private sector range from INR 500 to 2000 (US$ 7–28) depending on the location, and the basic outpatient diagnostic workup (routine blood tests, MRI, electrophysiology) costs INR 12,000 to 20,000 (US$ 165–280). Currently, there is no government-based program for the genetic diagnosis of ALS in India, and patients bear its full costs, which range from INR 15,000 to 40,000 (US$165–550) depending upon the set of tests requested. The guidelines for testing of the relatives, as adopted by geneticists, are no different from those generally existing in other countries, and to our knowledge, there are no national consensus guidelines on this subject.

Since ALS is an incurable disease, patients who can afford to usually seek multiple opinions to check on the diagnostic and therapeutic options. Edaravone and riluzole are both available to patients and have been freely used in the therapy of ALS in India. Riluzole has been distributed on neurologists' prescriptions by a local generic pharmaceutical firm (Sun Pharma) for the past two decades as a charitable service, and most patients do try it for a few years. Edaravone (30 mg vial, INR 300–500 per vial (US$4–8)) was made available by multiple generic manufacturers about seven years ago, and in the last two years or so, most patients will try a few ten to fourteen-day cycles of IV therapy. Stem cell clinics with no scientific provenance have set up shop in all large cities, and it is a challenge for the neurology community to protect our patients from being preyed on by them.

Most Indian neurologists are unaware of the scope and potential of their responsibility once the diagnosis is made. Cases 2 and 3 exemplify this. With no training in communication skills or the basics of palliative medicine, the general tendency is to inform only the family of the diagnosis, and that begins the slippery slope of collusion and abandonment. Bringing neurologists and palliative care physicians together is possible in the large cities, and putting it all together at least for ALS/MND is low-hanging fruit for the emerging subspecialty of neuropalliative care (Gursahani 2016).

A LACK OF ALS/MND-SPECIFIC FACILITIES

To our knowledge, no dedicated service exists for care, teaching or research of ALS/MND in either the public or private sector. Public awareness is also minimal, with no coverage in print media, television or films. The federal and some state governments have published policy documents for palliative care in general with only a passing mention of MND/ALS, but the implementation, if any, has been patchy. To our knowledge, the first patient and family support group for MND/ALS began functioning only early in 2019, with both the authors involved as consultants.

Institutional care is not available, and almost all patients are cared for at home, unless they are admitted in crisis toward the end. General paid caregiving is available with costs ranging from INR 300 to 3000 (US$4–40) per day depending on location and level of training. Paid caregiving is becoming the norm especially in the middle class and above, but this is basically self-financed without any public or insurance support. Assistive technologies available commercially elsewhere are generally available for sale in India by e-commerce. As mentioned earlier, stem cell therapies, homeopathy and other alternative therapies are all available commercially without effective regulation. Recently, a system of relatively stringent drug trial regulations has been introduced. Right-to-try legislation is probably unnecessary at present.

Palliative and rehabilitative care are particularly underdeveloped in India. Thus, even someone who is quite wealthy can end up having a particularly poor quality of life when affected by serious illness or toward the last year of life (Gursahani and Mani 2016). The authors know of individuals who are wealthy by global standards but who end up having terrible deaths. The legal system has only just begun to recognize advance directives, and the basic constitutional right to autonomy in health care choices was instituted only in 2018 (Gursahani and Khadilkar 2018). Moreover, an inclusive system for advance care planning is non-existent, and medical aid in dying may not be considered for at least two decades. Opioid usage was severely constrained until a few years ago because of worries of misuse, but systematic and monitored prescription of morphine is now possible in most states.

Hospice facilities are available only for cancer patients and only in large cities, although the first general hospices are now being established. These are essentially charitable, and there is no government or policy support for hospice care. Home hospice is patchy and again dependent on non-profit organizations. The bright spot is the state of Kerala where community involvement is widespread and non-oncology diagnoses are also accepted for home care.

Like other Asian societies, discussion of death and dying is taboo in India, and as exemplified in the cases, this has proven to be a major barrier in provision of palliative care. There is active resistance to the idea of truth-telling, and collusion is the rule. On the other hand, only about 5 percent of Indians live on their own, and most patients will be cared for at home. Because of the poor linkage between palliative care and neurology, and without appropriate counseling, most MND patients in the middle class and above end up with invasive ventilation in the last few years of life, while patients with limited financial resources, like our first patient, die. Painful deaths seem to be the norm.

To our minds, the biggest barrier is the lack of awareness and training in the medical profession about palliative and end-of-life care. This is now being addressed in the medical curriculum and awaits widespread implementation. With no formal training in communication skills, most Indian doctors find it difficult to discuss serious illness or manage shared decision-making. It has been estimated that there are only about 200 physicians trained in palliative care for all of India. Moreover, until recently, there has been an almost exclusive focus on cancer patients, but this is beginning to change gradually.

ROAD MAP FOR THE FUTURE

1. *Patient awareness and support groups.* Our experience with the first support group has been very positive, especially in restoring a sense of agency to the carers. As of now only occasional patients attend. The main tool has been an online (WhatsApp) group which allows members, again mainly family carers, to converse and advise each other. This group, based out of Mumbai, was initiated by the son of an ALS patient after his mother died. Regular meetings have been held to disseminate information, and it is open to any Indian patient or carer. Similar groups can be set up in other cities. Another online resource that seems to be used quite frequently in India is ALS Worldwide. Our support group will need hand-holding and fund-raising to become an active patient advocacy organization.

2. *Clinician training and orientation.* At this stage, ALS care cannot be separated from the broader field of neuropalliative care. Neurologist training in the basics of palliative care allows us to learn communication skills and symptom management for our own patients. Collusion is best tackled when the neurologist who first makes a definitive diagnosis of ALS/MND also divulges it sensitively to the patient and family. For Indians, we suggest a minor tweak of the SPIKES (Gursahani and Mani 2016) or similar protocols: at the first consultation, the patient and family are jointly asked to decide who will take the discussion forward, as part of a 'warning shot'. Similarly, palliative care physicians need to be oriented to symptom identification and management for neurology patients. Both specialties need facilitation to form local alliances that can lead to multidisciplinary teams for all neurology patients or even specifically for patients with MND/ALS. Concerned neurologists and palliative care physicians can then jointly target uniform and appropriate counseling for MND patients and for patient and family choice regarding percutaneous endoscopic gastrostomy and non-invasive and invasive ventilation at the onset of bulbar symptoms and respiratory weakness.

3. *Advocacy*. Neuropalliative care cannot be separated from advocacy for appropriate legislation, government support and public awareness of the entire fields of palliative and end-of-life care. Advance care planning needs to be institutionalized so that it becomes the norm rather than the exception. ALS is the most common neurologic disease for which physician-assisted suicide is used in the United States. For India, this stage is realistically still a couple of decades away.

REFERENCES

Gourie-Devi, M., V.N. Rao and R. Prakashi (1987). Neuroepidemiological study in semi-urban and rural areas in South India: Pattern of Neurological Disorders including Motor Neurone Disease. In M. Gourie-Devi, ed. *Motor Neurone Disease: Global Clinical Patterns and International Research*. New Delhi: Oxford and IBH; pp. 11–21.

Gursahani, R. (2016). Palliative care and the Indian neurologist. *Annals of the Indian Academy of Neurology* 19: S40–44.

Gursahani, R. and S.V. Khadilkar (2018). Death and dying in India: Circa 2018: What the conscientious physician needs to know. *J Assoc Phy Ind* 66: 11–12.

Gursahani, R. and R.K. Mani (2016). India: Not a country to die in. *Indian Journal of Medical Ethics* 13: 30.

Nalini, A., K. Thennarasu, M. Gourie-Devi, S. Shenoy and D. Kulshreshtha (2008). Clinical characteristics and survival patterns of 1153 patients with ALS: Experience over 30 years from India. *Journal of Neurological Sciences* 272: 60–70.

Wikipedia: Healthcare in India. (2019). Permanent link https://en.wikipedia.org/w/index.php?title=Healthcare_in_India&oldid=920613699

World Bank Group (2017). Maharashtra: Poverty, Growth and Inequality. http://documents.worldbank.org/curated/en/806671504171811149/pdf/119254-BRI-P157572-Maharashtra-Poverty.pdf.

CHAPTER 9

The Experience of Amyotrophic Lateral Sclerosis in Ireland

Orla Hardiman, Stela Lefter, and Miriam Galvin

Abstract The Irish Republic (population 4.9 million) has 150 new cases of ALS each year and 380 individuals living with the condition. There is one specialist public multidisciplinary service for ALS in the country, linking closely with the voluntary organization (IMNDA) and providing care for all Irish citizens.

Patients are reviewed at six-week intervals and care is coordinated with community-based professionals and palliative care services. The clinical service is linked to a large research group based at Trinity College Dublin. The research group curates the population-based ALS Register and engages in clinical research in epidemiology, phenotyping, genomics, imaging, neuroelectric signal analysis, health services research and clinical trials. Although efficient, cost effective and quality of life enhancing, the

O. Hardiman (✉) • M. Galvin
Trinity College Dublin, Dublin, Ireland
e-mail: hardimao@tcd.ie; galvinmi@tcd.ie

S. Lefter
Southmead Hospital, Bristol, UK

Beaumont Hospital, Dublin, Ireland
e-mail: stela_lefter@yahoo.com

© The Author(s) 2021
R. H. Blank et al. (eds.), *Public Policy in ALS/MND Care*,
https://doi.org/10.1007/978-981-15-5840-5_9

Irish ALS service relies heavily on philanthropic and research grant support. A detailed evidence-based business has been generated to provide sustainable long-term funding for holistic integrated care, underpinned by high-quality clinical research.

Keywords ALS • Population-based register • Multidisciplinary care • Palliative care • Quality of life • Caregiver burden • End-of-life decision making • Clinical research

ALS in the Irish Healthcare System

The incidence of ALS in the Republic of Ireland is approximately 2.6/100,000 over 18 years of age, and the prevalence is approximately 8.0/100,000. Approximately 130 new cases of ALS/MND are diagnosed in Ireland each year—with approximately 350 patients living with ALS and 40 patients with primary lateral sclerosis (PLS). The mortality rates are close to the incidence rates.

A population-based Register of ALS/MND has been in continuous operation in Ireland since 1995. This Register collects demographic and clinical features of all patients with ALS/MND in the Republic of Ireland and is the longest running Register of its kind for ALS/MND in the world. It has had almost full patient ascertainment since its foundation and has tracked the patterns of over 2500 familial and sporadic ALS cases within the Republic of Ireland over the past 25 years. The Register has also enabled a number of population-based studies in epidemiology, genetics and phenotyping, including studies of cognition and behavior in ALS/MND and studies of patient and caregiver journeys (see http:// mnd.ie/current-research/). The Register is linked to a large repository of over 1500 samples of DNA from ALS patients, and 1000 controls, from which the genetic epidemiology of ALS in Ireland has been determined.

The data from the Irish Register is compliant with GDPR, and patients agree to the sharing of their codified data with other groups across Europe as part of a series of large European collaborations under the auspices of the European consortia of Project MinE (https://www.projectmine. com), ENCALS and TRICALS (https://www.tricals.org). The Register receives no state funding and is administered through funding from research grants and with philanthropic support.

ALS/MND Clinics

A national public clinic for ALS/MND was started in 1995 at the National Centre for Neuroscience (Beaumont Hospital, Dublin). This service has evolved to be one of the first multidisciplinary and cross-disciplinary neurological services in the country, and was the first in the world to demonstrate the survival benefit of multidisciplinary care in ALS/MND (Traynor et al. 2003; Rooney et al. 2015). As has been the case for many world class specialist services in the Republic of Ireland, the ALS/MND Centre evolved organically from a consultant-provided clinic that began in collaboration with the voluntary organization the Irish Motor Neuron Disease Association (IMNDA www.imnda.ie) in response to an unmet need for patients with ALS/MND.

The ALS/MND service now comprises a dynamic team of 20, including 2 senior neurologists, 4 clinical fellows, specialist clinical professional staff, specialist nurses, full-time clinical trial staff and basic scientists working closely with the IMNDA and the Irish ALS/MND Research Group (www.mnd.ie) on behalf of patients with ALS/MND and their families.

The specialist clinical professional staff within the clinic hold public sector contracts as hospital employees but are not formally recognized by the hospital as having a specialist role/expertise in ALS/MND. In many cases, additional time must be "bought out" by philanthropic and grant funding. This additional funding enables augmented clinic time for those with ALS/MND and can facilitate extensive outreach programs, teaching, training and research. However, this remains an unstable and unsustainable system that is overly dependent on a small number of "founder" individuals and the availability of ongoing charitable donations.

Notwithstanding the absence of official support by the publicly funded Health Service Executive (HSE), the Irish ALS/MND services has been formally recognized by the Department of Health and by the Royal College of Physicians in Ireland Rare Disease program as a national specialist service, and suitable for inclusion in the European Reference Network for Rare Diseases (http://www.ern-rnd.eu/news/). However, this recognition does not bring additional funding or resources.

In 2019, following conclusion of austerity measures within the public healthcare sector as a result of the financial crash in the 2000s, a detailed business case was submitted to the HSE outlining and justifying the need for a funding strategy for ALS/MND over the coming 5 years to include additional support for six new specialist nurses in ALS/MND and support for fully dedicated clinical professionals (physiotherapy, occupational therapy, speech and language therapy, dietetics and a full-time neuropsychologist). The business plan also includes a proposal to provide long-term sustainable funding for the ALS/MND Register, as well as to support an additional senior neurologist with expertise in ALS to render the national ALS/MND Clinic sustainable following retirement of key founder personnel. The HSE has agreed to fund two years of the proposal but cannot formally commit to funding thereafter as the Irish health service does not currently have facility for multi-annual budgeting.

OPERATION OF THE ALS/MND SERVICE

The national ALS/MND service currently operates a weekly publicly funded clinic and engages directly with over 80 percent of all ALS/MND patients and their families in the Republic of Ireland. The clinic also provides free-of-charge second opinions for patients from Northern Ireland and for patients traveling from other European countries. Two additional monthly, publicly funded satellite clinics operate in regional centers (Cork and Galway) respectively, providing local integrated care for those unwilling or unable to travel. Satellite clinics do not have a research component and do not engage in clinical trials. The entire system is integrated under a joint management structure (Fig. 9.1).

Two peer-reviewed studies have demonstrated a survival advantage of nine months for those attending the clinic and engaging with multidisciplinary care (Traynor et al. 2003; Rooney et al. 2015). Additional details of the operation, function and benefits of the multidisciplinary service have also been described in over 50 peer reviewed publications specifically relating to ALS/MND care (Traynor et al. 2003; Rooney et al. 2013, 2015; Burke et al. 2015, 2017a, b, 2018, 2019; Galvin et al. 2015, 2016, 2017b, 2018).

Diagnostic Pathway

Despite the availability of an established multidisciplinary service and enhanced knowledge of ALS/MND in the community, the median delay from first symptom to diagnosis of ALS/MND in Ireland is 11 months

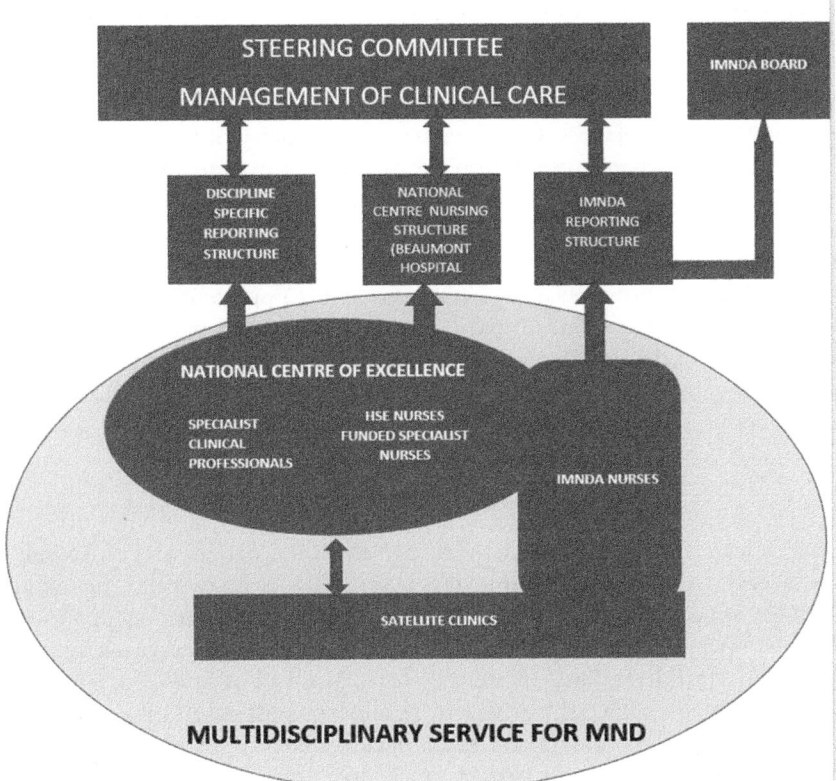

Fig. 9.1 Management structure of the ALS/MND services in Ireland

(Galvin et al. 2017b). A recent study has shown that the mean standard cost of an ALS diagnosis in Ireland should be €1414 (US$ 1565). This assumes the diagnostic journey consisted of consultations with a GP and neurologist, as well as lumbar puncture, blood tests, MRI of the brain and spine and neurophysiological testing. However, Irish patients with ALS/MND have an average of four contacts with healthcare professionals and 4.8 investigations/tests prior to diagnosis (Galvin et al. 2017b), leading to a mean cost of diagnosis of €3486 (US$ 3855). Avoidance of unnecessary consultations and interventions during the diagnostic journey could result in aggregated savings of €2072 (US$ 2290) per patient.

This assumes the diagnostic journey consisted of consultations with a GP and neurologist, as well as lumbar puncture, blood tests, MRI of the brain and spine and neurophysiological testing.

While most ALS patients attend their GP as the first point of engagement with health services, there remains a mean delay of five months from first symptom to first presentation for medical evaluation. A longer interval from first symptom to time of final diagnosis is also associated with a higher overall economic cost. The availability of high-quality MRI and detailed neurophysiologic studies reduces the rate of inappropriate surgical intervention; however, the occurrence of decompressive surgery of the cervical and lumbar spine in patients with ALS remains more common than a misdiagnosis of ALS in patients with cervical or lumbar compressive myelopathy, indicating that the misdiagnosis of ALS has a significant economic cost.

Operation of the Multidisciplinary Team Care

Once referred to the National ALS/MND clinic, patients receive same-day access to the multidisciplinary team. The team within the clinic includes specialists in neurology, nursing, physiotherapy, occupational therapy, speech and language therapy, dietetics and neuropsychology. However, staff attendance is neither formalized or ringfenced, and the hospital managers have the power to re-allocate staff based on competing needs within the system. There is no back up facility for professionals in the case of illness or longer periods of absence (e.g., maternity leave).

The ALS/MND service has a strong background and track record in cognitive and behavioral assessment (Phukan et al. 2012; Elamin et al. 2013; Burke et al. 2017b; Pinto-Grau et al. 2017; Elamin et al. 2017). The service routinely screens all ALS/MND patients for cognitive/behavioral changes in the clinic at the time of first visit and performs a three-monthly screening thereafter. This is funded by research grants and philanthropic support. Those with evidence of cognitive change on screening undergo full neuropsychological assessment as appropriate. The close attention to cognitive/behavioral change allows the service to provide extensive psychological support for patient and caregivers, including initiatives for recognition and management of caregiver burden. This program has been funded by the Health Research Board, the ALSA Association (USA) and the MND Association (UK).

Four nurses funded directly by the voluntary organization (IMNDA) also attend the National Clinic and satellite clinics in Cork and Galway. These nurses work closely with the multidisciplinary team within the hospitals and provide additional support and links between the satellite and national clinics, links to the community services, organize home visits and counseling support and facilitate the provision of specialist equipment free of charge, where necessary.

GENETIC TESTING

Until recently, Irish patients were not routinely offered genetic testing for known ALS genes. However, with the advent of potential new treatments for *C9orf72*-related ALS, a new policy has been instituted of offering genetic testing free of charge, subject to appropriate counseling. There is currently no formally established funding program for genomic testing in Ireland, and standard procedures that are embedded in public health systems of other countries (e.g. the use of gene panels, or whole genome sequencing) are currently not routinely possible in Ireland for budgetary reasons. At present, each *C9orf72* test must be individually negotiated with the laboratory managers.

Presymptomatic testing for known gene variants in ALS is not offered in Ireland, although a research ethics approved study is currently underway by the Irish ALS/MND Research Group (www.mnd.ie) to examine first-degree relatives of those with ALS to identify cognitive and neurological endophenotypes that may associate with the genotype. This study has been funded in part by the Health Research Board and in part by Science Foundation Ireland as part of a genomics project. Genomics researchers are provided with codified samples from consenting patients with no access to identifying information. Clinicians engaged in the delivery of care are not provided with genomic information about patients unless they have undergone formal genetic counseling followed by commercial testing.

MANAGEMENT OF ALS/MND

The ethos of the Irish ALS/MND service is to provide excellent evidence-based care, free of charge, in an out-patient cross-disciplinary setting and to facilitate and support the integration of hospital and community-based services with close links with specialist palliative care. Patients are reviewed within the multidisciplinary clinic at six-week intervals, with an "open door" policy for those requiring urgent attention. Care is coordinated by the integrated network of specialist nurses, of whom four are funded directly by the IMNDA and three by the publicly funded HSE (as part of a commitment to fund a five-year business plan for ALS/MND care). The ALS/MND service prioritizes management and care in the home where feasible. All ALS/MND nurses work as a team to undertake regular home visits and integrate care between the hospital and community services.

Additionally, respiratory management, including initiation and management of non-invasive ventilation (NIV), is undertaken at home through the activities of three HSE-funded senior Clinical Nurse Specialists in ALS/MND. These nurses provide this service for the entire country. This specialist nurse-led service also provides an opportunity to discuss end-of-life issues in a home setting, advise on advance care directives and incorporate educational secessions with community, hospital and hospice staff. This service was initiated in 2011 when 11 patients were commenced on NIV at home. In 2018, 60 patients were initiated with NIV at home obviating the need for hospitalization. This represents a cost saving of over €150,000 to public hospital services (based on a requirement of a minimum of three days admission) and a saving of a minimum of 180 bed days. This service also prevents emergency admissions and reduces the risk of unplanned/emergency invasive mechanical ventilation.

Gastrostomy is performed according to the existing standard of care (Andersen et al. 2012). Within the National Centre at Beaumont Hospital, most patients undergo radiology-inserted gastrostomy with an average length of stay of seven to ten days. Percutaneous endoscopy gastrostomy (PEG) is performed by satellite services. Approximately 30 percent of prevalent patients have gastrostomy in situ.

STATE BENEFITS FOR ALS/MND PATIENTS AND INFORMAL CARERS

Patients with ALS/MND in Ireland are not automatically entitled to free healthcare despite the severity of their diagnosis. Those who fulfill the stringent means-testing (based on low income) can access free GP and community services. The Irish healthcare system also operates a "hardship" program for those whose income/assets exceed the threshold for means-testing, but who are deemed to require free access to GP and community services. This decision is made by a dedicated unit within the HSE and is based on the diagnosis of an illness with a life expectancy of less than six months or the diagnosis of an illness that is likely to incur significant financial hardship. The fact that ALS/MND patients must apply for discretionary approval for free medical care based on these criteria creates a significant burden for patients and caregivers already grappling with a catastrophic life-changing diagnosis.

Those deemed eligible for free medical care (approximately 95 percent of ALS/MND are ultimately awarded free medical care, albeit with delays of three to six months in many instances) can avail of community-based services, including physiotherapy, occupational therapy and speech and language therapy, in addition to the free services of the GP and free medications. Patients are also entitled to the provision of enabling equipment (e.g. wheelchairs and walking aids). However, there are long waiting lists both for review by community occupational therapy and speech and language services, and for selection and approval of equipment, and once shipped, equipment is often not fully aligned to the needs of the patient. To address this gap, the voluntary organization (IMNDA) operates an extensive equipment bank for patients and provides larger items (beds, wheelchairs, stair lifts, communication devices, etc.) free of charge following approval by the relevant clinical professional within the specialist clinic.

Patients who require additional advanced technologies for assisted living are referred to a specialist center (Central Remedial Clinic) for assessment. Specialist equipment such communication enabled iPads, eye gaze technology and environmental controls are also provided and funded by the IMNDA. Patients who require non-invasive ventilation who are not eligible for free medical care can rent the appropriate equipment using a subsidy scheme in which they pay a maximum of €120 per month. However, once deemed eligible for the free medical scheme, the rental costs are covered by the state.

CARE SERVICES FOR ALS PATIENTS IN IRELAND

In Ireland, homecare assistance is provided through the Home Support Service of the HSE. There are also numerous private companies that provide care hours to patients in their own homes. State-supported funding for home care services is generally limited to a maximum of 20 to 28 hours per week. The IMNDA also provides additional financial assistance toward home care for people with ALS/MND and helps to arrange home care assistance.

Caregivers can claim a state benefit (Caregiver's Allowance) if the person receiving care is regarded as requiring full-time care and attention where:

- The person is so incapacitated as to require continuous supervision in order to avoid danger to him/herself or continual supervision and frequent assistance throughout the day in connection with normal bodily functions

     or

- The person so incapacitated as to be likely to require full-time care and attention for a period of at least 12 months

While claiming this allowance, caregivers must not be engaged in employment, self-employment, training or education courses outside the home for more than 15 hours a week.

This payment is means tested (i.e. the resources, property other than the family home and income of the spouse/partner are taken into consideration). In ALS/MND, when the means of caregivers are assessed as falling above the limit, a personal appeal is often made to local decision makers, and failing that, to local political representatives. The Respite Care Allowance is a cash payment made to caregivers by the Department of Social and Family Affairs in Ireland. Carers can use the grant in whatever way they wish. It is not necessary to use it to pay for respite care (https://imnda.ie/wp-content/uploads/2014/03/Carers+Brochure.pdf).

Patient and Caregiver Attitudes to Care

A series of studies of patient and caregiver attitudes toward their ALS/MND journey and experience of the multidisciplinary clinic have been recently undertaken using a Discrete Choice Experiment paradigm (Douglas et al. 2005). This experimental method seeks to determine underlying attitudes using a series of multiple choices. This work has shown that perspectives and attitudes toward the disease and engagement with multidisciplinary care differ between patients and caregivers from the time of diagnosis. For example, Irish caregivers ascribe greater value to the expertise of the multidisciplinary clinic than do patients. Throughout the patient journey, caregivers consistently express a greater desire for additional information about the disease trajectory, show more evidence of planning for the future and are more realistic about the likely trajectory of the disease than are patients.

Despite the evidence that (time limited) specialist palliative care can provide additional support from the time of diagnosis, Irish patients and caregivers consistently express negative attitudes toward palliative care, reflecting a perception that engagement with palliative/hospice care is an indication of entry to a terminal stage of disease rather than a positive quality-of-life enhancing intervention. Indeed, even when Irish patients are linked with palliative care services, they continue to express preferences that they should receive all their care in home rather than a hospice setting. Moreover, despite having engaged with palliative care services, Irish patients also remain negative toward direct home-based care by palliative care physicians. This may also indicate a perception that home visits signal a terminal stage of disease. By contrast, as their experience with palliative care services develops, Irish patients show evidence of recognition of the additional value of local hospice services.

Bereaved Irish caregivers exhibit different attitudes toward palliative care and respite care. In cases where the multidisciplinary team has had extensive input in the provision of respite care, the burden experienced by caregivers is lower. By contrast, those caregivers who have expressed high levels of burden during the illness consistently exhibit low opinions of their experience with palliative care.

While there is considerable geographical variability in the availability of palliative care in Ireland, particularly with respect to respite, the negative expression toward palliative care does not correlate with geographic location, but more likely reflects the unmet needs of the caregiver as a function of subjective perceptions of burden.

Formal and Informal Caregiving

Care of people with ALS/MND in Ireland largely takes place in the community, and the vast majority (over 80 percent) of patients dies at home. For most Irish patients, family caregivers are key figures in ALS/MND care, playing a central role in clinical decision making. Most of these informal caregivers are female and are spouses or partners of the patient. As is the case in most countries, caregivers inside the home cannot easily evade the care situation. Indeed, most Irish caregivers had not planned to be caregivers—this evolves from existing family relationships. As noted, informal care in Ireland is typically unpaid or partially supported by the Caregivers Allowance, which is generally subsistence level.

Irish caregivers identify both positive and negative caregiving experiences. Positive factors include reciprocity, reward, increased self-esteem and opportunity to learn new skills. Difficulties include watching decline of a loved one, the restriction on activities that contribute to the caregivers' own quality of life, changing role and relationships, effects on the household routine, care of children, disruption of relations within and outside the family and reduced hours of employment (Galvin et al. 2016).

Studies by Galvin and associates of caregiver burden in Ireland have also shown that heterogeneity of caregiver-patient relationships influences the burden experiences. In general, relationship strain between the patient and caregiver correlates with many factors, including the pre-morbid relationship quality of patients and caregivers. Loss of intimacy, reduced social contacts and the extent of change caused by the disease increase tension, worry and stressful situations for both patient and caregiver are important drivers of burden in Ireland.

Additionally, because of fragmentation of the Irish healthcare system, family members are often expected to perform complex tasks like those carried out by paid health or social service providers. This is often at great cost to their own well-being, but great benefit to their relatives and to society at large. For these reasons, Irish caregivers describe an experience of burden involving physical, psychological, emotional, social and practical challenges.

The factors contributing to caregiver burden are diverse and can vary significantly among different caregivers. Cognitive, behavioral and neuro-psychiatric symptoms experienced by patients are significant factors that contribute to caregiver burden and negatively impact on quality of life.

There is also evolving evidence among Irish families that caregivers' psychological status may also influence the mental and physical outcome of patients (Burke et al. 2015, 2017a, 2018; Galvin et al. 2016, 2017a, 2018). This suggests that attention to the mental health needs of caregivers may not only relieve caregivers' distress but also alleviate patient distress and improve quality of life. Irish caregivers were recently interviewed to identify their perceived needs and what they would find helpful to them across 12 to 18 months of the caregiving journey. While their needs were clearly identified, these changed with time and over the disease trajectories. Articulated needs include support from family, friends and healthcare professionals in managing practical tasks, navigating the health services and the emotional demands of caregiving. Most Irish caregivers stated that they could discuss their experiences and their needs with healthcare professionals in hospital and community services. Those who felt constrained in discussing their needs offered reasons including time limitations at the clinical encounter, not being asked about their concerns by healthcare professionals and not feeling it an appropriate thing for them to do since the focus is on the patient.

PALLIATIVE CARE AND END OF LIFE

Clinical indications for referral to palliative care are not clearly defined in Ireland and there remains a perception among healthcare professionals, patients and caregivers that palliative care occurs traditionally at "end-stage" disease. There is no widely accepted national standard of timing for referral of those with ALS/MND to specialist palliative care services. Recent work by the Irish ALS/MND Research Group has sought to identify points at which specialist palliative care intervention is beneficial prior to end of life: at the time of introduction of NIV; in the context of high levels of patient distress; or when there is evidence of psychosocial distress within families or experienced by the primary caregiver.

Clinical management at the end of life in Ireland aims to maximize quality of life of both the patient and caregiver and incorporates appropriate palliation of physical, psychosocial and existential distress (Connolly et al. 2015). However, as most Irish healthcare professionals are trained to promote and maintain life, they often have difficulty when faced with the often-rapid decline and death of people with terminal illnesses such as ALS/MND. The emotional burden of healthcare professionals caring for people with terminal neurological disease in Ireland is poorly recognized, and the moral and ethical challenges related to providing end-of-life care are not currently well characterized.

The IMNDA in collaboration with ALS/MND Centre Beaumont Hospital and the charity supporting palliative care services (Irish Hospice Foundation) support healthcare professionals and service providers when working with people with ALS/MND. To address this, the Irish ALS/MND service provides training of HCPs that include workshops in management ALS/MND and in providing skills that help to sensitively manage the rapid evolution of cognitive, behavioral and physical decline that is associated with ALS/MND.

Advance Directives and Invasive Mechanical Ventilation

Advance directives are encouraged but are not legally binding in Ireland. The ALS/MND clinic seeks to engage in early and open discussion of end-of-life issues with patients and families to allow time for reflection and planning, obviate the introduction of unwanted interventions or procedures, provide reassurance and alleviate fear. This is frequently undertaken in the home at the time of initiation of NIV. Those with evidence of early cognitive/behavioral change are encouraged to seek legal advice regarding an enduring power of attorney.

There is no formal state-funded structure that supports those wishing to pursue invasive mechanical ventilation. In the rare instances where patients have undergone elective tracheostomy (five patients in the past ten years), all but one remained hospitalized for the duration of their illness. The public hospitals are now reluctant to facilitate this procedure, as there are no long-term step-down facilities for patients using tracheostomy. As advance directives do not have legal status in Ireland, there is no legal mechanism to discontinue full mechanical ventilation in the event of a patient becoming totally "locked in." Physician-assisted suicide is illegal.

Applied Research and Generation of Standards

The ALS/MND services has embedded research into clinical practice and has implemented practice guidelines as part of an ongoing quality improvement cycle. Clinical intervention and outcome data are regularly reviewed and are subject to ongoing evaluation (e.g. stakeholder choice experiments, audit reviews, etc.). The service also undertakes regular self-audits of nursing and clinical professional activities, and quality-of-life measurement is embedded into the services. Examples of applied research and audit undertaken by staff within the ALS/MND clinic include:

- Longitudinal respiratory assessment to evaluate the predictive value of FVC, SVC, peak cough flow and sniff nasal inspiratory pressure (SNIP)
- Evaluation of the beneficial effects of clinic-based shoulder injection by physiotherapists for adhesive capsulitis in MND
- Evaluation of the beneficial use of cough assist in managing secretions
- Evaluation of beneficial effects of psychological intervention for caregiver burden
- Comparison of breath stacking versus cough assist in management of secretions
- Introduction and evaluation of the beneficial effects of voice banking
- Effects of dysphagia and gastrostomy feeding on quality of life in ALS/MND

The ALS/MND Clinic at the National Centre is closely linked with the Academic Unit of Neurology at Trinity College Dublin, which houses the Irish ALS/MND Research Group (www.mnd.ie). The Research Group is responsible for the ALS/MND Register and DNA bank.

The Academic Unit of Neurology at Trinity College Dublin has six main patient-oriented work streams, including epidemiology and deep phenotyping, biomarker development (imaging and neuroelectric signal analysis), genomics, outcome measures, health services research and clinical trials.

Detailed genetic epidemiologic studies of ALS in Ireland have provided information about the rates of familial ALS within the Irish population and information about the frequency of known mutations within the population. This work has been performed in a research setting and has demonstrated that *C9orf72* repeat expansions account for approximately 10 percent of all ALS cases in Ireland and 50 percent of known familial ALS. The remaining "known genes" (*SOD1*, *TDP43* and *FUS*) are rare in the Irish population.

The ALS/MND clinical and research group is leading a series of large European consortia that assess and evaluate the patient journey in ALS/MND and that determine the use of various respiratory-based measurements that increase the accuracy of outcome prediction and interventions (e.g. insufflation/exsufflation machines "cough assist" that reduce intercurrent infections and enhance quality of life).

FUTURE REQUIREMENTS TO IMPROVE CARE AND ADVANCE RESEARCH SUPPORT FOR ALS/MND

Although the Irish healthcare system is fragmented, the current care for those with ALS/MND in Ireland is of a high standard. This is primarily a function of the combined work of the Multidisciplinary Clinical Service at Beaumont Hospital (working closely with the IMNDA) and the Irish ALS/MND Research Group based at Trinity College Dublin.

However, the long-term sustainability of the clinical programs is at risk in the absence of a formal exchequer-provided funding stream. Although a five-year business plan for service development has been generated, the absence of multi-annual budgeting within the Irish public health system means that the sustainable funding of the service remains at risk over the coming years.

From a research perspective, the Irish ALS/MND Research Group has successfully tendered for competitive grant funding from both national and international funding agencies and is likely to continue to grow. The combined clinical and research arms of Irish ALS/MND have also successfully engaged in a series of Phase II and Phase III clinical trials of new compounds for ALS/MND, including an early phase antisense oligonucleotide for those carrying the *C9orf72* repeat expansion. The Irish ALS/MND Group is also a founding member of the recently formed European Treatment Initiative to Cure ALS (TRICALS) the purpose of which is to promote both commercial and investigator-led clinical trials of therapeutic agents in ALS/MND.

Finally, both the clinical and research programs have sought to attract young professionals to work in the field of ALS/MND. Both programs have grown from a single neurologist and specialist nurse, to two neurologists at the National Centre (with additional neurologists providing satellite services in the regional centers of Cork and Galway) and seven nurses providing a national network of care throughout the community. The ALS/MND Research Group now comprises 40 researchers. The National Clinic and Research Group have supported the training of specialists in physiotherapy, occupational therapy, speech and language therapy and dietetics. To ensure long-term sustainability, the service will require dedicated funding from the National Exchequer and the full integration between the clinic and research activities.

REFERENCES

Andersen, P. M., S. Abrahams, G. D. Borasio et al. (2012). EFNS guidelines on the clinical management of amyotrophic lateral sclerosis (MALS)—Revised report of an EFNS task force. *European Journal of Neurology* 19: 360–75.

Burke, T., M. Elamin, M. Galvin, O. Hardiman and N. Pender (2015). Caregiver burden in amyotrophic lateral sclerosis: A cross-sectional investigation of predictors. *Journal of Neurology* 262: 1526–32.

Burke, T., M. Galvin, M. Pinto-Grau, K. Lonergan et al. (2017a). Caregivers of patients with amyotrophic lateral sclerosis: investigating quality of life, caregiver burden, service engagement, and patient survival. *Journal of Neurology* 264: 898–904.

Burke, T., M. Pinto-Grau, K. Lonergan, P. Bede et al. (2017b). A Cross-sectional population-based investigation into behavioral change in amyotrophic lateral sclerosis: Subphenotypes, staging, cognitive predictors, and survival. *Ann Clin Transl Neurology*, 4: 305–17.

Burke, T., O. Hardiman, M. Pinto-Grau, K. Lonergan et al. (2018). Longitudinal predictors of caregiver burden in amyotrophic lateral sclerosis: A population-based cohort of patient-caregiver dyads. *Journal of Neurology* 265: 793–808.

Burke, T., J. Wilson O'Raghallaigh, S. Maguire, M. Galvin et al. (2019). Group interventions for amyotrophic lateral sclerosis caregivers in Ireland: A randomised controlled trial protocol. *BMJ Open* 9: e030684.

Connolly, S., M. Galvin and O. Hardiman (2015). End-of-life management in patients with amyotrophic lateral sclerosis. *Lancet Neurology* 14: 435–42.

Douglas, H. R., C. E. Normand, I. J. Higginson and D. M. Goodwin (2005). A new approach to eliciting patients' preferences for palliative day care: The choice experiment method. *Journal of Pain Symptom Management* 29: 435–45.

Elamin, M., P. Bede, S. Byrne, N. Jordan et al. (2013). Cognitive changes predict functional decline in ALS: A population-based longitudinal study. *Neurolog*, 80: 1590–97.

Elamin, M., M. Pinto-Grau, T. Burke, P. Bede et al. (2017). Identifying behavioural changes in ALS: Validation of the Beaumont Behavioural Inventory (BBI). *Amyotrophic Lateral Sclerosis and Frontotemporal Degeneration* 18: 68–73.

Galvin, M., C. Madden, S. Maguire, M. Heverin et al. (2015). Patient journey to a specialist amyotrophic lateral sclerosis multidisciplinary clinic: An exploratory study. *BMC Health Services Research* 15: 571.

Galvin, M., B. Corr, C. Madden, I. Mays et al. (2016). Caregiving in ALS—A mixed methods approach to the study of Burden. *BMC Palliative Care* 15: 81.

Galvin, M., R. Gaffney, B. Corr, I. Mays and O. Hardiman (2017a). From first symptoms to diagnosis of amyotrophic lateral sclerosis: Perspectives of an Irish informal caregiver cohort—A thematic analysis. *BMJ Open* 7: e014985–e85.

Galvin, M., P. Ryan, S. Maguire, M. Heverin, et al. (2017b). The path to specialist multidisciplinary care in amyotrophic lateral sclerosis: A population- based study of consultations, interventions and costs. *PLoS One* 12: e0179796.

Galvin, M., S. Carney, B. Corr, I. Mays, N. Pender and O. Hardiman (2018). Needs of informal caregivers across the caregiving course in amyotrophic lateral sclerosis: A qualitative analysis. *BMJ Open* 8: e018721.

Phukan, J., M. Elamin, P. Bede, N. Jordan, et al. (2012). The syndrome of cognitive impairment in amyotrophic lateral sclerosis: A population-based study. *Journal of Neurology, Neurosurgery and Psychiatry* 83: 102–8.

Pinto-Grau, M., E. Costello, S. O'Connor, M. Elamin et al. (2017). Assessing behavioural changes in ALS: Cross-validation of ALS-specific measures. *Journal of Neurology* 264: 1397–1401.

Rooney, J., S. Byrne, M. Heverin, B. Corr et al. (2013). Survival analysis of Irish amyotrophic lateral sclerosis patients diagnosed from 1995–2010. *PLoS One* 8: e74733.

Rooney, J., S. Byrne, M. Heverin, K. Tobin et al. (2015). A multidisciplinary clinic approach improves survival in ALS: A comparative study of ALS in Ireland and Northern Ireland. *Journal of Neurology, Neurosurgery and Psychiatry* 86: 496–501.

Traynor, B. J., M. Alexander, B. Corr, E. Frost and O. Hardiman (2003). Effect of a multidisciplinary amyotrophic lateral sclerosis (ALS) clinic on ALS survival: A population based study, 1996–2000. *Journal of Neurology, Neurosurgery and Psychiatry* 74: 1258–61.

CHAPTER 10

Public Policy of ALS Care in Israel

Marc Gotkine and Efrat Carmi

Abstract Israel has a population of 9 million people, with an estimated 120 to 150 people diagnosed each year and around 600 people living with ALS. There is no population-based national ALS registry, but the Israel ALS Research association (IsrALS) manages its own database. There are two major ALS clinics operating within academic institutions in Israel; however, full multidisciplinary care in a single center is not available locally for most patients. Most patients stay at home at all stages of the disease, even on home ventilation, with many employing one or more foreign care workers. Religious and cultural issues unique to Israel are critical factors which have shaped public policy for end-of-life care. Palliative sedation and withholding of mechanical ventilation are legal in Israel; however, any form of active euthanasia or assisted suicide is illegal. The IsrALS was established in 2004 and has dramatically improved public perception, government policy and funding of clinical and research care.

M. Gotkine (✉)
Hebrew University-Hadassah Medical Center, Jerusalem, Israel
e-mail: marc@gotkine.com

E. Carmi
The Israeli ALS Research Association, Haifa, Israel
e-mail: info@israls.org.il

R. H. Blank et al. (eds.), *Public Policy in ALS/MND Care*,
https://doi.org/10.1007/978-981-15-5840-5_10

Keywords ALS • IsrALS • Assistive technology • Judaism • Israel • Invasive ventilation

INCIDENCE AND PREVALENCE AND DEATHS OF ALS IN ISRAEL

As of 2019, Israel has a population of nine million with a median age of around 30 years, reflecting its highest fertility rate in the OECD (2017) (3.1 children per woman). Thus, ALS incidence and prevalence rates should be interpreted within the context of these demographic data, which are skewed toward a younger population. There are estimated to be around 600 people with ALS in Israel, and around 120 to 150 people are diagnosed per year (IsrALS).

THE ISRAEL ALS RESEARCH ASSOCIATION

The Israel ALS Research Association (IsrALS) IsrALS Website. (n.d.) was established in 2004 and is active in patient and family support at an individual level, as well as in research funding and coordination. The CEO is Efrat Carmi, the co-author of this chapter. IsrALS supports people with ALS and their family: they describe their vision as: "To create a world where ALS is a treatable and manageable disease, and ALS patients can enjoy an optimal quality of life." The IsrALS is active in several fields.

Promoting ALS Research in Israel

Until 2005 there was no coordinated ALS research in Israel. When IsrALS was established, the first aim was to fundraise for research and, in parallel, to recruit active investigators in the field of ALS research. At this time, IsrALS has distributed over 15 million NIS (4.3 million USD) to fund ALS research in Israel. There are now ALS research groups in all major academic institutions in the country.

The IsrALS holds an annual scientific conference, bringing together researchers, clinicians and members of the pharmaceutical industry. The IsrALS supports eligible post-doctorates who are returning from overseas and wish to establish their own ALS research group.

When the IsrALS was established, there was only one ALS clinic within the country. The IsrALS helped to establish a new ALS clinic in the Hadassah University Hospital, Jerusalem, with a view to providing multi-disciplinary care and serving as an additional research hub for researchers throughout the country. The Hadassah University Hospital ALS clinic is currently running two first-in-human clinical trials (one drug-based and one stem-cell based). The IsrALS is also coordinating a collaborative study between the Israeli ALS clinics and the NY Genome Center in order to allow whole genome sequencing of all consenting Israeli people with ALS.

Supporting ALS Patients and Their Family Members

IsrALS has a team of social workers who cover the entire country and meet every new patient as soon as possible after diagnosis. The team is available for any questions regarding benefits, emotional coping and family support and has access to clinical and para-clinical professionals who are familiar with the disease.

IsrALS has numerous specific programs:

(a) An assistive technology service (see below)
(b) A transportation service with a specially adapted vehicle
(c) A dedicated program for ALS patients and their families within the Arab sector
(d) A program for families (with a specific program focused on the support of younger children)
(e) An informative/educational program for patients before they decide whether to use invasive ventilation

IsrALS publishes an annual magazine with updated information regarding both research and clinical/para-clinical care, and it holds events for fundraising and raising awareness of the disease.

The organization also works with governmental entities to improve the benefits of ALS patients in Israel and is prominent in the media.

GOVERNMENTAL ACTION ON ALS

We are unaware of any dedicated reports or actions regarding ALS prior to the establishment of the IsrALS in 2004. During the 15 years since the IsrALS was established, the organization has worked closely with many governmental entities in order to improve the status of ALS patients in Israel.

The Israeli healthcare system is based on the National Health Insurance law, which mandates all resident citizens to join one of the four official health insurance organizations (HIOs) known as "Kupot Holim." These HIOs are run as non-profit organizations and are mandated, by law, to accept membership from any Israeli resident, irrespective of pre-existing conditions. Although these are not government agencies per se, they are bound by law to provide medical care to all their members according to the government-defined "health basket." Thus, when riluzole became available within the health basket, each of the HIOs was mandated to cover the cost of this drug. The health basket is updated annually to allow introduction of new drugs and technologies; this is implemented through a dedicated sub-committee, which consults with experts in the relevant field.

The IsrALS is in contact with the HIOs regarding organization of services for people with ALS, as well as the government agencies themselves, to improve public policy on ALS.

Meetings between the IsrALS and government agencies have dealt with the following issues:

- Israel Ministry of Health Website. (n.d.): The IsrALS is involved in lobbying for introduction of new drugs and assistive technologies into the health basket.
- National Insurance Ministry: The IsrALS presented the needs of ALS patients. Specifically, they raised awareness regarding the importance of "fast-tracking" claims from them so that their application for support can be processed within a timeframe that is relevant to the pace of their disease. The dialogue with the Social Security management is an ongoing one, with services continuing to improve. The IsrALS co-authored a publication with the National Insurance Ministry detailing the rights of people with ALS and how to navigate the process on a practical level.
- IsrALS met with the Population and Immigration Authority regarding the complex subject of foreign paid caregivers. There is a severe lack of qualified paid caregivers within Israel, thus many Israeli ALS patients are reliant on foreign paid caregivers (e.g., from the Philippines) and need to navigate the procedures imposed by the Authority. This is often the rate-limiting factor for ALS patients and

their families to be able to receive the help of a professional caregiver. Although the laws have improved, this discussion with the Authority is an ongoing process.

- IsrALS is an active member of the Rare Diseases Coalition, which is fighting to promote awareness and benefits for the sufferers of several rare diseases in Israel. This coalition formed a "Rare Diseases" lobby in the Knesset (parliament). The goal of this lobby is to promote governmental activities and laws to benefit those unique populations of patients.

FUNDING OF ALS RESEARCH AND PATIENT CARE

Research

The IsrALS is currently the only charity-based organization within Israel that is dedicated to funding ALS research. Between 2007 and 2018, an organization called Prize4Life was active in funding ALS research within Israel and internationally. In 2018 Prize4Life stopped working independently and transferred US-based assets to ALSA.

Sources of public funding for ALS research in Israel include the Israel Ministry of Health Website (n.d.), the Israel Science Foundation Website (n.d.) and the Israel Ministry of Science and Technology (MOST) (n.d.). There is no systematic annual funding for ALS from these bodies. ALS research projects are often awarded grants within broader categories such as neuroscience, neurodegenerative diseases or regenerative medicine. Specific focus areas are often designated (changing each year), and ALS research is selected every few years for funding.

Some research grants are specifically awarded for collaborative research between Israel and partner countries; for example, the MOST funded two binational grants with Italy in 2016 specifically for ALS. In addition, collaborative research with other countries has been funded by organizations based solely in the partner country; for example, the UK-based MNDA funded a collaborative genetic study among the Israeli population—a joint effort between researchers in the Hadassah University Hospital (part of the Hebrew University) and King's College, London.

Public funding for ALS research in Israel is insufficient to sustain the research community and is supplemented from other sources. Israel is known for having a vibrant startup culture, which extends to the biomedical field. The Israel Innovation Authority Website (n.d.) is an independent publicly funded agency that works in a variety of spheres, including bio-medical startups. It facilitates the development of international collaborative partnerships and is involved in generating funding. They have also been active in supporting biomedical companies with a focus on ALS. In addition, an established pharmaceutical company, TEVA, has funded academic research within some of Israel's academic institutions. Donations to academic institutions within Israel are another important source of funding.

Patient Care

Public funding for patient care is insufficient. There is no differentiation of reimbursement based on the complexity of cases seen in a neurology clinic. Thus, the amount of money that a hospital receives for a clinic visit for initial ALS diagnosis is the same as that received for a follow-up visit of someone with stable migraines.

There is no public funding of multidisciplinary clinics. As such the burden of funding for many aspects of care of ALS patients rests on the IsrALS. As a non-profit organization that is also committed to funding research, the IsrALS does not have sufficient funds to establish a full multidisciplinary clinic.

The government does provide funding for caregivers, but it is partial and needs supplementation. The government recently approved public funding for assistive technology, but the assessments necessary to prove eligibility for this are not covered by public funding and the IsrALS funds this aspect.

PUBLIC/MEDIA/COMMERCIAL PERCEPTIONS OF ALS

One of the first strategic missions of the IsrALS was to raise awareness of the disease in order to increase the funds invested in research and patient care. The IsrALS makes sustained efforts to engage the media and to publicize fundraising events and other activities. The media often run stories about individual patients coping with the disease and publicize scientific breakthroughs from Israel and around the globe. There is no doubt that awareness has increased substantially over the last decade. Most of the Israel population has heard about the disease through the Ice Bucket Challenge, as well as media depictions of prominent persons with ALS within Israel and elsewhere.

The increased media attention and awareness of the symptoms of ALS through the Internet may also have had some less desirable consequences; we have noticed a significant increase in consultations of people who fear they have ALS, despite having no neurological dysfunction. Often, they have noticed fasciculations, and may recall hearing that this is often a symptom of ALS or come to that conclusion after an Internet search.

Curiously, the way that ALS is often translated, at least colloquially, into the Hebrew language remains a point of confusion. Most laypersons refer to ALS in Hebrew as "muscle degeneration," which is the same term given to muscular dystrophy. This results in frequent appearances of muscular dystrophy patients in the ALS clinic.

Long-Term Care of Persons with ALS

At the early stages of the disease, most families take care of the patients by themselves. Usually the spouse is the main caregiver with the help of other family members and friends. Israeli society is more family oriented than other developed countries, and families tend to be larger, which can be helpful for sharing the load among family members. Additionally, Israeli society has more of an expectation that families will be heavily involved in patient care, often much more than is reasonable, given the challenges of caring for those with ALS.

As the disease progresses, most families require paid help. Most families employ a foreign worker, who receives a permit to work in Israel as a caregiver. Most foreign caregivers in Israel come from the Philippines, India, Nepal or the former Soviet Union. Some families find that employing one paid caregiver is enough if they share the burden of care themselves. Other families find it impossible to handle the care with only one paid caregiver and choose to employ two or three caregivers. Employing two or three paid caregivers covers 24/7 care and can allow the family to integrate care of the ALS patient with their other commitments. Many families cannot afford the expense of full-time care—in many cases, the cost of the caregiver outweighs the income they would receive from going to work. As a result, the family member may often decide to give up employment in order to care for the person with ALS.

Most paid caregivers are live-in employees. The family provides lodging in their own home, provides food and covers other living expenses. The family gets financial help from the government for the employment of the first paid caregiver, but when they choose to employ more than one care-giver, the additional expense is paid out of their own pocket.

We estimate that less than 5 percent of ALS patients in Israel live in institutional care. Most of the patients continue to live at home through all stages of the disease, even when they are ventilated invasively. There is no respite care policy in Israel. Family caregivers can use their own sick leave in order to miss workdays and take care of the ALS patient, but this benefit is negligible, given the length of the disease. Some employers are amenable to allowing family caregivers to work from home, if practical; however, this is not part of public policy. In some parts of the country, family caregivers can be recognized as employed caregivers and get a mini-mal pay for their time.

ACCESS TO ASSISTIVE TECHNOLOGIES

Until 2015, assistive technology was not provided by government agen-cies and IsrALS had prioritized access to communication devices to allow all ALS patients access to this technology. IsrALS established an assistive technology service in 2012 that employs four occupational therapists (OTs) who specialize in assistive technology. Every ALS patient who feels that his/her ability to communicate is deteriorating is eligible for a home or workplace visit by an OT. During the visit, the OT performs an evalua-tion of the person's condition and recommends the best technology for the stage of the disease. Until 2015, ALS patients who wished to retain communication were forced to fund all devices out of their own pocket. Since the cost of many of these devices is high, many patients could not bear the costs and were left with antiquated, low-tech methods for communication.

In 2015, after years of lobbying by the IsrALS, the government passed a law which added all communication devices to the health basket budget. This is considered one of the main achievements of the IsrALS. As a result, every ALS patient, after being evaluated by IsrALS's team, gets any devices needed for communication paid for by the Health Ministry. This break-through has enabled many patients who were previously unable to com-municate to return to their families and social circles. Unfortunately, the cost of the evaluations themselves is still not covered within the health basket, and IsrALS is still funding them.

STATUS OF MULTIDISCIPLINARY TEAM CARE AND CLINICS

There are now four ALS clinics in Israel: in Jerusalem, Tel Aviv, Haifa and Zfat. The Jerusalem and Tel Aviv ALS clinics are situated in tertiary referral centers and are involved in academic research and clinical trials. We estimate that most persons with ALS in the country are seen at some stage in either the Jerusalem or Tel Aviv clinic even if they also use one of the other smaller clinics. All clinics are headed by a neurologist. The Jerusalem ALS clinic offers access to a pulmonologist and pulmonary function tests on the same day; however, the patient must obtain separate coverage by their HOI for each of the assessments. Separate rehabilitation clinics with multidisciplinary teams do exist; however, the only one with a focus on ALS is in Haifa, which offers occupational therapy, physiotherapy and nutritional consultation. In addition, there is a palliative care home care or "home-hospice" team, which is usually covered by the HOIs, and has extensive experience with patients in the later stages of ALS.

ACCESS TO UNAPPROVED DRUGS

Israel does not have right to try legislation; however, Israeli physicians are allowed to prescribe medications as off-label treatments with committee-based approval. An example of this would be mexiletine for muscle cramps in ALS. In addition, medications approved by other major drug approval authorities around the world, such as the FDA, can be prescribed. For example, edaravone is not within the health basket; however, it may be prescribed (pending committee approval) to any ALS patient and is invariably approved by the committee. As a rule, the HIOs do not cover the cost of the drug itself; however, some patients do receive reimbursement from private insurance agencies or, in certain cases, if they purchased additional insurance cover from the HIOs prior to diagnosis.

GENETIC TESTING OF PATIENTS WITH ALS

Genetic testing is offered to all ALS patients attending the Jerusalem ALS clinic as part of a research program. The cost of this is covered by research grants, including support from the IsrALS. Routine genetic testing is offered to all persons with ALS who have a definite or possible family history of ALS or FTD, but this will, in general, only be covered by the HIO for patients of child-bearing age. In this scenario, unaffected relatives of a person with ALS with an identified mutation will also be offered genetic testing, if desired, and the cost of this will usually be covered by the HIO. The results in all cases are confidential. Reports from the genetics clinic are only accessible by the genetics staff; even the treating neurologist cannot see the results in the electronic patient records. The results reach the treating neurologist in paper form. Genetic counseling is usually offered to all people with a family history before genetic testing is undertaken and on receipt of the results. ALS patients who agree to have genetic testing as part of a research program are counseled by the neurology team during consent and can decide if they wish to receive positive results. In such cases, we choose to involve a genetic counselor in the process, although this is not mandated by law.

End-of-Life Decision Making

Most ALS patients in Israel die at home. This is usually defined as a "home hospice" and is a service covered by all the HIOs. Only 5 percent spend the last stage of their life in a nursing facility. Some patients die in hospital when they are being treated for acute deterioration, usually pneumonia with worsening respiratory failure. There are no data regarding the incidence of hospital deaths from ALS; however, we estimate that this is a very small proportion of patients, probably less than 3 percent.

Access to Palliative and Hospice Care

Over the last ten years, there has been an exponential growth of palliative care services in Israel. Before this, there was little in the way of palliative care outside of oncology. The vast improvement in this area was the result of policy changes instituted after years of lobbying.

Today, ALS patients are eligible for palliative care in the form of a home hospice if they suffer from respiratory distress but choose *not* to receive ventilation via tracheostomy. In these cases, they continue to receive non-invasive ventilation and are treated by a hospice team that includes a palliative care doctor and a nurse. As ventilation failure progresses and they begin to suffer from symptoms related to respiratory distress, they are offered palliative sedation. Our estimation is that 25 to 35 percent of the patients choose this option and make an active choice to opt for palliative care toward the end of their lives.

In cases where the ALS patient chooses long-term invasive ventilation, the HIO provides visits from a home invasive ventilation team, which deals with the care of chronically ventilated patients in general. All symptomatic care is coordinated by this team, and ventilated patients are not seen by the palliative care team.

Advance Directives and Withholding or Withdrawing Mechanical Ventilation

The factors influencing the legal status in Israel regarding advance directives and withdrawal of ventilation are very complex. The complexity arises from numerous religious, social and cultural factors that are detailed in the next section.

Although withholding mechanical ventilation is permitted, withdrawing ventilation is prohibited. Advance directives are permitted and commonly used, and healthcare professionals are mandated by law to follow them, irrespective of their own religious views. Having said that, in cases where advance directives are unclear to the medical team (usually in the setting of an emergency), there is a tendency of many doctors to default toward ventilation, even for people with ALS. If a patient has been ventilated, they cannot demand withdrawal of ventilation. This is the case even if they had written an advance directive not to be ventilated that was unavailable to the medical team at the time of ventilation.

Over the last 15 years, the IsrALS has been educating ALS patients regarding long-term invasive ventilation. Before this campaign, the default situation was for almost all patients to receive a tracheostomy. Since then, most ALS patients have been made aware of the option to refuse invasive ventilation and are advised to fill out advance directives relatively early in the disease. They are encouraged to inform their family and friends about their wishes and the location of the documents detailing them. We estimate that, currently, around 50 to 60 percent of ALS patients choose invasive ventilation in Israel. Palliative sedation is legal in a hospice care environment. Euthanasia and assisted suicide are illegal in Israel.

FACTORS UNIQUE TO ISRAEL CRITICAL FOR UNDERSTANDING DECISION MAKING FOR ALS

There are several unique factors active within Israeli society that affect decisions of patients and their families and the public policy surrounding ALS.

Religious

A significant proportion of the population in Israel follow a religious lifestyle, whether Jewish or Muslim. Even within each religious group, there are many subgroups, each accepting varying levels of stringency regarding end-of-life care issues. Judaism is the official national religion, and religious Jewish political parties serve in the government and hold cabinet positions. As such, religious considerations are certainly taken into account in the development of public policy. Euthanasia is considered akin to murder in Judaism. Actively withdrawing ventilation would also fall within this category, whereas withholding ventilation from a terminal patient would not be considered as such. The legal status of these scenarios reflects this differentiation.

On a philosophical level, disease is often considered by the more spiritual persons with ALS to be "their challenge" and they are empowered by a feeling of religious purpose in life, which leads them to choose invasive ventilation. The predominant spiritual view within Judaism is that life has a purpose, and so long as the person is alive, they can fulfill their purpose. This is a good example where assistive technologies have made a significant change—many religious ALS patients feel they are able to have a fulfilled life while ventilated because they are able to continue to learn religious material and even continue to teach students.

Cultural and Social

In addition to religious tradition and beliefs, Israeli culture is shaped by events in recent history. The experience of the Holocaust, Israeli wars, terrorist attacks and even biblical stories have engrained within Israeli culture an almost mythical value of survival of the people and the individual despite suffering and hardship. The culture values "life" at the center and cherishes life over death, even in the face of suffering. ALS patients will often say they wish to be ventilated to live to attend the wedding of a child or the birth of a grandchild.

Family Structure and Commitment

In Israel it is almost taken for granted that family members should act as caregivers. This involves extended families, friends and neighbors. This is distinctive from a desire not to "become a burden." The geography of Israel also facilitates this: Israel is a small country, with most of the population living within one to two hours' drive of each other. Furthermore, families often tend to live near their parents.

Israel has the highest fertility rate in the OECD (3.1 children per woman). People start families at a younger age and have more children. The corollary is that a person with ALS will have more family members who can help in some way, thus often allowing for the load to be spread to some extent. Interestingly, the presence of large families, coupled with a tendency for some sectors to marry within their own extended families (consanguinity), has been beneficial in terms of genetic research in general and specifically the study of ALS genetics.

Government Support

When patients are on invasive ventilation, they require full-time care. The law in Israel allows families to get financial help for one paid caregiver, which makes home ventilation a financially viable option. Employing foreign paid caregivers is very common in Israel and there is an established, although not always efficient, process set up for finding, hiring and employing them.

RECOMMENDED CHANGES IN POLICY TO IMPROVE CARE OF ALS PATIENTS

There is no doubt that Israel requires a significant injection of money into the health service in general and for care of persons with ALS specifically. There is a critical need to increase the funding of multidisciplinary clinics as well as research support for academic institutions. Streamlining the process of foreign worker placement is a priority that would incur minimal expense.

In terms of medical therapy, it is too soon to conclude as to whether adding edaravone to the health basket should be considered a priority. Medical cannabis is legal in Israel, and it is estimated that around 60 to 70 percent of ALS patients benefit from this. With the expansion of indications for medical cannabis, the approval process has become more difficult in recent years for some patients. A fast-track should be developed for medical cannabis approval for ALS patients.

Finally, the process by which advanced directives are made and communicated to medical teams should be made more efficient and secure, such that if a person with ALS has made a directive to avoid invasive ventilation, this should automatically appear within electronic patient records at any emergency room or medical facility in the country.

REFERENCES

OECD. (2017). Social and Welfare Statistics Family Indicators. https://www.oecd-ilibrary.org/social-issues-migration-health/data/oecd-social-and-welfare-statistics/family-indicators-edition-2017_7bb8ed6f-en

Israel Ministry of Health Website. (n.d.). https://www.health.gov.il/English/Pages/HomePage.aspx

Israel Science Foundation Website. (n.d.). https://www.isf.org.il

Israel Ministry of Science and Technology. (n.d.). https://www.gov.il/en/departments/ministry_of_science_and_technology

IsrALS Website. (n.d.). http://en.israls.org.il/

Israel Innovation Authority Website. (n.d.). https://innovationisrael.org.il/en/

CHAPTER 11

Public Policy in ALS Care: The Italian Situation

Simone Veronese and Andrea Calvo

Abstract ALS care in Italy is mainly managed by specialist neurological centers, often hospital based, working as hubs linked to other specialist services involved in the care process. Because the Italian National Health Service is regionalized, locally different models of care can occur. A National Research Programme promotes the integration of public and private sectors on research priorities and opportunities. Patients' associations play a substantial role advocating for legal rights, adequate service provision and support for carers. National and regional laws guarantee benefits for ALS patients and their carers by means of economic support and device provision. Palliative care in ALS is developing fast in Italy. There are research groups involving neurologists, rehabilitation specialists and palliative specialists, and recommendations were recently released on this topic. End-of-life care is regulated by specific national laws; patients have

S. Veronese (✉)
Fondazione FARO, Turin, Italy
e-mail: simone.veronese@fondazionefaro.it

A. Calvo
ALS Turin Center, University of Turin, Turin, Italy
e-mail: andrea.calvo@unito.it

© The Author(s) 2021
R. H. Blank et al. (eds.), *Public Policy in ALS/MND Care*,
https://doi.org/10.1007/978-981-15-5840-5_11

the right to decide on withholding or withdrawing treatments. Euthanasia and assisted suicide remain illegal, even though there is a social movement toward more permissive legislation.

Keywords ALS\MND • Palliative care • End-of-life care • Models of care • Multidisciplinary care • Integration • Patients' rights

EPIDEMIOLOGY OF ALS IN ITALY

The epidemiology of ALS in Italy has been evaluated over time and many population-based registers are active. The Piemonte and Valle d'Aosta Register for ALS (PARALS) was established in 1995 to assess the epidemiology of the disease in two regions of northwestern Italy. The mean annual crude incidence rate in this period was 3.03/100,000 population, which increased from 2.83/100,000 in the 1995/2004 decade to 3.23/100,000 in the 2005/2014 decade, a 14 percent increase. The prevalence rate of ALS in PARALS on December 31, 2014, was 10.5/100,000 population, one of the highest reported in the literature, and 34 percent more compared with that on December 31, 2004 (7.9/100,000) (Chiò et al. 2017).

Other active prospective registers in Italy include the Emilia Romagna Registry for ALS (ERRALS), with a crude incidence rate of 2.63/100,000/ year, characterized by a micro-geographic heterogeneity throughout this region, with higher incidence rates in the low density population (3.27/100,000) (Mandrioli et al. 2014); the Liguria Amyotrophic Lateral Sclerosis Registry (LIGALS) that found a standardized incidence, age and gender adjusted to the 2001 Italian population, of 2.51/100,000 (Bandettini di Poggio et al. 2013); Sclerosi Laterale Amiotrofica—Puglia (SLAP) Registry reported an annual crude incidence for ALS in Puglia for the two-year period 1998–1999 of 1.6/100000 (Logroscino et al. 2005). In another study based on a retrospective survey in the Friuli-Venezia Giulia (FVG) region, the authors found a crude incidence of 2.81/100,000 person-years and a prevalence of 8.36 (6.74–9.97)/100,000 (Palese et al. 2019).

NATIONAL POLICIES, FUNDING STRATEGIES AND USER INVOLVEMENT

In Italy, there is no single centralized organization or association for ALS patients, but there are many national or local associations. The biggest of these is the Associazione Italiana per la SLA (AISLA), but many other groups are also very active in advocacy field. The work of these associations has produced important benefits for patients and families, particularly economic care supports. Although it varies from region to region, ALS patients receive a monthly monetary contribution for care assistance dependent on the stage of disease.

The instrument that identifies strategies and priorities for Italy's research system is the National Research Programme (NRP). The primary goal is to promote the progressive integration of public and private research. The NRP was drawn up by the Ministry of Education, University and Research (MIUR) through broad consultation with the scientific and academic community, economic forces and relevant administrative entities and is approved by the Inter-ministerial Committee for Economic Programming (CIPE). There are different competitive research programs, such as Ordinary Fund for Research Institutes and Bodies (FOE), Fund for Investments in Basic Research (FIRB), Research Support Fund (FAR) and Research Projects of National Interest (PRIN). There are also research foundations that are to some extent focused on ALS research including Telethon, ARISLA, Compagnia di San Paolo and Fondazione Cariplo e Fondazione CRT, all of which are private organizations that finance different competitive grants.

Research funding for ALS is increasing in Italy but is still insufficient, especially in the palliative care field. In the last two decades, the social media impact for ALS has been incredibly strong, in part because of the efforts of the patients' associations but even more because of the causal association between ALS and professional athletes (Chiò et al. 2009). The recent law about living wills and informed consent (Law 219 of 2017) caused a huge media coverage, with a consequence of a constant presence of information on each medium, though sometimes distorted and dangerous.

The Italian Model of ALS Care

To date, there has been a heterogeneous level of ALS care over the Italian peninsula. Despite this, in recent years there has been a significant improvement in the standard of care, at a significantly more competent and efficacious level. The model of care adopted by the ALS centers is that of multidisciplinary care, developed by the ALS centers in the early 1980s. In Italy there are different types of systems, depending on the involvement of the territory. In Piedmont, for example, there are two well-established ALS expert centers: they are grounded on interdisciplinary collaboration within hospital services, outpatient specialities and general practitioner collaborations (Chiò et al. 2006). Since 2009, in this very efficient system, palliative care is a main resource.

The care of people with ALS in Italy varies significantly due to individual economic differences as well as divergent regional habits. Most ALS patients die at home. For instance, within the Piemonte and Valle d'Aosta Registry, 75 percent die at home, 10 percent in hospital, 6 percent in hospice and 9 percent in nursing or long-term care facilities (data prom PARALS, not published). Every patient has an opportunity to benefit from augmentative alternative communication. Throughout Italy, speech therapy consultation is available to perform an extensive evaluation for the best type of assisted communication device, with the possibility for the patients to obtain those instruments free under the national health system.

Palliative Care for Patients with ALS in Italy

Palliative care in neurology has seen a progressive growth in Italy over the last decade. ALS has always been considered a paradigm of a neurological condition requiring palliative care. In 2000 the subgroup of study for bioethics and palliative of the Italian National Society of Neurology (SIN) published its first position paper focusing on the need to provide palliative care to patients dying with neurological conditions such as ALS (De Fanti 2000). The same group analyzed who should receive palliative care, how these services should be delivered and integrated in the national care system, and what timing would best address the impelling needs and adopted ALS care as a theoretical model to be used as a model for other neurological conditions (Causarano 2005). In the same period a charity organization, Gilberto Cominetta AGC-PCN, organized the first palliative care education course for neurologists. The aim of this initiative was to provide education to specialized physicians on the principles of palliative care, the paradigm shift from cure to care, the paramount importance of symptom control, the role of advance care planning and the need of family carers.

Unfortunately, despite these initiatives from the Italian neurological field, patients with ALS and other progressive neurological conditions did not have access to palliative care. Hospices and palliative care teams (PCT) were available, with exceptions, for cancer patients only. In 2005 the Italian Society for Palliative Care (SICP) published in its official journal the Italian translation and adaptation of a seminal paper about the role of palliative care in ALS. It was an incentive to provide education to palliative care providers on the nature of this disease, its course, main decision points, principles of symptom control, role of the multidisciplinary care, importance of communication and the care in the terminal phase (Borasio et al. 2005).

In the following years, research projects aimed at exploring the palliative care needs of patients with conditions like ALS were conducted (Veronese et al. 2015a), and the first Italian prospective RCT evaluating the impact of specialist palliative care for neurological patients was published (Veronese et al. 2015b). These promising results induced the SICP to start a collaboration with SIN in order to publish a joint position document with the goal of developing new pathways of care for people suffering from progressive neurological disorders, paying particular attention to the families and the professional carers (SICP-SIN 2018). The Italian government followed this scientific and education movement, passing a national law that extends the right to receive palliative care to all patients affected by a chronic, incurable condition regardless of diagnosis (Legge 38 2010). It is now a right for patients with ALS (and their families) to receive comprehensive palliative care services, deliverable throughout all the course of the disease, in any setting of care, based on their needs and according to their preference of care.

The unsolved issue is now at an organizational level. Since in Italy most of ALS care is organized according to the tertiary clinic model which showed the best results for patients' outcomes (Chiò et al. 2006), best practice seems to be the integration of palliative care services into the network of these services, serving as hubs of the care network. The uneven distribution of the services across the nation does not allow an equal distribution of this network. Where no connection between palliative care and neurological services exists, the provision of adequate palliative care for ALS patients remains uncoordinated and is left to local initiatives. SIN and SICP are both providing a strong effort to enhance collaboration and support initiatives aimed at improving the quality of care for neurological patients.

Very recently, a European online survey, under the auspices of the European Academy of Neurology (EAN) and European Association for Palliative Care (EAPC), that explored the relationship between neurology and palliative care in 22 European countries, had responses from 142 Italian palliative care professionals and 71 neurologists (by far the highest response rate on the continent). This result was obtained thanks to the involvement of national scientific societies that actively sponsored the survey in national conferences and on the websites. ALS and brain tumors are the conditions with the highest rate of collaboration (31 to 45% and 33 to 36%, respectively) between palliative care and neurology. Collaboration is described as useful in 75–93 percent of respondents depending on the specialties. Barriers to better coordinated service provision are due to financial issues and to the lack of local palliative care teams as well as some resistance by primary healthcare teams to care for patients with ALS and other neurological disorders (Oliver et al. 2019).

END-OF-LIFE CARE IN ITALY

ALS remains an incurable disorder, and the terminal phase of the disease is a huge challenge to the systems of care. Patients report many fears, such as choking to death, dying in hospital or in other settings not desired, feeling a burden for their families and not having their choices at the end of life respected. Family carers are often exhausted by very long caregiving tasks, having to fight to receive adequate care and support (above all at home), and they are afraid of what may happen during the dying phase and at the death of their beloved one. Most of them must leave their jobs in order to look after their ill relative, and financial issues are common. Professionals face a challenge to recognize the end-of-life phase in ALS patients and struggle to obtain home care or long-term facility services, and sometimes do not have specific education and competence for managing the last days or weeks of life of their patients.

In Italy most ALS patients want to die at home, cared for by their families. They want a conservative approach at the end of life and do not want life-prolonging treatments, such as tracheostomy and invasive mechanical ventilation (IV). The percentage of ALS patients in IV varies in Italy by region, and no national data are available to date. In Piedmont (Northwest region of Italy) 10.6 percent of patients with ALS underwent tracheostomy in a ten-year period (Chiò et al. 2010). In other areas of the country, the percentage is as high as 30 percent of all ALS patients. For this group of patients, the quality of death and dying, the recognition of the dying phase and the provision of palliative at the end-of-life care are still underdeveloped (Veronese et al. 2014). The proportion of ALS patients dying in a palliative care setting (hospice care or home palliative care services) is not available at a national level, but at the ALS Centre in Turin, palliative care is guaranteed for all the patients who want these services. Within the FARO Foundation, one of the main palliative care providers of the northwestern region of Italy, ALS patients make up 8 to 10 percent of the patient numbers under their care at any time. This care includes home care, hospice admissions, education and research on end of life in ALS. This is just an example of local initiatives that are spreading out throughout Italy.

Advance Directives and Withholding or Withdrawing Life-Extending Interventions

Italy has long been considered very controversial regarding end-of-life decisions in Europe (Van der Heide et al. 2003). Legislation was deemed insufficient regarding withdrawing treatments, and clinical practice showed that even withholding undesired measures was not assured for ALS patients. A qualitative study exploring the last stages of life of ALS invasive ventilated patients found that while the vast majority did not want to receive IV, in the end they often consented because there was a lack of alternatives. Moreover, decisions were often made with little time for discussion in an emergency setting (Veronese et al. 2014).

The Italian Constitution since 1948 has declared that personal liberty is inviolable and Italian citizens cannot be forced to any medical treatment without their informed consent. The Physicians Code of Ethics has confirmed this principle. Unfortunately, there is evidence that these fundamental rights were not always adhered to in Italian medical settings and many ALS patients received unwanted treatment and could not obtain the withdrawal of treatment, the excuse often used that there was no clear legislation. The main reasons for this were attributed to the Catholic Church's ethical stance of the sacredness of life, which would not allow any option of withholding or withdrawing treatments that could shorten life, medical paternalism or the general fear that these actions represented the introduction of euthanasia.

AISLA (Associazione Italiana Sclerosi Laterale Amiotrofica, the ALS patients' association) published on their website an advance directive that clearly stated the right of ALS patients to refuse any undesired treatment and have any life-support measure withdrawn under specific conditions such as locked-in syndrome, when all communication is lost. This position paper was gradually adopted by different ALS centers, all of which agreed on the right to refuse any unwanted treatment, although some did not offer the chance of withdrawing IV.

The EAPC published a position paper clarifying the differences between euthanasia, assisted suicide and non-treatment decisions which were adopted by the Italian Palliative Care Society (Radbruch, L., et al. Board Members of EAPC 2016). After long political, ethical, social and medical debates, triggered by numerous cases that appeared in the news, finally at the end of 2017 a national law on the end-of-life decision was passed by the Parliament. This compromise regulation was reached after widespread agreement by the political parties, medical associations and even the Catholic Church. At the time of the passage of this law, the Pope released a statement for the European Regional Meeting of the World Medical Association on end-of-life issues, held in the Vatican in conjunction with the Pontifical Academy for Life. The Holy Father wrote:

> It has also become possible nowadays to extend life by means that were inconceivable in the past. Surgery and other medical interventions have become ever more effective, but they are not always beneficial: they can sustain, or even replace, failing vital functions, but that is not the same as promoting health.

Then, recalling a notorious statement from Pope Pius XII of 1957, he reiterated that: It is "morally licit to decide not to adopt therapeutic measures, or to discontinue them, when their use does not meet that ethical and humanistic standard that would later be called 'due proportion in the use of remedies.'" In order to make clear the difference between withdrawing or withholding an undesired treatment and euthanasia, he added:

> Here one does not will to cause death; one's inability to impede it is merely accepted (Catechism of the Catholic Church, No. 2278). This difference of perspective restores humanity to the accompaniment of the dying, while not attempting to justify the suppression of the living. It is clear that not adopt-

ing, or else suspending, disproportionate measures, means avoiding over-zealous treatment; from an ethical standpoint, it is completely different from euthanasia, which is always wrong, in that the intent of euthanasia is to end life and cause death. (Pope Francesco 2017)

This law, Rules on Informed Consent and Advance Directives of Treatment 219–2017, declares the right of any Italian citizen to decide in advance on possible therapeutic options, provides a process of identifying a surrogate who can decide on behalf of the patient in case of loss of capacity and affirms the right of a patient to withhold or withdraw any medical treatment including nutrition, hydration and respiratory support. The same law advocates for palliative care as the best option for people severely affected by relentless conditions and confirms palliative sedation as an appropriate treatment for refractory symptoms. Any request for voluntary hastening of death (euthanasia or assisted suicide) remains illegal.

Following the release of this law, numerous patients requested to be withdrawn from invasive mechanical ventilation. Unfortunately, to date it is not possible to quantify how many people have taken this action, but in our unit four patients requested and obtained a removal of the respiratory tube. The procedure was done according to the Withdrawal of Assisted Ventilation at the Request of a Patient with Motor Neurone Disease professional guidelines published by the Association for Palliative Medicine of Great Britain and Ireland (APM, 2015). It took on average two to three months from the moment of the request to the act of withdrawal, during which time a thorough palliative care assessment was provided, secondary reversible causes of suffering were explored, options were proposed and family support was facilitated. At the end of this process, patients who confirmed their decision were sedated and the unwanted respiratory support was withdrawn. They all died within an hour without any sign of suffering, and their carers received bereavement support.

This recent law defines the right of refusing treatments, but does not clarify who, where and how the withdrawal of life-supporting measures must happen. In theory the physicians who obtain an informed consent to start a treatment are the same as those who should remove it once it is no longer desired. This would mean that pulmonary or resuscitation specialists would be involved. However, often neurologists are the professionals more involved in the care of the patient and know well their stories, their families and the process of the choices. Some Italian neurological departments offer the possibility to be admitted in the neurological ward to be withdrawn from mechanical ventilation, and this is part of the informed consent form signed, or video recorded, by the patient.

In most cases, palliative care services are involved in this process due to the specific skills of PCTs in terms of palliative sedation and end-of-life choices. Although clearly end-of-life care is a task of PCTs, the professionals in this field do not want to be considered as the team who would switch off machinery when this has been prescribed by other team members at the patient's request. In order to avoid this, the SICP-SIN document (SICP-SIN 2018) adopting the recommendations suggested by the EAPC-EAN reference group for palliative care in neurology, encourages and advocates for an early involvement of PCT during the trajectory course (Oliver et al. 2016). This is particularly true for ALS, where various triggers of deterioration and clinical turning points have been highlighted and can be used to start conversation about end-of-life decisions and begin an advanced plan of care.

Legal Status of Palliative Sedation, Euthanasia and Physician-Assisted Suicide

The role of palliative sedation for patients affected by incurable conditions like ALS, facing unbearable and refractory symptoms, has been described earlier in the chapter. Palliative sedation in such conditions is legal, encouraged as a therapeutic option and considered as a right of the patient as well as a duty for the caring teams. Any other form of voluntarily hastening of death is illegal and punished by the Italian law.

Public debate is now very active on these end-of-life issues. Recently an official statement of the Italian Committee for Bioethics expressed a favorable opinion for assisted suicide. In September 2019 the Constitutional Court pronounced a sentence stating that in specific conditions, helping a person affected by an irreversible condition and kept alive by life-sustaining measures, to terminate his or her own life may be not punishable by law. This issue must be evaluated case by case by a judge, and a specific law is required to clarify these situations.

CONCLUSIONS

Palliative care in ALS in Italy is moving toward important changes and challenges. In the last decade there has been a linear increase in the involvement of PC in the end-of-life phase of ALS. More recently the collaboration between PC and ALS centers has improved, and there is now a tendency toward early PC interventions based on patients' and families' unmet needs rather than prognosis. The model of ALS centers as hubs with a network of satellite services drawn around users' needs seems to be a good pathway of care for ALS in Italy.

Among the many barriers that prevent access to palliative care for ALS patients is the reluctancy of some PC services to serve neurological patients and a lack of confidence of some neurologists in palliative care. Also, the lack of resources is an important constraint since many parts of the country do not have enough services or staff to fulfill this need. However, collaboration between specialties is improving and the national scientific bodies are initiating several efforts to enhance mutual education and shared clinical practices. Numerous academic educational programs have been started to improve the palliative culture in young Italian physicians.

End-of-life issues are changing rapidly, and many rights are now recognized through Italian legislation, although some organizational steps are yet to be completed. Ethical issues surrounding the anticipation of death are now a hot topic in Italy. The closeness to Switzerland, where assisted suicide is tolerated and where some ALS patients have paid to go and die by assisted suicide, has raised the topic on the news, and some civil rights associations are now pushing to introduce the right to die.

There is need for better integration and implementation of good practice according to the evidence of benefits of early integrated palliative care on patients' and families' outcomes published in the literature.

References

APM (2015). Withdrawal of Assisted Ventilation at the Request of a Patient with Motor Neurone Disease. Retrieved from https://apmonline.org/wp-content/uploads/2015/02/APM-Guidance-on-Withdrawal-of-Assisted-Ventilation-Consultation-1st-May-2015.pdf

Borasio, G.D., R. Voltz and R.G. Miller (2005). *Le cure palliative nella Sclerosi Laterale Amiotrofica. Rivista Italiana di Cure Palliative.* Numero 2 estate 2005. Translated from the same authors, *Palliative care in amyotrophic lateral sclerosis. Neurologic Clinics* 2001; 19: 829–47.

Bandettini di Poggio, M., et al. (2013). Clinical epidemiology of ALS in Liguria, Italy. *Amyotrophic Lateral Sclerosis and Frontotemporal Degeneration* 14 (1): 52–57.

Chiò, A., et al. (2006). Positive effects of tertiary centres for amyotrophic lateral sclerosis on outcome and use of hospital facilities. *Journal of Neurology, Neurosurgery and Psychiatry* 77 (8): 948–50.

Chiò, A., et al. (2009). ALS in Italian professional soccer players: The risk is still present and could be soccer-specific. *Amyotrophic Lateral Sclerosis* 10 (4): 205–09.

Chiò, A., et al. (2010). Tracheostomy in amyotrophic lateral sclerosis: A 10-year population-based study in Italy. *Journal of Neurology, Neurosurgery and Psychiatry* 81: 1141–43, https://doi.org/10.1136/jnnp.2009.175984

Chiò, A., et al. (2017). Piemonte and Valle d'Aosta Register for ALS (PARALS). Secular trends of amyotrophic lateral sclerosis: The Piemonte and Valle d'Aosta Register. *JAMA Neurology* 74 (9): 1097–04.

Causarano, I.R. (2005). Le cure palliative in neurologia: Come, dove e quando. *Neurological Sciences* 26: S127–S131.

De Fanti, C.A. (2000). Gruppo di Studio per la Bioetica e le Cure Palliative in Neurologia: documento programmatico. *Neurological Science* 21: 266–71.

Legge 38 (2010). Retrieved from https://www.gazzettaufficiale.it/gunewsletter/dettaglio.jsp?service=1&datagu=2010-03-19&task=dettaglio&numgu=65&redaz=010G0056&tmstp=1269600292070

Logroscino, G., et al. (2005). Incidence of amyotrophic lateral sclerosis in southern Italy: A population-based study. *Journal of Neurology, Neurosurgery and Psychiatry* 76 (8): 1094–98.

Mandrioli, J., et al. (2014). Epidemiology of amyotrophic lateral sclerosis in Emilia Romagna Region (Italy): A population-based study. *Amyotrophic Lateral Sclerosis and Frontotemporal Degeneration* 15 (3–4): 262–68.

Oliver, D., et al. (2016). A consensus review on the development of palliative care for patients with chronic and progressive neurological disease. European Journal of Neurology 23 (1): 30–38.

Oliver, D., et al. (2019). EURO-NEURO survey: Collaboration between neurology and palliative care: A European survey. Poster at the 5th Congress of the European Academy of Neurology, Oslo.

Palese, F., et al. (2019). Epidemiology of amyotrophic lateral sclerosis in Friuli-Venezia Giulia, North-Eastern Italy, 2002–2014: A retrospective population-based study. Amyotrophic Lateral Sclerosis and Frontotemporal Degeneration 20 (1–2): 90–99.

Pope Francesco (2017) Messaggio del Santo Padre al Presidente della Pontificia Accademia per la Vita in occasione del Meeting Regionale Europeo della "World Medical Association" sulle questioni del "fine-vita". Vaticano, 16.11.2017 ret from https://press.vatican.va/content/salastampa/it/bollettino/pubblico/2017/11/16/0794/01721.html#en

Radbruch, L. et al., Board Members of EAPC. (2016) Euthanasia and physician-assisted suicide: A white paper from the European Association for Palliative Care. *Palliative Medicine* 30 (2): 104–16. https://doi.org/10.1177/0269216315616524.

SICP-SIN. (2018). Le cure palliative per il malato neurologico. Retrieved from https://www.sicp.it/documenti/sicp/2018/10/le-cure-palliative-nel-malato-neurologico-documento-intersocietario-sicp-sin/

Van der Heide, A., et al. (2003). End-of-life decision-making in six European countries: Descriptive study. *Lancet* 362 (9381): 345–50.

Veronese, S., et al. (2014). The last months of life of people with amyotrophic lateral sclerosis in mechanical invasive ventilation: A qualitative study. *Amyotrophic Lateral Sclerosis and Frontotemporal Degeneration* 15 (7–8): 499–504.

Veronese, S., et al. (2015a). The palliative care needs of people severely affected by neurodegenerative disorders: A qualitative study. *Progress in Palliative Care* 23 (6): 331–42.

Veronese, S., et al. (2015b). Specialist palliative care improves the quality of life in advanced neurodegenerative disorders: NE-PAL, a pilot randomised controlled study. *BMJ Supportive & Palliative Care* 0:1–9. https://doi.org/10.1136/bmjspcare-2014-000788

CHAPTER 12

ALS Policy: A Japanese Perspective

Mieko Ogino and Tamerlan Babayev

Abstract The prevalence of ALS and the age at onset in Japan have been increasing in recent years. Japan has various insurance systems for incurable diseases, and financial assistance for medical care and care is generous. In some areas, there are long-term hospitalization facilities, but home medical care is substantial and many patients stay at home. The proportion of patients selecting tracheostomy ventilators is higher than in Western countries. Patients have access to any physician under public insurance and can participate in treatment trials. Large-scale ALS centers are difficult to establish, but multidisciplinary medical care is covered by insurance. The withdrawal of ventilators is not routinely performed in Japan and can be problematic in patients with advanced tracheostomy ventilators. The challenge is to train medical professionals who specialize in ALS.

Keywords ALS • Intractable disease • Japan Agency for Medical Research and Development (AMED) • The Japanese Consortium for ALS (JaCALS)

M. Ogino (✉) • T. Babayev
International University of Health and Welfare, Narita, Japan
e-mail: ogino@iuhw.ac.jp; babayev@iuhw.sc.jp

© The Author(s) 2021
R. H. Blank et al. (eds.), *Public Policy in ALS/MND Care*,
https://doi.org/10.1007/978-981-15-5840-5_12

177

INCIDENCE, PREVALENCE AND MORTALITY OF ALS

In Japan, ALS is recognized as a designated intractable disease, and patients can receive support with their medical expenses. For this reason, patients usually report their diagnosis and receive a beneficiary certificate, enabling the government to gather population statistics on the number of ALS patients in Japan, by prefecture (the administrative areas in Japan) and by age (https://www.nanbyou.or.jp/entry/5354). However, if the patient can receive medical expense subsidies through alternative pathways such as welfare or disability certificates, he/she may not apply, so the number of patients is thought to be slightly higher than the number of beneficiary recipients. It is estimated that there is a prevalence of 7 to 8/100,000, and an incidence of about 1/100,000 in Japan. Comparing prefectures, the prevalence is higher in those with older populations and in general as patient age increases (https://www.nanbyou.or.jp/entry/5354; https://www8.cao.go.jp/kourei/whitepaper/w-2018/html/zenbun/s1_1_4.html).

GOVERNMENTAL INVOLVEMENT IN ALS CARE AND RESEARCH

In 1972, the guidelines for the treatment of intractable diseases were finalized, and research funding and medical expenses subsidies for patients began. Thereafter, the number of target diseases gradually increased, and in 1974, ALS was added. The increasing number of patients and rising medical expenses made it difficult to expand the target diseases, but this created a disparity among incurable diseases, and it was felt that legislation should be enforced to ensure fairness and secure budgets. Therefore, a new intractable disease law came into effect on January 1, 2015. Unlike the previous system, only severe cases could apply and mildly ill patients were no longer accepted, thus reducing the number of beneficiaries. However, if the treatment cost is high, patients can apply if they meet additional criteria. With ALS, using riluzole or edaravone can be costly, and thus patients can apply for subsidy after three months of treatment.

All health systems in Japan are designated as national, but they are implemented by prefectures and carried out by municipalities. There is a system that encompasses medical expenses subsidies and care and a system for coverage of persons with disabilities when they have a disability certificate. There is high-cost medical treatment system through medical insurance (the maximum amount of self-pay for medical expenses is set by income) and a long-term care insurance system for care executed by municipalities.

The upper limit of support is set according to the severity of a patient's condition, and the arrangement of various services is performed either by a care manager in the long-term care insurance system when required or by a consultation support specialist (the Disability Independence Support Law). Basically, the user cost is 10 percent, depending on household income. In addition, there is a public health nurse in charge of intractable diseases at each public health center. They are responsible for visiting patients in the area when patients apply for designated intractable disease support, to assess their condition, offer appropriate medical advice and provide information to medical institutions when necessary. Due to the enforcement of the Intractable Diseases Law, the system for providing intractable disease medical care has been changed, and it is currently under restructuring.

Intractable disease consultation support centers have been set up in each prefecture, and consultation support staffs provide advice to patients. Recently, a new intractable disease medical treatment coordinator and medical treatment counselor have been established at the base hospital where patients from intractable disease consultation have been placed. They will be consulted and will be responsible for their support.

Like the National Institutes of Health in the United States, the Japan Agency for Medical Research and Development (AMED) reviews research proposals that meet research guidelines. The Ministry of Health, Labor and Welfare solicits and conducts research directly related to policy. Although there are private organizations not specialized in ALS that accept solicitations for research funds, they are often small compared to the grants from AMED. ALS-related research funding by AMED is difficult to estimate, but the total research funding for designated intractable diseases, including ALS, was about US$98.6 million in 2019.

ALS ASSOCIATIONS AND ADVOCACY GROUPS

The ALS Association of Japan is the most established organization that is active in Japan. However, the regional differences are large, and the participation rate overall is low with less than 20 percent of all patients involved. Often those patients on ventilators who can participate for a long time form the bulk of the membership. They participate in ALS/

MND international symposia as a representative of the patient association of Japan. There are numerous other groups including END ALS and WITH ALS launched by relatively younger generations of ALS patients primarily through Internet communication. In addition, there are associations organized mainly by caregivers and bereaved families and patient associations organized by facilities, all of which are small.

PUBLIC AND MEDIA PERCEPTIONS OF ALS

ALS is a relatively "hot" disease in terms of the attention it receives. Documentaries about ALS have been broadcast frequently, including by Japan's public broadcaster NHK. In 2014, during the Golden Hour, a drama was broadcast on the theme of ALS, which featured a popular actor as the main character. The Ice Bucket Challenge was well known in Japan and increased donations to patient groups. In the animated cartoon world, the authors of the Space Brothers feature ALS in the cartoons, although none of them continued beyond one-off publications.

WHERE ALS PATIENTS LIVE

Accurate research has not been conducted for nationwide data on the proportion of home versus institutional care for patients with ALS/MND in the last decade. Prior to the enforcement of the Act on Intractable Diseases, a 2005 personal questionnaire reported that 13.2 percent of patients were at work or school, 58.2 percent were under home care, 27.5 percent were in a hospital and 2.4 percent were in a nursing-care facility. Of patients using a tracheostomy ventilator, 42 percent were being cared for at home and 57 percent were admitted or hospitalized (Atsuta et al. 2009). However, this is likely to include shorter term hospitalization for complications and respite, so more patients are likely to be largely living at home.

In preparing the response to this question, the author made requests and investigated the situation in each prefecture and found great differences by region. In prefectures with hospital wards where long-term hospitalization is available, there was a tendency for more medical treatment at facilities. In urban areas 80–90 percent seem to be living at home. Inpatient facilities are paid higher medical fees if they are equipped with ventilators. Although there are a small number of wards that can hospitalize a patient long term, few facilities accept non-respiratory patients.

Perhaps only 10 percent of patients who do not use a tracheostomy are at facilities because there are few that will accept them.

COMPOSITION AND SUPPORT OF CAREGIVERS

Caregivers are often family members, but they can request home helpers through the long-term care insurance system or the independence support system for persons with disabilities (severity-based visit system). The limit is determined by the severity of the disease, and any extra costs are covered by the patient. There are care support systems such as day services and day care, but there are differences in the number of hours paid by local governments. In some prefectures, patients who use a ventilator and live alone can receive 24-hour care. Despite the funding system being common throughout the country, there are large regional differences in the extent to which establishments undertake it.

As a national countermeasure against incurable diseases, a main hospital for intractable disease medical care and a cooperating hospital for intractable disease medical care have been established, and legislative systems are being developed to strengthen diagnosis and respite care. Although there are no direct payments to patients or caregivers for incurable diseases, there is a subsidy for medical expenses, and long-term care insurance can reduce the burden of care. In most prefectures, there is a respite care system for incurable diseases, but unfortunately the number of beds is inadequate, and the quality of care is not comparable with home life. If a family cares at home without using the system at all, there is a monthly cash payment of 20,000 yen (US$182).

ACCESS TO ASSISTIVE TECHNOLOGIES

Information on communication devices can be obtained from occupational therapists in hospitals or home visits, public health nurses in public health centers, doctors in hospitals, visiting physicians or private organizations of patient associations such as ICT rescue teams. There is a limit in the independence support system for persons with disabilities, but it is covered. The level of entitlement paid according to the degree of disability. The ALS Association headquarters/branches have a rental system for equipment which has been donated by patients who have died. Communication equipment is provided as a tool for daily living with a maximum limit of 500,000 yen (US$4566) as stipulated by the Act on Comprehensive Independence for the Disabled.

STATUS OF MULTIDISCIPLINARY TEAM CARE AND CLINICS

In Japan, medical care is covered by universal insurance, so any patient can receive medical care from multiple professionals such as doctors, rehabilitation specialists and medical social workers if necessary. Early-stage ALS patients are typically seen in relatively large hospitals where multidisciplinary teams work together to provide care.

Although they are not necessarily named ALS clinics, since the 1990s medical treatment in multidisciplinary teams like those in Europe and the United States has been established in many locations across Japan. However, there is not much of a culture of donation, and financial support for the medical treatment from patient associations cannot be expected. Also, it is difficult to secure continuous research funding with limited public funding research budgets that are about one-tenth the size of those in the United States. Moreover, it is difficult to secure adequate full-time human resources as a multidisciplinary team because the income from clinical trials is often considered revenue by hospitals and is not necessarily available to ALS specialists.

In Japan, where the number of outpatients per physician is ten times higher than in the United States, the time available for outpatient care is limited but medical fees are low (less than US$100 per ALS patient), therefore a clinic that only serves ALS patients would not be cost efficient. As described earlier, it is difficult to operate an organization that specializes only in ALS mainly due to financial problems, and thus ALS is seen along with many other diseases.

The approximately ten hospitals that most ALS patients use employ systems of intensively treating ALS on fixed days of the week. Multiple medical specialists are available, such as medical engineers, clinical psychologists, medical social workers, dieticians, pharmacists, dentists, dental hygienists, public health nurses, physical therapists, speech therapists, occupational therapists, nurses, rehabilitation doctors and neurologists.

The author ran an ALS clinic, likely the largest such clinic in Japan, but the number of patients was still only about 120 annually. In 2015, a survey of neurologists found that 66 percent had three or fewer ALS consultations per year, 94 percent had fewer than ten and only 0.4 percent had forty or more such consultations (Ogino et al. 2015). It appears that patients rely on seeing specialists in a decentralized manner rather than concentrating in a large ALS center.

CLINICAL TRIALS AND USE OF UNAPPROVED DRUGS

In Japan, mixed medical funding of care by public health insurance and private payment is banned in principle, but there is an officially selected medical treatment fee system. If an application is approved, even drugs that have not yet been formally approved can be used with public medical insurance. Moreover, many people have private medical insurance to cover unapproved drugs. If research is conducted at an individual medical institution, it can be used with insurance medical treatment at the expense of the medical institution with the approval of the Ethics Committee. In addition, clinical trials of a new drug must comply with national laws, but are usually conducted by multiple institutions nationwide, so that any patient who meets the criteria can enter the trial.

GENETIC TESTING OF PATIENTS WITH ALS

Genetic diagnosis of designated intractable diseases is accepted as a medical fee covered by national health insurance. However, because a genetic diagnosis kit has not been approved for ALS, application for medical fees has not yet been approved. This is recognized as a problem, and we are working to resolve it. Currently, when performing the genetic testing, if the patient is registered with the Japanese Consortium for ALS (JaCALS), a patient registry system with 33 institutes nationwide provides genetic analysis, including for patients with sporadic ALS, free of charge. Otherwise, it depends on the medical institution; it may be paid by the institution or by the patient.

It is recommended that genetic counseling be performed when making a genetic diagnosis during which the method of notifying the individual or relatives will be discussed. There are cases where patients want their data used for research but do not want to know the results himself/herself. Similarly, there are patients who do not want to tell their relatives, and these issues are considered case by case. The Japanese Society of Neurology does not recommend pre-symptomatic genetic testing for ALS because the most frequent mutation found in ALS patients in Japan is the *SOD1* mutation in which penetration is not often high. If a person who is at risk of familial ALS wants to be tested, he/she will definitely needs to have genetic counseling.

Where ALS Patients in Japan Die

There are no data on places of ALS deaths across Japan, but in our own experience, 36 percent were attended to at home and others in neurology wards in hospitals. Having this relatively large proportion of ALS patients dying at home is probably not representative of the usual situation in Japan. Taking care of end-of-life patients at home is not typically part of the neurologist's role in Japan, so many ALS specialists have limited experience providing end-of-life care outside of the hospital setting. In my case, being dual-specialized in neurology and home care means that we are able to offer substantial home medical care, thereby likely increasing the proportion of patients cared for at home. There are very few nursing homes that can care for ALS patients at the end of life. In Japan, hospice is still indicated for cancer or AIDS due to national health insurance, and ALS is not covered. On the other hand, we have an excellent home care system which includes home visiting doctors, nurses, rehabilitation therapists, pharmacists, dieticians, dentists and other healthcare professionals covered by national health insurance. Despite this, in general (not only in the case of ALS) in 2016, 75.8 percent of patients died in hospitals, 9.2 percent at nursing facilities and only 13 percent at home (E-Stat 2016).

Access to Palliative and Hospice Care

As mentioned earlier, admission to hospice is limited to cancer or AIDS patients in Japan. There are some facilities where palliative care teams can provide consultation even if medical fees are not paid, but they are few. Therefore, in practice, a neurologist or a home physician often looks after their patients until the end. In Japan, nurses cannot prescribe and have limited authority, so there are many situations where doctors themselves must consult. There are no national data on the extent to which palliative sedation (not simply sedation, but comprehensive palliative care) is provided for ALS patients in Japan. A 2015 survey asked neurologists about how much they had used in opioids in palliative ALS patients, and only 35 percent said they had ever used it (Ogino et al. 2015). However, 87 percent of neurologists treat less than three cases of end-stage ALS annually, and it has been reported that only 50 percent of end-stage ALS patients require opioids. Thus, there are limited opportunities for neurologists to gain experience using them in this setting.

Although there are no data on how many patients with ALS receive palliative care including opioids in home care, it appears that this has been steadily increasing since opioids were covered by ALS insurance in 2011. All patients receive palliative care in our practice, and 48 percent needed opioids, a percentage that increased to 55 percent when patients use non-invasive ventilation more than 22 hours a day.

ADVANCE DIRECTIVES AND WITHHOLDING OR WITHDRAWING LIFE-EXTENDING INTERVENTIONS

Although Japan does not have a specific law on end-of-life decision-making, it has national guidelines that play a role as a soft law. According to these guidelines, death is based on the individual's autonomous decision-making, and the medical and care team continuously discuss it and records it when an agreement is reached. Due to the extensive system of home ventilation and home care covered by national health insurance, most patients do not need to give up the tracheostomy ventilator for financial reasons, although it may be difficult to secure trained caregivers in some areas.

Withholding of a tracheostomy ventilator has been practiced in many patients and has not been a problem in Japan, but once it has been started, discontinuing it is generally not practiced. Although no law exists that prohibits the suspension of respirators and it remains a matter of interpretation, it has not been practiced conventionally. Moreover, withdrawal has strong opposition from the ALS Association of Japan and organizations of persons with disabilities worried about the slippery slope they feel that this represents. A 2009 survey about this topic found that 25 percent of neurologists felt that they should not accept the practice of discontinuing ventilation in patients (Ogino et al. 2009). Recently, guidelines from various academic societies and others have stated that the right to discontinue life-saving treatment has been granted (Guidelines 2012, 2014). The situation is gradually changing.

There is great variation in the use of respirators in different regions. Some prefectures in the Kyushu area and the Tohoku area have places where the tracheostomy ventilator usage rate was more than 60 percent of all patients with ALS. On the other hand, it was about 30 percent in urban areas such as Tokyo and Osaka (based on personal communications and unpublished data). The trend was higher in areas where facilities that accept long-term hospitalization were more substantial. Reasons for this regional difference might include the ease of securing caregivers such as a large family system, the local medical treatment environment such as facilities for long-term medical care, differences in the discussion and explanation of the issues and attitudes of medical personnel.

LEGAL STATUS OF PALLIATIVE SEDATION, EUTHANASIA AND PHYSICIAN-ASSISTED SUICIDE

Palliative sedation is generally accepted as part of palliative care. However, it is rare that active palliative sedation with midazolam or the like is necessary in ALS. As a result, a sedative effect may be obtained with CO_2 narcosis. On the other hand, euthanasia and assisted suicide are illegal in Japan. Clear interpretations have not been established for the discontinuation of tracheostomy ventilators in the chronic phase, and this is not commonly performed because doctors cannot be sure that they will not be indicted for murder or assisted suicide. In the acute setting, the discontinuation of ventilators has become more accepted, as described previously (Guidelines 2014).

In 2008, an ALS patient who had been living on a ventilator for twelve years while the paralysis of the body was progressing requested that his attending physician remove the ventilator and let him die when he reached the totally locked-in state. His request was sent to the hospital and accepted by the hospital's ethics committee and the expanded ethics committee of out-of-hospital ethics and legal experts, but the hospital director rejected the patient's wishes because he thought it was too early for Japanese society to accept such an action. It was taken up by NHK and became a social issue, but the situation has not changed much since then.

FACTORS UNIQUE TO JAPAN THAT INFLUENCE ALS POLICY

One of the most difficult decisions relates to ventilator support for the patient with ALS. Japan has the highest rate along with Italy (Spataro et al. 2012). Other Asian countries including Taiwan and South Korea also have high rates compared to most Western countries (Tsai et al. 2015; Bae et al. 2012). A recent study on this topic compared five ALS centers in the United States to six in Japan. The same questionnaire was sent to the ALS patients, their families and neurologists (Rabkin et al. 2013, 2014; Christodoulou et al. 2015). From the results of the patient survey, Japanese patients are more likely to refuse a tracheostomy ventilator (TV) at the early stage of the disease; meanwhile, the proportion of patients who agree to use it does not differ between the United States and Japan at this stage. The big difference is that if an uncertain patient progresses in the United States, TV will not be used forcibly.

In the caregivers' responses, however, there were big differences. More Japanese caregivers knew someone utilizing TV (32 percent) than American caregivers (6 percent), and caregivers who knew someone utilizing TV showed a greater degree of acceptance. More Japanese caregivers were in favor of TV (56 percent) compared to American caregivers (33 percent), and it is likely that caregivers can have a significant effect on eventual utilization (Christodoulou et al. 2015). In Japan, families often want tracheostomy ventilation used for their relatives, but not for themselves if they were affected. One could say this represents the selfishness of the family, but the Japanese patient often accepts this. We could say that there is no one who dies because he wants to die. This is one of the cultural ways of thinking, focusing on family units over individuals, family happiness being important more than individual happiness.

From the result of neurologists' survey, we found the same percentage of US and Japanese doctors would choose tracheostomy ventilator for themselves. US doctors recommend TV to their patients at the same rate that they themselves would choose it, whereas Japanese doctors were more likely to make the recommendation for their patients (Rabkin et al. 2013). Several questions arise from this result. Do US doctors impose the idea that a poor quality of life is inevitable? Are Japanese doctors paternalistic in suggesting that their patients do what they themselves would not do?

Therefore, from the patients' and the families' perspectives, many patients in Japan choose ventilation and state that they are happy. Personal body independence may not be considered as important as in the West because Japanese patients have a less negative view of disability. The activities of patient associations in Japan also have great influence on attitudes to tracheostomy ventilation. From the neurologists' perspective, doctors are conscious of such values in Japan even if they do not think so themselves. So, as doctors we try to keep a fair balance of both sides. But still we must always ask ourselves, is it easier to treat or do nothing? Is it easier for us to encourage patients to live on? Are doctors responsible for the patient's life afterwards?

Recommended ALS Policy Changes in Japan

There is a need in Japan to provide patients greater authority than they have been afforded in making treatment decisions, including that of discontinuing treatment. This should be done through developing guidelines informed by the law, which either reflect a national consensus on the matter, or at least encourage public opinion to accept these changes. Moreover, patient associations should give stronger endorsement of the right to live, especially with tracheostomy ventilation. To this end, the government needs to provide 24-hour independent care. Currently, this can only be provided in limited areas. Under these circumstances, many patients simply give up trying to live. Furthermore, there is a need to provide appropriate information and perform collaborative decision-making across Japan. Recently, advance care planning has become more common because Japan is the fastest aging country in the world, and many people including elderly people, themselves, are aware that it is critical. If the atmosphere of the society respects the will and autonomy of the individual person, this way of thinking about ALS may change.

This year we will perform several clinical trials simultaneously, and it is predicted that recruiting patients will be difficult. Clearly, Japan needs better registration systems for enrollment of patients into clinical trials. Patient associations, too, need to play a more central role in providing information. Also, we must work to organize large-scale ALS centers to provide good-quality ALS care and easy access to clinical trials. This requires an effort to make the field attractive to many healthcare professionals, especially physicians. In that sense, more funds need to be allocated to ALS including clinical research on care, providing financial support to establish multidisciplinary ALS clinics like those in the United States and Europe and deregulating monitoring to facilitate clinical trials.

References

Atsuta, N., H. Watanabe, M. Ito, et al. (2009). Age at onset influences on wide-ranged clinical features of sporadic amyotrophic lateral sclerosis. *Journal of the Neurological Sciences* 276: 163–69.

Bae, J.S., Y.H. Hong, W. Baek, E.H. Sohn et al. (2012). Current status of the diagnosis and management of amyotrophic lateral sclerosis in Korea: A multicenter cross-sectional study. *Journal of Clinical Neurology* 8: 293–300.

Christodoulou, G., R. Goetz, M. Ogino, H. Mitsumoto and J. Rabkin (2015). Opinions of Japanese and American ALS caregivers regarding tracheostomy with invasive ventilation (TIV). *Amyotrophic Lateral Sclerosis Frontotemporal Degeneration* 17 (1–2): 47–51.

E-Stat (2016). https://www.e-stat.go.jp/stat-search/files?page=1&layout=datali st&toukei=00450011&tstat=000001028897&cycle=7&year=20160&mont h=0&tclass1=000001053058&tclass2=000001053061&tcl ass3=000001053065

Guidelines. (2012). The guidelines for process of decision making of care for elderly person, especially about artificial nutrition. The Japan Geriatrics Society, June 2012 (in Japanese). https://www.jpn-geriat-soc.or.jp/proposal/guideline.html

Guidelines. (2014). The guidelines of the end of life in the emergency and intensive care. Japanese Association for Acute Medicine, The Japanese Society of Intensive Care Medicine, The Japanese Circulation Society, November 2014 (in Japanese). http://www.jaam.jp/html/info/2014/info-20141104_02.htm

Ogino, M., Y. Ogino and J. Hamada (2009). The survey report of the ALS physicians in Japan. *Amyotrophic Lateral Sclerosis* 10 (Suppl. 1): 48.

Ogino, M., N. Tominaga, A. Uchino, K. Takahashi et al. (2015). Did morphine usage become more popular in Japan? *Amyotrophic Lateral Sclerosis Frontotemporal Degeneration* 16 (Suppl. 1): 71.

Rabkin, J., M. Ogino, R. Goetz, M. McElhiney et al. (2013). Tracheostomy with invasive ventilation for ALS patients: Neurologists' roles in the US and Japan. *Amyotrophic Lateral Sclerosis* 14: 116–23.

Rabkin, J., M. Ogino, R. Goetz, M. McElhiney et al. (2014). Japanese and American ALS patient preferences regarding TIV (tracheostomy with invasive ventilation): A cross-national survey. *Amyotrophic Lateral Sclerosis Frontotemporal Degeneration* 15: 185–91.

Spataro, R, V. Bono, S. Marchese and V. La Bella (2012). Tracheostomy mechanical ventilation in patients with amyotrophic lateral sclerosis: Clinical features and survival analysis. *Journal of Neurological Science* 323: 66–70.

Tsai, C-P., K-C. Wang, C-S. Hwang, I-T. Lee and C.T-C. Lee (2015). Incidence, prevalence, and medical expenditures of classical amyotrophic lateral sclerosis in Taiwan, 1999–2008. *Journal of the Formosan Medical Association* 114 (7): 612–19.

CHAPTER 13

ALS Policy in Mexico

Ildefonso Rodriguez-Leyva

Abstract As in many parts of the world, lack of education, poverty and insufficient public health resources in Mexico result in the inability to make early and timely diagnoses. The new public health system (INSABI) offers free and universal support, but much work is needed to achieve this goal and ensure that patients with ALS have quality care. In private hospitals, care for patients with ALS, especially for those with resources, is possibly as good as in the best places in the first world. Neurology programs in Mexico are not sufficient to meet the country's needs. Palliative measures, ventilation and nutrition support must be improved, and thanatology services in the country should be increased. Mexico continues as a place of opportunities where there is much to be done.

Keywords ALS in Mexico • UNELA • IMSS • ISSSTE • INSABI

I. Rodriguez-Leyva (✉)
Autonomous University of San Luis Potosí,
San Luis Potosi, México
e-mail: ildefonso.rodriguez@uaslp.mx

© The Author(s) 2021
R. H. Blank et al. (eds.), *Public Policy in ALS/MND Care*,
https://doi.org/10.1007/978-981-15-5840-5_13

ALS INCIDENCE AND PREVALENCE IN MEXICO

There is no specific knowledge on the incidence and prevalence of ALS in Mexico. Olivares et al. (1972) reported an incidence of 0.4/100,000 and a prevalence of 1.44/100,000 population, but Kurtzke (1982) observed that case-selection bias could exist in Mexico. In a more recent study, Martínez et al. (2011) report a predominant male over female ratio of 1.8:1, with an onset age of 47.5 ± 10.5 years and an interval period of 12 months from the start of the disease to the diagnosis. There is spinal presentation in most (66 percent), and the phenotype was upper motoneuron in 53 percent of 61 analyzed subjects. The average survival time was 68.6 months. In the landmark report from Saeed et al. (2009), the authors used a control group of twelve Hispanic people without finding the mutation of *SOD1 A4V*. However, the number of identified mutations and polymorphisms is growing, and more genetic studies are needed in the Mexican population. Recently, the government has included in its official web page an explanation directed to the general public about ALS and its main characteristics (5 percent genetic and 95 percent sporadic) and the ways it can present itself (bulbar and spinal) (Mexican Government 2019).

ALS SUPPORT GROUPS

There currently are a variety of support groups for patients with ALS in Mexico. A key group is Gila (https://www.ela.org.mx/) through which the affected person, his/her family and any interested person can have access to different specialists all over the country. Moreover, Gila has an alliance with various associations including the International Alliance of ALS/MND Associations, the Union of Associations of ALS in Latin-America (UNELA), Cemefi (Mexican center for philanthropy), the Mexican Federation of Rare Diseases (FEMEXER) and Familiares de ELA (ALS's families). Gila directs many of its efforts on providing information about existing clinical trials and the various ways to obtain help. The government's website (Mexican Government 2019) cites the possible prevalence of 6000 cases in Mexico with an ALS diagnosis, marks the date of 21 June as the World Day of ALS and encourages readers to visit Gila AC's web page.

There is also another organization named FYADENMAC, which was formed by families and friends of patients with ALS disease (Mexican Association against ALS; http://www.fyadenmac.org/). This organization reaches out and gives education and clinical support to patients, including wheelchairs, communications systems, hospital beds, follow-ups and even respiratory therapy. The organization functions with donations and shares information and photos of patients to raise awareness and support the disease. These associations represent some of the most important sources for ALS care, with the rest covered by the public or private hospitals.

THE HEALTHCARE SYSTEM AND ALS

Mexico currently spends roughly 6.2 percent of its budget on healthcare, one of the lowest rates in the OECD and well below the average of 9.6 percent. This limited budget is directly reflected on the healthcare system. In Mexico, two-thirds of the hospitals (2988 institutions) are private institutions, but only 10 percent of the Mexican population has private insurance coverage. Most of the population is covered by public hospitals, with much variability in the level of care. The predominant institutions are general hospitals, and only a few are national health institutes or highly specialized institutions. In Mexico, about 50 percent of the population has Social Security, and 28 percent had Popular Security. However, now with the Institute for Health Welfare (INSABI), more than 31 million people without any insurance will receive support from the government using population taxes (Douglas and Borasio 2007).

Mexico's private sector is booming. New clinics and specialized hospitals are proliferating in Mexico City, Guadalajara and especially Monterrey. Monterrey and Tijuana are becoming massive centers for medical tourism, particularly for Americans trying to escape their expensive healthcare system. The cost of treatment in Mexico can be anywhere from 36 to 89 percent less expensive than in the United States.

In 2012, the Mexican government created the "Seguro Popular", which is a type of universal healthcare system to cover 40 million Mexican people. Mexican children receive the same childhood vaccinations as those in Canada, but indigenous and poor people have limited access to decent medical care aside from these vaccines. With about 120,000,000 inhabitants (51.2 percent females), life expectancy in Mexico is as high as that in first-world countries and at least 25 percent of the population will be elderly by 2050 (Gómez Dantés et al. 2011). The average life expectancy increased from 70 years in 1990 to 75 years in 2011.

President Peña Nieto's National Development Plan put great emphasis on prevention programs to reduce the morbidity and mortality of non-communicable diseases such as diabetes, hypertension and heart and cerebrovascular diseases. Unfortunately, many diseases like ALS were not included in this program.

With the new government in December 2018, several policy changes have been made, but the treatment and care for ALS patients is not considered as a priority in any of the various healthcare programs. The Article 4 of the Constitution states that public care is guaranteed to all Mexican citizens. Therefore, through Seguro Popular, the Secretariat of Health offers healthcare coverage to Mexicans who are not formally employed, covering over 50 million people. There is also an institution called Instituto Mexicano del Seguro Social (IMSS) that has 279 hospitals and covers all formal employees. Another institution is the Institute for Social Security and Services for State Workers (IMSS) that serves seven million people in 115 hospitals. The Secretariat of Health has the most extensive healthcare system in the country and serves around 50 million people in 809 hospitals. Other govermental facilities cover around three million people: Secretariat of National Defense, Mexican Navy, Mexican Oil Company ("Petróleos Mexicanos") and the Red Cross (with 279 hospitals).

As noted earlier, even though Article 4 of the Mexican Constitution states that every person has the right to healthcare, there are different levels of treatment depending on the payment capacity or whether there is an affiliation to a private or public institution. When seeking proper healthcare, many persons will not have the adequate and needed support, and the adequacy will be even lower for a disease like ALS. At least 20 percent of the population has a deficient socioeconomic level, and around 25 percent of the population has no access even to hypertension and diabetes detection programs (Torres-Arreola et al. 2006).

The Mexican institutions with resources for ALS are the National Institutes of Health through their Neurology Residency Programs. Within these are the National Institute of Neurology and Neurosurgery (Manuel Velazco Suárez) and the National Institute of Medical Sciences and Nutrition (Salvador Zubiran). Besides these, there is the General Hospital of Mexico, Juarez Hospital of Mexico, Mexican National Center "SXXI", Mexican National Center "La Raza", Occidental Mexican National Center (Guadalajara), ISSSTE "20 de Noviembre" National Center, Military Central Hospital, Central Hospital in San Luis Potosi, the Hospital of the

University of Nuevo León and the Technological Institute of Monterrey (single private program).

ALS RESEARCH AND AWARENESS

Unfortunately, at present there is not enough support and investment toward research on ALS in Mexico. Limited trials are conducted by both by public or private means, but clinical research in Mexico is limited as support is only given through pharmaceutical companies and as part of international clinical trials that need authorization from the hospitals with which they are working.

Because it is not economically attractive and there are not enough programs to help patients, most Mexicans do not understand about ALS. Moreover, the media has not provided enough coverage to inform the population about it. One of the most significant problems in Mexico is education, and learning about more obscure diseases is limited. Most of the investments made by the government in healthcare are directed toward preventing diseases and raising awareness on vaccinations and the importance of maintaining a healthy lifestyle to prevent obesity, hypertension and diabetes. Education on ALS is rare, and it often is only known as the disease that affected prominent people such as Stephen Hawking, Lou Gehrig and Morrie Schwartz. Undoubtedly, there is a need to educate our population so that not only it is able not only to recognize the early manifestations of this disease but also they can help and work on raising awareness and establishing prevention programs.

Sadly, the educational condition is worse in some sectors of the population, especially in the indigenous areas, where the bilingual education programs are insufficient to offer even primary education. With this we can see that there are many more goals to pursue before working on educating our people on diseases like ALS.

ALS PATIENT CARE IN MEXICO

Mexico is limited in its available infrastructure to support people with ALS, either at home or in institutions, and only Gilas has made it possible for patients and families to receive minimal support. The Mexican government recently decided to end the Seguro Popular and initiate a program called Instituto para el Bienestar de la Salud, which has the objective to reinforce the primary health system. Unfortunately, it will be a challenge to include diseases such as ALS in this kind of program which is directed to the poorest people in our country who do not have social security by either IMSS, ISSSTE, SEDENA (military health system), Petroleos or other health programs supported by the government. Therefore, most patients suffering from ALS need to be attended in their own homes, and very few of them are cared for in hospitals or in long-term care institutions, which are rare in Mexico.

Today there are many professional caregivers in Mexico, most of whom have a specialty in rehabilitation or have partial training in this area or a nursing foundation where they learn to support and help people who are suffering from ALS. Caregivers are paid by the patient's family, although some of the aforementioned organizations can provide partial economic and nursing help. There are few specialized centers and training for supporting ALS in the country. Although there is no specific economic or care support from the government for ALS patients, they can be medically attended in the public system in any near and adequate hospital when they suffer a comorbidity problem, such as pneumonia. Those fortunate patients who were able to acquire private medical insurance before diagnosis have access to more resources depending on the kind of support that the insurance company offers.

In Mexico, access to assistive technologies such as electronic communication devices is available only to patients who have the economic means to acquire it. Fortunately, some electronic devices are inexpensive and can at least help the patient and the caregivers temporarily. In a country like Mexico, there are some very wealthy people who can go to the best places in the world to receive treatment and who can also have all the available resources in their own home or be cared for in an institution. Middle-class people can attempt to obtain respiratory and gastrostomy procedures but with limited possibilities of nursing and rehabilitation support needed for this kind of disease. In contrast, people that live in poverty will deteriorate quickly without help from a neurologist or gastroenterologist, many of them without even a diagnosis of the disease. The available palliative, spiritual, psychosocial, respiratory distress and language support for many are limited and inaccessible (Douglas and Borasio 2007).

Most of the second- and third-level hospitals in Mexico have specialists in pulmonology, rehabilitation, gastroenterology, psychotherapy, nutrition and neurology to offer adequate support to the patients with ALS. Multidisciplinary collaboration is growing in Mexico, but it increases the cost of the treatment and makes it more difficult to access by the patient.

There is legislation about the use of drugs in Mexico, and the Federal Commission for the Protection Against Sanitary Risk (COFEPRIS) must approve all the new products and drugs. The process is complicated, but if a product shows reliability and safety, it will be approved. There are drug stores that can help in obtaining pharmaceutical products that are available in the United States but not in Mexico. As in other countries, there are many "natural supplements" and products that people without scruples market as cures with little control by the government.

Nationals Institutes of Health have genetic departments that directly, within their institution, or indirectly, by sending to partners organizations, offer the genetic test to ALS patients with family history. The Massachusetts General Hospital for several years offered a free genetic study for ALS patients.

END-OF-LIFE ISSUES FOR ALS IN MEXICO

There are no exact numbers, but at least 80 percent of ALS sufferers die at home and both the patient and his/her family know it is nearing the end of life. To lengthen the life expectancy, many patients have CPAP and gastrostomy support or receive thanatology support. Unfortunately, there are not enough resources like hospice care or palliative support to help ALS patients. Only people with economic resources can access better care system support.

In July 2019, the Mexican Senate approved assisted death for individuals who are suffering from diseases such as ALS and who choose to take this path. This law is already a reality in Mexico City, but it will expand to the rest of the country soon. Euthanasia and assisted death are possibilities now with legal approbation but are only available with a modification of the Article 4 of the Mexican Constitution. However, there is a public debate about the importance of assisted death in Mexico accompanied by increased knowledge about palliative care in chronic and terminal diseases like ALS (Neudert et al. 2001).

Mexico is a Roman Catholic country (77.4 percent), and most think that the fight for life is an obligation. Considerable education is needed to change existing views toward health and convince the population that the quality of life and the right to die with dignity and without suffering are acceptable. Palliative measures at the end stage of ALS are not always available, few have access to mechanical ventilation or gastrostomy, and sometimes the ending is painful. Fortunately, the increase in the study of thanatology and the knowledge of palliative measures can help many patients (Cossío-Díaz et al. 2015).

Conclusions: Where to Go from Here?

It is a great advantage that information from around the world has become easily and quickly available, thanks to the Internet and satellite news. However, we must recognize that since everyone is allowed to make use of the Internet and post or spread new information, there can also be some misleading or confusing data that can give false hope to families, patients and even physicians that are looking for resources to help ALS patients.

To better our chances on fighting this disease it is necessary to form more multidisciplinary ALS healthcare centers in Mexico. Currently, there are two of them within the National Institutes of Health of Mexico (National Institute of Neurology and Neurosurgery and the National Institute of Medical Sciences and Nutrition) in Mexico City. The National Medical Centers of the IMSS and the ISSSTE provide multidisciplinary work and offer the best diagnostic, therapeutic, rehabilitation and support to these patients.

In Monterrey, Nuevo León, the Institute of Neurology and Neurosurgery of Tecnológico de Monterrey is a referral center with a very successful interactive group. These groups include neurophysiologists, pulmonologists, physiotherapists, diabetologists, gastroenterologists, neuroimmunologists and neurologists who work together, seeking maximum benefit for the patient. Currently, we are working on creating more centers where the specialists can work together to achieve the most significant benefit of these patients. There are countless areas of opportunity in Mexico to develop integral care centers with multidisciplinary management that help address a problem that is challenging and that incapacitates the individual and shortens his/her life. We hope to expand the number of excellence centers that can care for the patient at the development stage of the disease and in the various stages of ALS with an interdisciplinary approach, psychosocial evaluation, spiritual support and proactive caregiver programs that provide the best quality of help and care in this disease (Mitsumoto et al. 2006).

References

Cossío-Díaz, J.R., J.F.F. González-Salas, D. Kershenobich-Stalnikowitz et al. (2015). "Regulación de los cuidados paliativos y muerte asistida." *Gaceta medica de México* 151 (1): 119–30.

Douglas, M.J. and G. Domenico Borasio (2007). Amyotrophic lateral sclerosis. *The Lancet* 369 (9578): 2031–41.

Gómez Dantés, O., S. Sesma, V.M. Becerril et al. (2011). Sistema de salud de México. Salud Pública de México, [S.l.], v. 53, mar. 2011. ISSN 1606-7916. Disponible en: <http://saludpublica.mx/index.php/spm/article/view/5043/10023>. Fecha de acceso: 29 oct. 2019

Kurtzke, J.F. (1982). Epidemiology of amyotrophic lateral sclerosis. *Advances in Neurology* 36: 281–302.

Martínez, H.R., J.F. Molina-López, L. Cantú-Martínez et al. (2011). Survival and clinical features in Hispanic amyotrophic lateral sclerosis patients. *Amyotrophic Lateral Sclerosis* 12 (3): 199–205.

Mexican Government (2019). La esclerosis lateral amiotrófica (ELA), https://www.gob.mx/conadis/es/articulos/la-esclerosis-lateral-amiotrofica-ela?idiom=es#targetText=La%20Esclerosis%20Lateral%20Amiotr%C3%B3fica%20(abreviadamente,y%20de%20la%20m%C3%A9dula%20espinal.

Mitsumoto, H., et al. (2006). Promoting excellence in end-of-life care in ALS. *Amyotrophic Lateral Sclerosis* 6 (3): 145–54.

Neudert, C., D. Oliver, M. Wasner and G.D. Borasio (2001). The course of the terminal phase in patients with amyotrophic lateral sclerosis. *Journal of Neurology* 248 (7): 612–16.

Olivares, L., E. San Esteban and M. Alter (1972). Mexican resistance to amyotrophic lateral sclerosis. *Archives of Neurology* 27 (5): 397–402.

Saeed, M., Y. Yang, H.-X. Deng et al. (2009). Age and founder effect of SOD1 A4V mutation causing ALS. *Neurology* 72 (19): 1634–39.

Torres-Arreola, L.P., et al. (2006). Study of primary care health needs through family health diagnosis. *Atencion Primaria* 38 (7): 381–86.

CHAPTER 14

Public Policy in MND Care: Nigerian Perspective

Yomi Ogun and Babawale Arabambi

Abstract There is paucity of epidemiological data on motor neuron disease (MND) in Nigeria. MND is an additional financial burden on the inadequate health services in Nigeria, but there have been no governmental action/reports/committees to date. Most patients live at home, and the caregivers are family/paid caregivers. Effective MND management is available in few centers, partly due to bad planning of health-delivery system to meet "the demands" of the people rather than their "needs." There is multidisciplinary-care approach to management, but with limited access to assistive technologies/communication devices. In conclusion, there is suboptimal low standardized level of MND community knowledge and neuro-care in Nigeria, and scaling-up community recognition, management, care and rehabilitation are needed to improve outcomes. Knowledge on telemedicine to manage patients in rural/remote centers may be helpful in extending care throughout Nigeria.

Y. Ogun (✉) • B. Arabambi
Lagos State University Teaching Hospital, Ikeja, Lagos, Nigeria
e-mail: yomiogun2002@yahoo.com; babawale.arabambi@gmail.com

© The Author(s) 2021
R. H. Blank et al. (eds.), *Public Policy in ALS/MND Care*,
https://doi.org/10.1007/978-981-15-5840-5_14

Keywords Motor neuron disease • Nigeria • MND management
• Limited access • Cultural constraints

INCIDENCE AND PREVALENCE OF MND IN NIGERIA

The consideration of chronic diseases globally suggests that all populations are susceptible to neurological disorders, and variation in rates exists because of differential exposures to environmental causes, disparities in healthcare-seeking cultural practices, differential inequalities in access to neurological services and care, inadequate resources, socioeconomic differences, the influence of underlying differences in genetic factors and lifestyle modifications (Ogun et al. 2019). There is paucity of epidemiological data on motor neuron disease (MND) in Nigeria, with most of the available studies hospital-based and published years ago. A retrospective hospital-based study found an approximate prevalence of 21/100,000 hospital population between 1958 and 1973 with a male-to-female ratio of 3:1. The most common variant identified was amyotrophic lateral sclerosis (ALS), which accounted for 79 percent of the patients during the study period. The mortality rate by the end of this study was 15.1 percent (Osuntokun et al. 1974). A community-based prevalence study in 1987 found a crude point prevalence ratio 15/100,000 population (Osuntokun et al. 1987). Another study in southeastern Nigeria found that MND accounted for 0.8 percent of all neurological admissions between 2003 and 2007 (Ekenze et al. 2010). A retrospective review of neurology patients seen between 1980 and 1999 at a tertiary hospital in southwest Nigeria identified a total of 21 patients with MND. Of these cases, the records of 16 patients were reviewed. All the studied cases were the ALS variant (Imam and Ogunniyi 2004).

LIMITED GOVERNMENTAL AND NON-GOVERNMENTAL SUPPORT AND ACTION

At the time of the compilation of this chapter, there are no known actions, reports or committees set up by the Nigerian government relating to the care of MND in both private and non-governmental organizations. MND is not well known to the public, which may be due to the relatively low prevalence of the condition. More resources should be devoted by the government to the research, treatment and public education for this condition (Quansah and Karikari 2015).

Although data to back this up are not readily accessible, it is rational to conclude that most patients with MND live at home. Presentations to the hospital are typically due to complications such as respiratory distress, aspiration pneumonitis, urinary tract infections or decubitus/pressure ulcers. Moreover, "Nigeria still lags in hospice and palliative care provision" ("Nigeria behind in palliative care provision—Minister" 2017). Caregivers comprise a combination of family and paid caregivers, with some private companies providing the latter. There is no known governmental aid provided for family caregivers. Established non-governmental organizations (NGOs) exist to support other neurological disorders such as stroke, epilepsy, Parkinson's disease/multiple system atrophy, but none for MND.

Furthermore, there is limited access to assistive technologies or communication devices. Patients who can afford them end up paying for these devices out of pocket. In the tertiary hospitals and a few secondary facilities, there is a multidisciplinary care approach to management of patients. The team includes neurologists, physiotherapists, psychiatrists, psychologists, occupational therapists, speech and language therapists, dietitians and social workers. Nurses are also available, but they are not typically specialist neurology nurses. The team is close to that recommended by the National Institute for Health and Care Excellence (2016), despite the major problem of a low medical staff to patient ratio.

Drug trials that concern MND have not yet been extended to Nigeria. When it eventually happens, advocacy for the "right to try" legislation can be pushed through the major stakeholders involved in patient care and governmental policies. Payment for genetic testing and most of the other evaluations required in the patients are usually out of pocket by the patient. In a few selected cases, charity organizations and insurance companies pay for these investigations.

Advance directives of the patients are respected. In the absence of one, the next of kin's decision determines the end-of-life care of the patient. Euthanasia and physician-assisted suicide are not legal in Nigeria at this time ("Nigeria, five others reject physician-assisted suicide, euthanasia" 2018).

MND Services in Nigeria

Effective management of MND requires well-established guidelines, which include dedicated neurology units, neurologists, neurosurgeons, specialist nurses, relevant radiology services, neuro/electrophysiological studies, physiotherapists, speech and language specialists, occupational therapists and social workers, among others. Such services are available in only a very few centers in Nigeria, partly due to bad planning of the health delivery system to meet "the demands" of the people rather than their "needs."

MND services in Nigeria vary from no formal care, to established neurological care with residency training and ancillary equipment. More often, health care systems are liberal, private sector driven, with inefficient models of universal national/state health insurance coverage with relatively high cost of care out of pocket. There is poor community awareness of MND and stunted and inadequate manpower development with limited local training. Resources, personnel and neurologists are centralized in or near the big cities. Furthermore, abundant data, knowledge, service and treatment gaps, a lack of political will and a low priority of MND on the political agenda are obstacles to policy development, implementation of appropriate responses and adequate government funding. This has resulted in an inadequate resource allocation to health and lack of needed information systems.

Barriers for MND Care in Nigeria

Overall, the health systems in Nigeria are characterized in disparity by patients' location, financial inaccessibility, poverty, socioeconomic status and education; a rapid turnover of people in key positions; a lack of continuity in policy; a lack of resources; poor management and implementation of available resources; and religious and cultural beliefs of "spiritual attack." These peculiarities in Nigeria pose a challenge to the management of MND. There are many difficult issues including the unavailability of trained healthcare practitioners, inaccessibility to appropriate healthcare facilities, the high personal cost of healthcare and the lack of governmental support for patient care/research. Many Nigerians still believe that most illnesses are due to spiritual problems, and they would preferably present at religious centers than at the hospitals (Ekanem and Asira 2006).

Challenges and Opportunities in the Treatment and Care of Neurological Disorders in Nigeria: The Way Forward

It is evident that much still needs to be done at different levels to get better outcomes for patients with MND. First, there should be an MND association, composed of healthcare practitioners who take care of these patients along with other stakeholders. Their goals should include advocacy, public education and provision of state and national guidelines for standard practice. The media will also play a significant role in public health education and in the push for more governmental and private involvement in the care of MND patients. The government through the Ministry of Health needs to provide more funding for health-related research and patient care. The legislative assembly needs to pass specific laws relating to the treatment of these patients, specifically those concerned with the "right to try." Finally, more attention needs to be given to the provision of palliative care and rehabilitation.

Globally, neurological services and care in Nigeria cannot match the rapid progress in the developed world. Contributory socioeconomic factors include an inadequate infrastructure and equipment, healthcare personnel/workforce inefficiency, weak neurology training programs and lack of research facilities, publications in high-impact neurology journals and community health education/awareness programs. There are also issues of the stigma associated with neurological disease, security issues in some parts of the country and low healthcare funding within the background of the increasing burden of communicable and non-communicable diseases. Moreover, neurologists trained in the developed world prefer to stay overseas rather than return to their home countries, partly because of inadequate remuneration (brain-drain/double-burden inverse-relationship) (Ogun et al. 2019).

Multidisciplinary rehabilitation team management is difficult because of dearth of paramedical staff, physiotherapists, occupational therapists and specialist nurses, among others. Efforts are being made to resolve those challenges, as more centers actively try to establish neurology units. There is a drive to encourage young doctors to specialize in the field of neurology and practice in the specialist-deprived subregions of Nigeria.

Overall, a low standard level of care is widespread, and MND management in Nigeria is suboptimal, especially in the face of seemingly increasing incidence and prevalence. Most patients settle for physiotherapy and use of medications, such as free radical scavengers, anti-platelet treatment because of relative immobility and riluzole when affordable (Ogun et al. 2019). The training of more neurology specialists, research sponsorship, health-friendly government policies, health awareness programs and patient education could lead to better outcomes for patients with MND.

Furthermore, there is need to establish regional training centers and institutes of excellence for brain-disorder research, contributing to capacity building, with-NIGERIA, for-NIGERIA, as overseas training is not always adapted to the national and local needs. Moreover, there is need to optimize patient care; improve the clinical skills of general practitioners; establish an effective two-way referral national health insurance scheme to reduce social inequalities; and create platforms for reflection, education and exchange of information between Nigerian and Western colleagues as well as Nigerian and other African colleagues. This may be possible through the development of collaboration across Africa and internationally, involving policy makers, members of government, civil society and patient associations such as the ALS/MND International Alliance, African Academy of Neurology and the World Federation of Neurology. Assistance to Nigerian professionals to participate in international meetings and cooperate with industrialized world neuroscientists is crucial to improve the Nigerian research infrastructure.

We need to convert "brain-drain" to "brain-gain" and ensure Nigerian doctors remain in the country after education overseas, by offering them attractive and better remuneration. Moreover, there is need for support and increasing participation of service users, including neurologists and people with MND in policy making and service planning. Standards of practice should be developed and encouraged together with the increase of MND awareness, health education with public and private collaborations and facilitating MND research advocacy.

SHORT- AND LONG-TERM STRATEGIES TO IMPROVE MND OUTCOME IN NIGERIA

It is reasonable to implement the World Health Organization Strategy on Research for Health. These include:

1. Organization: Strengthening of the education and research culture
2. Priorities: Focusing globally on priority health needs
3. Standards: Helping to strengthen national systems for health care

4. Promoting good practice
5. Translation: Strengthening links between health research and health services from "Bench to Bedside" and "Bedside to Bench"

To improve the care of patients with MND, the organization of the neurological teams is necessary with the main targets areas such as developing a population strategy for MND care by public awareness programs, clarifying the role of the physician in a care strategy, developing clear management strategies for patient care and expanding the role of rehabilitation. Also there is a need for capacity building by training health care workers, the development of protocols and local and national guidelines and the creation of treatment networks at the subregions/national levels. We must also develop a research strategy that includes appropriate acute care rehabilitation, epidemiological studies and clinical trials to test various widely used, but unconventional, therapeutic interventions. The establishment of basic neuro-critical units with comprehensive specialist MND acute care, rehabilitation and palliative care services is crucial. Telemedicine may be helpful to manage patients in rural/remote centers.

REFERENCES

Ekanem, S. A. and A.E. Asira (2006). Religion and medicine in the 21st century Nigeria. *Sophia: An African Journal of Philosophy,* 9 (1): 56–61.

Ekenze, O.S., I.O. Onwuekwe and B.A. Ezeala Adikaibe (2010). Profile of neurological admissions at the University of Nigeria Teaching Hospital Enugu. *Nigerian Journal of Medicine* 19 (4): 419–22.

Imam, I. and A. Ogunniyi (2004). What is happening to motor neuron disease in Nigeria?

Nigeria behind in palliative care provision—Minister (2017, 2017/07/19/T17:36:28+00:00). *P.M. News.* Retrieved from https://www.pmnewsnigeria.com/2017/07/19/nigeria-behind-palliative-care-minister/.

Nigeria, five others reject physician-assisted suicide, euthanasia (2018, 2018/02/04/T03:00:52+00:00). *The Guardian Nigeria News—Nigeria and World News.* Retrieved from https://guardian.ng/features/nigeria-five-others-reject-physician-assisted-suicide-euthanasia/.

Ogun, S., O. Oshinaike, H. Ogun and A. Ogun (2019). Global disease burden: Neurological disorders in Africa. *Neuroepidemiology* 52: 10–11. https://doi.org/10.1159/000495016.

Osuntokun, B.O., A.O. Adeuja, B.S. Schoenberg, O. Bademosi et al. (1987). Neurological disorders in Nigerian Africans: a community-based study. *Acta Neurol Scand* 75 (1): 13–21. https://doi.org/10.1111/j.1600-0404.1987. tb07883.x.

Osuntokun, B.O., A.O.G. Adeuja and O. Bademosi (1974). The prognosis of motor neuron disease in Nigerian Africans: A prospective study of 92 patients. *Brain* 97 (1): 385–94. https://doi.org/10.1093/brain/97.1.385.

Quansah, E. and T.K. Karikari (2015). Motor neuron diseases in Sub-Saharan Africa: The need for more population-based studies. *BioMed Research International* 9. https://doi.org/10.1155/2015/298409.

Your MND multidisciplinary team Information for the public Motor neurone disease: assessment and management Guidance NICE. (2016). Retrieved from https://www.nice.org.uk/guidance/ng42/ifp/chapter/Your-MND-multidisciplinary-team.

CHAPTER 15

Public Policy of ALS: A Pakistani Perspective

Asfandyar Khan Niazi, Aqdas Kazi, and Arsalan Ahmad

Abstract Pakistan is forecast to have an increase in the incidence of ALS, but healthcare resources are not increasing correspondingly. As a result, access to specialist care is often difficult because of physical distance, long waiting hours, limited resources and high out-of-pocket payments. Neurorehabilitation is inaccessible to most people, but the situation is improving. There is a dearth of specialist palliative care services, with no government-funded hospices or nursing homes. Caregiver support is available from domestic help and housemaids. Medical assistive devices are expensive and not commonly available. Advance directives and euthanasia do not have a legal basis in Pakistan. Despite difficulties in the infrastructure and socioeconomic and cultural obstacles, things are improving in terms of the research output and healthcare facilities for patients with ALS in Pakistan.

Keywords Amyotrophic lateral sclerosis • ALS • Pakistan
• Palliative care

A. K. Niazi • A. Kazi • A. Ahmad (✉)
Shifa International Hospital, Shifa Tameer-e-Millat University,
Islamabad, Pakistan
e-mail: niazi.asfand@gmail.com; aqdaskazi@yahoo.com;
arsalan.ahmad@shifa.com.pk

© The Author(s) 2021
R. H. Blank et al. (eds.), *Public Policy in ALS/MND Care*,
https://doi.org/10.1007/978-981-15-5840-5_15

INTRODUCTION

Pakistan is the fifth most populous country of the world (World Bank 2019a). It is on the list of countries forecasted to have a rapid increase in the life expectancy with a resultant increase in the incidence of neurodegenerative disorders, including amyotrophic lateral sclerosis (ALS) (Logroscino and Piccininni 2019). Unfortunately, the country seems poorly prepared to confront this rapidly approaching problem in current circumstances. Much work remains to be done in order to facilitate research, healthcare and advocacy for patients with ALS. Accurate data on the epidemiology of ALS in Pakistan is limited. Population-based ALS registries have been instrumental in identifying the epidemiology and clinical characteristics of ALS in other countries (Logroscino and Piccininni 2019), but no such registry is currently in place in Pakistan. Shifa International Hospital in Islamabad does maintain an outpatient database of neurology patients which includes ALS patients. This database includes data on the demographic information, symptoms, treatment and outcomes of patients with ALS.

EPIDEMIOLOGY OF ALS

The best estimate of the epidemiology of ALS in Pakistan comes from the Global Burden of Disease study 2016, which suggested a prevalence of 3448 patients (1.44/100,000) (GBD 2017). This represented an increase of 7 percent over the prevalence of ALS in 1990. There were 223 deaths each year from ALS in Pakistan, and this increased by 66 percent between 1990 and 2016. There was a loss of 8950 Disability Adjusted Life Years (DALYs) in 2016, which represented a 48 percent increase over that in 1990. Despite this rapid increase in the prevalence and incidence of deaths from ALS in Pakistan, the healthcare resources have not increased to a corresponding degree. As a result, patients with ALS have limited access to neurologists, physiotherapists, rehabilitation specialists, speech therapists, pulmonologists and palliative care specialists.

GOVERNMENT ACTIVITY IN ALS

There have not been any governmental reports or committees on ALS. The National Health Vision 2016–2025 is the Pakistani government's guiding document for health strategy (Ministry of National Health Services 2016).

This document does not make any mention of neurodegenerative diseases in general or ALS specifically. This striking lack of focus on neurodegenerative diseases and ALS from the government's policy documents translates to reduced financing and strategic planning for healthcare of patients with ALS. Therefore, it is not surprising that as of 2014, the total expenditure on health per capita in Pakistan was only 129 USD, which represented 2.6 percent of the GDP (WHO 2019).

Pakistan is an Islamic country, and public attitude toward healthcare is shaped by religious and cultural views (Khan 2017). Diseases are accepted as will of God as a test. Euthanasia is not accepted. There are no organized palliative care units in Pakistan. It is widely believed that the time and manner of one's death is preordained. At the same time, it is thought that discussing negative outcomes may bring on their occurrence. Families are very close-knit in the Pakistani society, and diseases are considered family affairs instead of personal ones. Relatives of the patient expect to be informed about the diagnosis, prognosis and treatment options before the patient, and then they decide whether and how much to inform the patient. The concept of advance directives is neither covered in the Pakistani law nor widely practiced (Zaman et al. 2019).

The Pakistani government provides healthcare delivered at primary, secondary and tertiary healthcare centers (Hassan et al. 2017). Primary and secondary care centers are responsible for provision of basic medical care and for referral of patients to tertiary care centers for complex specialist care. Additionally, there are private clinics and hospitals that provide varying levels of complexity of care. Access to specialist care in government tertiary centers is often difficult because of physical distance from the patient's place of residence, long waiting times and limited resources. Private clinics and hospitals are often better equipped and are easier to access, but payments must be made out-of-pocket by the patients. Estimates suggest that almost 70 percent of healthcare across Pakistan is delivered by the private healthcare system and the remaining 30 percent by the government healthcare system (Hassan et al. 2017).

The Pakistani government has introduced the Prime Minister's Health Program, which allows people living under 2 USD a day to receive treatment for up to 3600 USD free of cost (Sehat Sahulat Program 2019). However, this program is available for residents in only 23 of the 154 districts. People with a monthly earning of less than 92 USD are also eligible for government assistance from the Bait-ul-Mal fund, created specifically for people with very poor social conditions (Bait-ul-Mal board 2019).

Assistance can be requested for healthcare costs including for obtaining medical equipment. Several non-governmental organizations are available to assist people with disabilities in financing their healthcare and obtaining medical equipment.

Almost 67 percent of the healthcare expenditure in Pakistan is through out-of-pocket payments (Thaver and Ahmad 2018; Malik and Azam 2012). This places a significant burden on the Pakistani population since Pakistan is a lower-middle-income country with a per capita gross national in 2018 (World Bank 2019b). Patients with ALS have direct (doctor fees, hospital fees, medications, medical equipment) and indirect (loss of productivity due to disability, loss of productivity of caregiver, caregiver stress) healthcare costs.

Advocacy and Awareness of ALS in Pakistan

Advocacy for ALS in Pakistan is still in its infancy. The Pakistan ALS Foundation was formed in 2018 to provide support to the patients with ALS and advocate for their rights (Pakistan ALS Foundation 2019). This is the only organization dedicated for working for ALS in Pakistan. The Pakistan Society of Neurology (PSN) also has a dedicated section on neurorehabilitation which focuses on rehabilitation of all neurological diseases in general (Pakistan Society of Neurology 2019a). Similarly, the Pakistan Society of Neurorehabilitation is working toward improving access to rehabilitation for patients with neurological diseases (Pakistan Society of Neurology 2019b).

There has been very little media coverage for patients with ALS. Studies have shown very poor awareness of ALS in the Pakistani society (Naveed et al. 2015). Despite the lack of resources and awareness, a study conducted between 2009 and 2013 showed a mean time from symptom onset to diagnosis of almost one year (Brohi et al. 2014). This time delay is comparable to that from developed countries.

ALS Research Funding

Funding for research in Pakistan comes from governmental and nongovernmental organizations. The Pakistan Health Research Council is the governmental organization responsible for supporting research in medicine and healthcare (Ministry of National Health Services 2019). Other departments of the government including the Higher Education

Commission also provide research grants (Higher Education Commission 2019). These grants are competitive and are available for both medical and non-medical research. Research funding in Pakistan stands at a tiny 0.25 percent of the GDP (World Bank 2019b). This funding includes grants for both medical and non-medical research.

Most non-governmental funding comes from universities and university hospitals. There are some private organizations dedicated to promoting scientific research that also provide research grants, for example, the Pakistan Academy of Sciences (2019). Unfortunately, there are no dedicated institutions for research on ALS. Despite these challenges, recent data from Pakistan has shown that funding for medical research has doubled over the past decade, and research publications have increased by almost seven times (Ahmed 2018).

CARE OF ALS PATIENTS

The primary caregiver for a large proportion of patients is their immediate family, and it is very uncommon for patients to be sent to nursing homes. This leads to significant indirect costs because of lost productivity from the family members who assume the role of a caregiver. Previously, the female members of the household were primarily responsible for being the caregivers of sick individuals, but with the progressive increase in the number of females entering the workforce, the family support system is becoming less reliable (Zaman et al. 2019).

Some families choose to employ untrained housemaids for taking care of the patients. The costs for employing such help are also directly paid by the patients or their family. A previous study on people caring for patients with stroke in Pakistan showed a high level of stress (Ain et al. 2014). This emotional and physical stress leads to caregiver burn-out in family members and housemaids who are not trained for caring for a person with disability and do not receive any social support.

Support from housemaids in caring for the patients is very important for reducing caregiver stress. In the absence of staff trained in caring for patients with neurological diseases, these housemaids can be given basic training to care for patients with ALS. As a similar example, traditional birth attendants in Pakistan have been used for reproductive and obstetric care (Islam and Malik 2001). These traditional birth attendants were given basic obstetric training. Their involvement in obstetric care in areas without qualified obstetricians has shown improvement in the healthcare outcomes as well as patient satisfaction.

Neurorehabilitation is inaccessible for most people living in Pakistan (Rathore and Manzoor 2016). There are very few rehabilitation medicine specialists in Pakistan, and most of them work in a single rehabilitation center. There is no postgraduate training program for specialized neurorehabilitation. However, there has recently been an increase in the number of physiotherapists. This increase may be partly attributed to the earthquake in Pakistan in 2005, after which there was a sudden increase in the requirement of rehabilitation services. Additionally, there has also been a recent increase in the awareness of the role of neurorehabilitation in the management of neurological diseases.

Medical assistive devices are not commonly available for people with disabilities in Pakistan (Safdar et al. 2019). They are also very expensive. A few non-governmental organizations and Pakistan Bait-ul-Mal provide aids for people requiring medical assistive devices (Bait-ul-Mal Board 2019). However, there is still very limited availability and utilization of medical assistive devices.

END-OF-LIFE ISSUES FOR ALS PATIENTS

Euthanasia has no basis in the Pakistani law, and most studies have found that healthcare professionals consider it to be unethical and do not favor its legalization (Khan et al. 2012). It is widely viewed to be against the principles of Islam, which state that God is the only authority to grant or take away life. Therefore, euthanasia is not practiced in Pakistan even for the terminally ill patients. In such a scenario, it is important to offer the best possible palliative care services to patients.

Palliative care as an established specialty is offered at three major institutions of Pakistan, and one of these is a cancer center. The dearth of specialist palliative care services can be demonstrated from the fact that there are only three trained palliative care consultants in all of Pakistan. There are no government-funded hospices or nursing homes to support these patients or to offer respite to their caregivers. The patients are looked after by their families, domestic help and private nurses, which is a huge financial burden. There are some charities that may support ALS patients, but they work at an individual level and there is no formal guidance for patients once a patient is diagnosed with this debilitating disease.

Policy Changes Needed for ALS

The way forward would be to have registries for ALS/MND patients at all government and private hospitals. Once there are accurate local epidemiologic data, multidisciplinary teams of neurologists, palliative care physicians, neurorehabilitation specialists, nurses, physiotherapists, occupational therapists and speech therapists could be developed, allowing collaborative meetings to identify patients' problems and find solutions. These meetings could be undertaken by video conferences and can benefit numerous patients, but each region will need a coordinator to organize these meetings and ensure that the plans are implemented. This requires a network of general practitioners (GPs) in the community to care for these patients on a day-to-day basis and address general medical problems like chest infections and pressure sores. These GPs will also be ideally placed to do home visits and provide home medical care. This capacity building must start at the grassroots level after accepting that specialty-trained consultants can only provide support at an advisory level through tertiary care centers, but these patients need to be managed at home by a trained, efficient and compassionate workforce, especially their GPs. Unless we empower and train the GPs, we cannot look after these patients. The trained workforce can work toward advance directives that have a legal status and are enforced and implemented as part of the advance care planning.

Despite the difficulties in the infrastructure and socioeconomic and cultural obstacles, things are improving in terms of the research output and healthcare facilities for patients with ALS in Pakistan. However, there is still a long way to go. Funding for research needs to be increased. Palliative care and neurorehabilitation services need to be improved. Policy changes are required to facilitate advance directives for patients with ALS.

References

Ahmed, I. (2018). Medical research in Pakistan. *Isra Medical Journal* 10 (6): 325–326.

Ain, Q.U., N.Z. Dar, A. Ahmad, S. Munzar and A.W. Yousafzai (2014). Caregiver stress in stroke survivor: data from a tertiary care hospital: A cross sectional survey. *BMC Psychology* 2 (1): 49.

Bait-ul-Mal Board. Pakistan Bait-ul-Mal. Available from http://www.pbm.gov.pk/pbm.html (Accessed on 29/06/2019).

Brohi, H., N.U. Ahmed, R. Khatri and I. Asghar (2014). Delay in diagnosis of motor neuron disease: A tertiary care experience. *Pakistan Journal of Neurological Sciences* 9 (1): 4.

Global Burden of Disease (GBD) (2017). Global, regional and national incidence, prevalence, and years lived with disability for 328 diseases and injuries for 195 countries, 1990–2016: a systematic analysis for the Study. *Lancet* 390 (10100): 1211–59.

Hassan, A., K. Mahmood and H.A. Bukhsh (2017). Healthcare System of Pakistan. *International Journal of Advanced Research and Publications* 1 (4): 170–73.

Higher Education Commission (2019). Research and development. Available from https://www.hec.gov.pk/english/services/Pages/RnD.aspx. (Accessed on 21/06/2019).

Islam, A. and F.A. Malik (2001). Role of traditional birth attendants in improving reproductive health: lessons from the family health project, *Sindh. Journal of Pakistan Medical Association* 51 (6):218–22.

Khan, R.I. (2017). Palliative care in Pakistan. *Indian Journal of Medical Ethics* 2 (1): 37–42.

Khan, A, S.M. Hasan and M. Hussain (2012). Euthanasia: Perspectives of Pakistani medical students and practitioners: A survey. *Professional Medical Journal* 19 (1): 112–16.

Logroscino, G. and M. Piccininni (2019). Amyotrophic lateral sclerosis descriptive epidemiology: The origin of geographic difference. *Neuroepidemiology* 52: 93–103

Malik, M.A. and S. Azam (2012). Socio-economic determinants of household out-of-pocket payments on healthcare in Pakistan. *International Journal of Equity Health* 11: 51.

Ministry of National Health Services (2016). National health vision 2016–2025. Available at http://www.nationalplanningcycles.org/sites/default/files/planning_cycle_repository/pakistan/national_health_vision_2016-25_30-08-2016.pdf (Accessed on 17/06/2019).

Ministry of National Health Services, Regulations and Coordination. Pakistan Health Research Council. Available from http://phrc.org.pk/. (Accessed on 21/06/2019).

Naveed, S., A. Hameed and S.M. Nadeem (2015). Knowledge of Amyotrophic Lateral Sclerosis (ALS) in pharmacy students. *Brain Disorders Therapy* 4: 1.

Pakistan Academy of Sciences (2019). Research grants. Available from http://www.paspk.org/research-grants/ (Accessed on 29/06/2019).

Pakistan ALS Foundation (2019), Mission Statement. Available from https://www.alspakistan.org/mission-statement (Accessed on 21/06/2019).

Pakistan Society of Neurology (2019a). Executive committee. Available from http://pakneurology.com /pages/OfficeExeComm.asp. (Accessed on 29/06/2019).

Pakistan Society of Neurology (2019b). Affiliated societies. Available from http:// pakneurology.com/pages/AffiliatedSocieties.asp. (Accessed on 29/06/2019).

Rathore, F.A. and S.N. Manzoor (2016). Neurorehabilitation in Pakistan: Needs, challenges and opportunities. *Khyber Medical University Journal* 8 (2): 59–60.

Safdar, S., S.A. Khan, N. Azam, H. Mahmood and F. Pervaiz (2019). Need assessment of assistive technology in children with multiple disabilities. *Pakistan Armed Forces Medical Journal* 69 (Suppl-2): S229–34.

Sehat Sahulat Program (2019). Introduction. Available from https://www. pmhealthprogram.gov.pk/ (Accessed on 29/06/2019).

Thaver, A. and A. Ahmad (2018). Economic perspective of dementia care in Pakistan. *Neurology* 90 (11): e993-e994.

World Bank (2019a). Population 2018. Available from: https://databank.worldbank.org/data/download/POP.pdf (Accessed on 24/07/2019).

World Bank (2019b). Pakistan. Available from: https://data.worldbank.org/country/pakistan (Accessed on 29/06/2019).

World Bank (2019c). Research and development expenditure. Available from https://data.worldbank.org/indicator/gb.xpd.rsdv.gd.zs   (Accessed   on 29/06/2019).

World Health Organization (2019). Pakistan. Available from https://www.who. int/countries/pak/en/ (Accessed on 29/06/2019).

Zaman, Q., M. Siddiqui and Z.I. Malik (2019). Dementia in Pakistan: An unprecedented challenge and local cultural beliefs, problems and actions required. *Pakistan Journal of Neurological Sciences* 14 (1): 45–51.

CHAPTER 16

Public Policy in ALS Care: The Polish Perspective

Anna Adamczyk and Wojciech Leppert

Abstract ALS prevalence in Poland is like that of other European countries. Patients diagnosed with ALS have a right to access all medical procedures which are reimbursed by the government and to the delivery of supportive measures from public funds. ALS patients may benefit from a social support system in which the scope and method of financing are regulated by the ministers. In the symptomatic management of ALS, drugs commonly used in palliative care for other patient groups are available. In the case of intractable symptoms, the use of palliative sedation is acceptable after fulfilling required criteria, including the patient's consent. Euthanasia and assisted suicide are forbidden by law. Improvement of quality of care for patients with ALS in Poland requires elaborating a uniform strategy of diagnostic, treatment and caring approaches that account for personal and financial resources possibilities.

A. Adamczyk
Ludwik Rydygier Collegium Medicum, Bydgoszcz, Poland
e-mail: anulaadamczyk@poczta.onet.pl

W. Leppert (✉)
Poznan University of Medical Sciences, Poznan, Poland
e-mail: wojciechleppert@wp.pl

© The Author(s) 2021
R. H. Blank et al. (eds.), *Public Policy in ALS/MND Care*,
https://doi.org/10.1007/978-981-15-5840-5_16

Keywords Amyotrophic lateral sclerosis • Diagnosis • Palliative care
• Symptom management

PREVALENCE

Data regarding prevalence and mortality of ALS patients are collected by
a Main Statistical Office (Statistics Poland—Główny Urząd Statystyczny),
but they are not published in separate reports. In Poland the prevalence of
ALS appears to be similar to other European countries, but data regarding
direct causes of death in ALS patients are not published in Poland.

SOCIAL SUPPORT FOR ALS PATIENTS

Patients diagnosed with ALS are provided with specific medical care in
Poland. They have a right to access all medical procedures which are provided by and reimbursed by a government. The diagnosis of ALS is usually
undertaken at the neurology departments by neurologists working in outpatient clinics. There is no requirement to confirm diagnosis in specialist
neurology centers as there are no special departments dedicated exclusively to patients diagnosed with ALS in Poland.

Patients diagnosed with ALS, as all patients defined as "disabled," may
benefit from a social support system, the range of which and method of
financing are regulated by the law (acts and decrees) issued by ministers in
the government. The level of reimbursement for this care depends on the
degree of disability, the presence or lack of caregivers and the patient's
income. The provision of care for patients at their homes usually depends
on the presence of family members or caregivers, and the governmental
care reimburses only an average of two hours a day of professional care for
patients at home.

Patients who have no family carers may be referred to nursing homes,
but the payment for this is expected to be primarily from their resources,
up to 70 percent of their income, supported by the local social care system. The access to such care is limited, as there are only a small number of
beds in these long-term care facilities. Some patients benefit from care in
private institutions, but this is associated with high costs. Patients diagnosed with ALS, who are unable to work, have a right to a pension from

the social insurance system and the amount provided depends on the previous contributions made to the social insurance system while they had been working.

Provision of Equipment

Patients have a right to the provision of support from the government, including wheelchairs, mattresses, anti-decubitus pillows, continence aids and catheters. Other devices such as specialist beds and electronic devices for communication are partly reimbursed from public resources, but the amount of support depends on the availability of the local social welfare funding and income of the patient and their family. The provision of electronic devices, such as communication aids, may be limited due to cost, and patients are often dependent on the provision from non-governmental organizations and public donations. Overall the public resources are insufficient for delivery of an appropriate level of care for patients with ALS, although there are no data available indicating the extent of a private sector participation and costs covered by patients and families.

Support for Caregivers

If the care is provided at home, family caregivers of patients with ALS may apply for an allowance, provided that they have been actively working and need to resign from work in order to provide care for the patient. The amount of allowance is lower than the lowest income that the government regulations state as a basic wage. The majority of caregivers are close family, mainly spouses and children. Paid caregivers typically support families for a few hours daily but this care is costly.

The only organization which is specifically devoted to care for patients with ALS is a non-governmental association Dignitas Doletium, which was initiated by patients and families, and it is not a scientific organization. It supports patients and their families through education about the disease, diagnostic and therapeutic procedures. It also offers financial support once or twice a year and lends medical equipment. The Association has a website in Polish: www.mnd.pl and it is not a member of any European or world organization.

Provision of Medication

The only drug registered in Poland for the management of patients diagnosed with ALS is riluzole. The use of all other drugs, substances or precursor cells for the treatment of ALS is deemed a medical experiment and there is a procedure to gain the informed consent of patients for any study. The medication for symptomatic management in ALS is commonly used in palliative care for other patient groups (Bede et al. 2011).

Palliative Sedation

If there are intractable symptoms in patients with ALS, as in all other palliative care patients, the use of palliative sedation after fulfilling the required criteria, including patients' consent for this procedure, is acceptable.

RESEARCH

Research into ALS is not coordinated in Poland and solely depends on the initiatives of scientists, who may apply for scientific grants in competitive fields for resources from national and European institutions. The private sector does not finance research in Poland.

GENETIC TESTING

Patients with ALS have an opportunity to undergo genetic tests that are funded from public resources. Patients are referred to genetic out-patient clinics by a physician and the range of testing is determined by the specialists in genetics. Access to genetic out-patient clinics is limited by the number of visits contracted by a public funding system (NHF). The mean waiting time for a visit is approximately a few months. The results of tests are presented to patients or persons who have been clearly designated by the patient. Genetic testing and the use of biological material cannot be used for research purposes without the patient's consent.

Public Awareness

In recent years in society and the media there has been an increase in the information about ALS, most commonly in the context of charity activities for individual patients, including fund-raising for alternative therapeutic methods.

Guidelines for Care of ALS Patients

The Polish Association of Neurology does not have its own recommendations concerning diagnosis and management of ALS patients. The clinical approach is based on recommendations of an Expert Working Group of European Federation of Neurology Associations published in 2011 (Andersen et al. 2012). In 2018 the Polish Association of Palliative Medicine (Polskie Towarzystwo Medycyny Paliatywnej—PAPM) issued recommendations regarding the qualification and extent of palliative care for patients with ALS in the context of current financing from public resources (Adamczyk et al. 2018).

In Poland there are no separate laws, regulations or financing regarding ALS. All diagnostics, treatment and care are financed by the government as a part of a specialist and palliative care. The gaps may be filled by non-governmental organizations such as Dignitas Doletium.

Patients with ALS may also receive support from enteral and parenteral nutrition units in all care settings. The care for patients with ALS may be provided concurrently with palliative care and invasive ventilatory support. Enteral nutrition costs including doctors and nurses from nutritional units, diet, devices and laboratory test costs are covered completely from public resources.

The care of home or stationary ventilatory units is also financed from public resources. The Poland National Health Fund (Narodowy Fundusz Zdrowia) requires that this care is provided within strict parameters, including the confirmation of respiratory failure in patients with ALS. The care for patients with ALS may include rehabilitation and they have the right to benefit from these types of medical care until the end of their life with no financial restrictions.

Palliative Care

Patients diagnosed with ALS may be qualified for palliative care, which is financed from public resources. However, the patient is not allowed to concurrently receive ventilation support at home and palliative home care (in Poland the so-called Home Hospice) or care within palliative care units or hospices. Patients may receive consultations with palliative medicine specialists in palliative medicine out-patient clinics. Patients in long-term facilities, financed from public resources, are excluded from concurrent access to palliative care in any form.

Multidisciplinary Care

Multidisciplinary care across different centers is not coordinated in any formal way in Poland. Specialists from separate units are not obliged to contact each other to establish a patient's management strategy. This leads to frequent unnecessary admissions to hospitals, particularly when there are symptoms of respiratory failure and invasive ventilatory support is introduced, without earlier discussions with the patient and, sometimes, even against the patient's will. At present, there is no law allowing the patient's statements regarding which therapeutic interventions are acceptable in the future. At present, no health-care professional is formally obliged by the law to comply with patients' oral or written declarations made in the past. In practice this means that if a patient at some point is unable to provide conscious consent for conducting a medical procedure, the physician may introduce lifesaving invasive interventions in critical situations.

ASSISTED DYING

In Poland euthanasia and assisted suicide are forbidden by a law. Assisted suicide is also illegal. Current law regulations forbid withdrawing invasive ventilatory support in patients until normal breathing returns or death of the brainstem is confirmed. This in practice means that patients with ALS on invasive ventilatory support will continue this treatment until death.

PLACE OF CARE AND DEATH

There are no data are available regarding place of care and death for people with ALS and there is no information on the percentage of patients receiving palliative care and invasive ventilatory support. It has been estimated that the percentage of patients with ALS in whom interventions prolonging survival are used in Poland is higher in comparison to other European countries (Hobson and McDermott 2016). This is associated with a society that considers that life is of the highest value and it requires protection at all costs. Over 90 percent of Poles declare themselves as belonging to Roman Catholic faith, and this may influence the views of these societies. Moreover, in Poland there has been no open public debate regarding quality of life, the use of potentially futile life-extending therapy, advance directives, medical decision-making with patients, or euthanasia or assisted suicide.

CONCLUSION

The improvement of the quality of care for patients with ALS in Poland requires the development of a clear national strategy for diagnosis, treatment and care that takes into account the personal views of patients and financial resources (Bede et al. 2011; Oliver 2019). Although there is access to interventions that prolong life, there is poor provision of care at patients' homes and in long-term care facilities. Extra attention is needed to develop financial support and respite care for caregivers at home and to provide palliative care at each stage of the disease and at the place where patients are living. The development of this strategy for patients with ALS requires the cooperation of governmental institutions and medical scientific associations.

REFERENCES

Adamczyk, A., M. Kwiatkowska and I. Filipczak-Bryniarska (2018). Polish Association for Palliative Medicine stand on qualification for palliative care and management of patients with amyotrophic lateral sclerosis and multiple sclerosis (in Polish). *Palliative Medicine* 10: 1150–30.

Andersen, P.M., S. Abrahams, G.D. Borasio et al. (2012). EFNS guidelines on the Clinical Management of Amyotrophic Lateral Sclerosis (ALS)—revised report of an EFNS task force. *European Journal of Neurology* 19: 360–75.

Bede, P., D. Oliver, J. Stodart et al. (2011). Palliative care in amyotrophic lateral sclerosis: A review of current international guidelines and initiatives. *Journal of Neurology, Neurosurgery and Psychiatry* 82: 413–18.

Hobson, E.V. and C.J. McDermott (2016). Supportive and symptomatic management of amyotrophic lateral sclerosis. *Nature Reviews Neurology* 12: 526–38.

Oliver, D.J. (2019). Palliative care in motor neurone disease: Where are we now? *Palliative Care: Research and Treatment* 12; https://doi.org/10.1177/1178224218813914.

CHAPTER 17

ALS Policy: A Russian Perspective

L. V. Brylev, D. V. Nevzorova, M. N. Zakharova,
and A. B. Guekht

Abstract Around 10,000 people in Russia live with ALS. People with ALS and their families have an overwhelming number of needs and most of them are addressed by the health-care system, social services and charity foundations, but the amount of support varies in different regions. The main challenge is implementation of standard of care across the country

L. V. Brylev (✉)
Institute of Higher Nervous Activity and Neurophysiology,
Russian Academy of Sciences, Moscow, Russia
e-mail: lev.brylev@gmail.com

Bujanov Moscow City Clinical Hospital, Moscow, Russia

D. V. Nevzorova
Sechenov First Moscow State Medical University, Moscow, Russia
e-mail: gyn_nevzorova@mail.ru

M. N. Zakharova
Research Center of Neurology, Moscow, Russia
e-mail: vincera@vincera.ru

A. B. Guekht
Russian National Research Medical University, Moscow, Russia
e-mail: guekht@gmail.com

© The Author(s) 2021
R. H. Blank et al. (eds.), *Public Policy in ALS/MND Care*,
https://doi.org/10.1007/978-981-15-5840-5_17

which includes multidisciplinary medical teams and social support. Recently, we have seen encouraging changes in palliative care support for people with ALS, but we still need to improve legislation in the field of end-of-life decisions and implement standards for end-of-life care.

Keywords Russia • ALS • Policy • Palliative care • End-of-life care • Live Now Foundation

INCIDENCE AND PREVALENCE

There have been few epidemiological studies on ALS in Russia. Davydova and colleagues (2007) calculated the annual incidence of ALS as 0.7/100,000 adult inhabitants while Skvortsova and associates (2009) estimated the prevalence of ALS in Moscow as 1.16/100,000 inhabitants in 2006–2007. Our data (forthcoming) show an incidence of 1.25/100,000/year. This is lower than in most other world countries (Marin et al. 2017) but is comparable to Estonia (1.27 (0.92–1.63) (Gross-Paju et al. 1998). Regional statistic departments group diseases by ICD-10 codes and only pooled data for G10–G12 codes (that include, among others, ALS) are available. From these figures it can be estimated that 1800 people are diagnosed with ALS every year in Russia. However, this may be an underestimate and experts suggest that there may be 10,000–15,000 people with ALS in Russia.

GOVERNMENTAL ACTION IN ALS CARE

Health-care legislation is provided by the Federal Ministry of Health, thus the medical care for ALS patients is covered mostly under the mechanism of compulsory health insurance from regional budgets, which vary across the country. The Parliament Committee on Health has an expert group on rare diseases that coordinates interaction between legislators, experts, the patient community and charitable organizations to facilitate the access to diagnostic procedures and treatment for patients with rare diseases. This is still being developed but such an approach should improve the care of people with ALS in the future.

Technical aids are funded by regional departments of social protection, but some devices specific for ALS (i.e., electronic communication devices) are not covered by the government. The amount of care and support differs among regions. As will be discussed shortly, Live Now provides a limited number of communication aids and ventilators for people who cannot afford them.

Professional caregivers who care for ALS patients at home generally lack specialized education and skill training programs; therefore, the care of patients is overwhelmingly covered by families, charity organizations and limited grants from the government.

Private ALS Organizations

The most active charitable organizations that care for people with ALS are Live Now, GAOORDI and Miloserdie. The Live Now Foundation (www. https://alsfund.ru/) is a member of International Alliance of ALS/MND Associations. It works with experts from the Scientific Center for Neurology, Buyanov City Hospital and the Center for Palliative Medicine to improve care services. It provides information to patients, raises awareness about ALS, funds medical care and research, and promotes changes in legislation and standards of care. It supports about 750 people with ALS and their families. In Moscow and St Petersburg, the charity provides people with equipment, including ventilators and communication aids, helps finance Centers for Assistance to ALS patients and provides caregivers to support families.

ALS Research in Russia

The Parliament Committee on Health expert group on rare diseases was recently joined by a specialist on ALS. Scientific projects in Russia are covered mostly by governmental grants and charitable organizations. The Moscow ALS center, with the support of Live Now, participates in international research projects in epidemiology and genetics of ALS. However, no disease-modifying drugs for ALS are approved in Russia and no international drug trials on ALS have ever been conducted in Russia.

Care of Patients with ALS

Pooled data (unpublished) show that more than 90 percent of patients stay at home and only about 30 percent of them are followed by general practitioners. Approximately 18 percent of ALS patients currently receive care from palliative care teams at home, 2 percent reside in hospices, about

15 percent get respiratory support through ventilators and only 1 percent receives morphine for pain and/or dyspnea.

Caregivers

Caregivers are supported by the government, but the amount of money they are paid is much lower than minimum wage. A draft bill to increase these payments is currently being considered by Parliament. Social workers, who visit patients at home several times per week, are provided by local departments of social protection. In addition, Live Now supports a very small number of families, up to ten at any one time.

Multidisciplinary Teams

A governmental initiative on implementation of clinical recommendations is aimed at standardizing the level of care across the country. Policy recommendations made by a group of experts on ALS policy are currently awaiting approval. If initiated, these recommendations will represent the next step in introducing a multidisciplinary approach to the care of ALS patients. Until now, only a few specialists in Moscow and Saint-Petersburg have experience in providing multidisciplinary care.

Right to Try

Although patients formally have a right to try unregistered drugs, very few are aware of this right so it is seldom used.

Genetic Testing

Genetic testing is not covered by compulsory health insurance; therefore, only a minority of patients, generally within specific research projects, undergoes any kind of genetic testing.

Palliative Care

About 18 percent of ALS patients are currently followed by palliative care teams at home and 2 percent stay in hospices. However, not all hospices are able to accept patients with ALS at the present time.

ADVANCE DIRECTIVES, EUTHANASIA AND PHYSICIAN-ASSISTED SUICIDE

There is no clear legal status of advance directives, of the withholding or withdrawing of mechanical ventilation and other life-extending interventions and mechanical support, or of palliative sedation. Because of the ambiguity of the law, the withdrawal of treatment occurs rarely. Moreover, euthanasia and physician-assisted suicide are strictly prohibited in Russia.

CONCLUSION: ALS POLICY CONTEXT IN RUSSIA

The services available for people with ALS and their caregivers in Russia are very limited. However, there have been recent policy developments that are encouraging and in the coming years it is hoped that a more coordinated approach will be developed, including increased emphasis on multidisciplinary team care.

REFERENCES

Marin, B., F. Boumédiene, G. Logroscino et al. (2017). Variation in worldwide incidence of amyotrophic lateral sclerosis: A meta-analysis. *International Journal of Epidemiology* 46 (1): 57–74.

Davydova, T.K. and T.A. Nikolaeva (2007). Amyotrophic lateral sclerosis in Yakutia. *The Siberian Medical Journal* 2: 23–25.

Samoshkina, O.I. (2007). Clinical and epidemiological picture of amyotrophic lateral sclerosis in Saint Petersburg.

Skvortsova, V.I., A.P. Smirnov, A.V. Alekhin and E.A. Kovrazhkina (2009). Clinical-epidemiological study of motor neuron disease in Moscow. *Zh Nevrol Psikhiatr Im S S Korsakova* 109 (3): 53–55.

Gross-Paju, K., M. Oöpik, S.M. Lüüs et al. (1998). Motor neurone disease in South Estonia: Diagnosis and incidence rate. *Acta Neurologica Scandinavica* 98: 22–28.

CHAPTER 18

Public Policy in ALS/MND Care: South African Perspective

Jeannine M. Heckmann and Alexandra S. Amaler

Abstract Suffering from a life-shortening illness such as amyotrophic lateral sclerosis (ALS) in a resource-constrained setting has its unique challenges and needs. These include poor access to specialist services, which can result in a delayed diagnosis of ALS. The Motor Neuron Disease (MND)/ALS Association of South Africa, a non-profit organization, provides substantial psychosocial support to patients and families and allows those without medical insurance to loan equipment not offered by the state, although this practice is confined to a few large cities. South Africans in the terminal phase of illness strongly prefer receiving comfort care to extreme life-extending measures. While the "right to die" narrative enters the public domain at intervals, many African cultures believe that the focus should be on having a "good death" with opportunities for family reconciliation. Nevertheless, there is a great need and opportunity to develop policies to support individuals with ALS and their caregivers, and we propose several avenues for the state and society to consider.

J. M. Heckmann (✉) • A. S. Amaler
University of Cape Town, Cape Town, South Africa
e-mail: jeanine.heckmann@uct.ac.za; Alexamaler01@gmail.com

© The Author(s) 2021
R. H. Blank et al. (eds.), *Public Policy in ALS/MND Care*,
https://doi.org/10.1007/978-981-15-5840-5_18

Keywords South Africa • ALS • Terminal • Good death • Palliation • Palliative care • Assisted suicide

Epidemiology of ALS in South Africa

Accurate epidemiological studies for amyotrophic lateral sclerosis (ALS) on the African continent are as yet unavailable. A recently completed four-year incidence study, performed in the Western Cape province of South Africa from 2014 to 2018, is expected to be reported soon (Henning et al., in preparation). In this region, which spans 129,462 km^2 (roughly the size of England) and is inhabited by 6.2 million people, most people classified themselves in the 2016 census as black African (35.7%), white or European-genetic ancestry (16.0%) or mixed African-genetic ancestry (Cape colored) (47.5%), which is the biggest subpopulation in the region (www.statssa.gov.za).

The highest incidence of ALS cases was observed in the white subpopulation which showed a very similar crude incidence rate to white European and American populations (Logroscino et al. 2010; Mehta et al. 2018). However, the incidence rates in the two largest subpopulations in the Western Cape Province, namely, mixed African-genetic and black subpopulations, were between three- and tenfold lower than those with European-genetic ancestry, respectively (Henning, et al. in preparation). Although a similar trend of twofold lower ALS prevalence among black Americans compared to white Americans was found in New Jersey (Mehta et al. 2018), the ALS risk among African Americans varied substantially according to socioeconomic status, with the highest ALS risk among the most affluent strata (Henry et al. 2015). While biological and epidemiological factors may be responsible for these discrepancies, it also raises the possibility of case under-ascertainment in socioeconomically deprived regions, such as Africa (see later).

Although the phenotypic spectrum of ALS appears similar among the different South African subpopulations, we have reported lower frequencies of bulbar onset ALS compared to reports in Europeans (Nel et al. 2019). In addition, those with black African-genetic ancestry had significantly younger symptom onset (Dekker et al. 2018; Nel et al. 2019). While the first genetic study in Africans with ALS found that the most well-known genetic cause for ALS among Europeans, the *C9orf72* expansion mutation, was not found among indigenous black Africans, the sample size was small (Nel et al. 2019). A Tanzanian hospital-based cohort reported a twofold higher prevalence of HIV infection rate among clinically identified ALS cases compared to the general population (Dekker et al. 2018). However, in South Africa, where 7 million people are living with HIV resulting in a prevalence rate of 13 percent, we have only encountered a few HIV-infected individuals diagnosed with ALS in the Western Cape region (Henning et al., in preparation) (https://statssa. gov.za).

The Tanzanian report emphasized the delay in the "presentation" of ALS patients from resource-constrained areas (Dekker et al. 2018). Indeed, universal access to health care remains a concern regarding under-ascertainment, and we have encountered at least six ALS patients over the past five years who either have died before they were able to attend their clinic appointment or were diagnosed with ALS in the intensive care setting after an emergency intubation in extremis (Heckmann, unpublished observations). Invariably these are patients with limited resources and poor access to specialist medical care, often from poorer areas, and who have experienced increasingly progressive symptoms for many months.

THE STATE OF HEALTH CARE IN SOUTH AFRICA

Health care in South Africa consists of a two-tiered system where the state is responsible for the health of over 80 percent of the population. While the public sector is poorly resourced, private sector health care, which services individuals who have medical insurance, is run on a commercial model catering for the middle- and high-income sectors (https://www. brandsouthafrica.com/south-africa-fast-facts/health-facts/health-care-in-south-africa). Implementing a national health insurance plan is a major goal of the present government, but these ideals are hampered by the fact that only a small proportion of the population contributes taxes, due to high unemployment, and the need to sustain the largest government-sponsored antiretroviral program worldwide. In addition, due to political instability in several sub-Saharan countries, such as Zimbabwe and the Democratic Republic of the Congo, many foreign citizens come and seek health care illegally in South Africa. Presently there is no official policy preventing illegal aliens from accessing such health care.

STATE OF PALLIATIVE CARE IN AFRICA

Africa has an enormous burden of life-threatening illnesses other than neurodegenerative diseases such as ALS, including human immunodeficiency virus (HIV) infections and tuberculosis infections (Centner et al. 2013), cancer and sickle cell associated strokes (Ddungu 2011). As alluded to earlier, an additional factor for ALS patients is the limitation of access to specialist neurology services in many areas in Africa; these patients are frequently incorrectly diagnosed at their primary care clinic and subsequently wait months to receive a more specialized service, if that is available. This delay in diagnosis is also seen in cancer sufferers where diagnoses are often made at an advanced stage (Ddungu 2011). Consequently, a delayed diagnosis of a life-shortening disease in a resource-poor African setting, where recognition of ALS is an ongoing need, stands in contrast with the palliative goals of the developed world, in which the individual's increasing disability accompanying advancing ALS can be alleviated by end-of-life ALS management policies and the health care system's support for patients and their families.

Experience in an African setting often reveals patients with unilateral weakness who have been misdiagnosed as "stroke" by primary or secondary health care facilities. An educational drive about ALS and related disorders in Africa is likely to substantially alter the present "prevalence" figures of ALS in Africa. Previously, a sizeable apparent increased incidence of myasthenia gravis was observed within a six-year period based on more widespread access to a diagnostic test ordered by neurologists (Mombaur and Heckmann 2015). Therefore, it is our assertion that ALS in Africa is underdiagnosed or recognized very late in the disease course.

Dr. John Weru from Kenya, in an opinion piece highlighting the need for palliative care in Africa, argued that access to palliative care for those with life-shortening illnesses is as much a fundamental a right as access to general health care (Weru 2017). However, palliative care in Africa is limited at best (Ddungu 2011). Although South Africa, Malawi, Rwanda, Swaziland and Uganda have recently integrated palliative care into their mainstream health care objectives, and while Kenya has expanded its hospice facilities across the country, most African countries have no palliative health care facilities (Ddungu 2011). The successful integration of palliative care requires, among others, formulation of policy, staff training and awareness, availability of drugs and other support measures, and recognition that partnerships between government, non-governmental and patient organizations is vital (The Kampala Declaration of 2016).

The in-hospital state-sponsored palliative paradigm in South Africa is striving to address the needs of patients and their families over the last 24 to 48 hours of life (Gwyther et al. 2018). In contrast, it is recognized in the developed world that the process of palliation should start as soon as possible after the diagnosis of a life-shortening disease such as ALS (Ddungu 2011). Nevertheless, the introduction of palliative care training programs for health professionals at the University of Cape Town and the Makerere University College of Health Sciences was an important advance in the goals of delivering palliative care to Africans (Ddungu 2011).

State of Palliative Care in South Africa

The South African National Health Council recently adopted the South Africa National Policy Framework and Strategy for Palliative Care (2017–2022; https://hpca.co.za). This was a significant step toward developing hospital palliative care services in South African public hospitals (Gwyther et al. 2018). Hospices were established in the 1980s, mainly in affluent communities able to support them. With the AIDS epidemic arriving in this country in the 1990s, and the government-sponsored anti-retroviral program rolling out only in 2003, the then-great need for community-based palliation for AIDS patients was absorbed by hospice facilities. However, the resources were, and remain, constrained, and patients with cancer, HIV and neurodegenerative diseases such as ALS largely receive their palliation at home from nurses, a few times per week (Gwyther et al. 2018). In certain areas with a high burden of AIDS cases requiring terminal care, very successful partnerships between hospice and government sectors were established which resulted in an integrated home-based care system that served the local community and highlighted to the state sector the benefits of such partnerships (Gwyther et al. 2018).

The first hospital-based palliative care program was established in 2001 at the Charlotte Maxeke Johannesburg Academic Hospital. Donations from Irish Aid (2003–2006) contributed to the development of the Gauteng Centre of Excellence for Palliative Care at the Chris Hani Baragwanath Hospital in Soweto. This public sector initiative started outreach visits to the large Soweto community (approximately 1.5 million residents), and it soon became apparent to health care administrators that it was also a cost-effective project as it reduced the burden on acute care in-patient beds (Gwyther et al. 2018).

In the Western Cape province, the first hospital-based palliative care facility, primarily for patients with life-limiting advanced organ failure, was established at Victoria Hospital in Cape Town, with seed funding from the Rotary Foundation (Gwyther et al. 2018). Although donor funding still largely supports this unit, the state sector has acknowledged the cost-effective nature of this facility, resulting in fewer admissions and increased home deaths. The state is now funding a part-time palliative nurse at this facility. At the University of Cape Town's Groote Schuur Hospital, a terminal care facility was introduced in 2011 where patients could be admitted if they were expected to die within 24 hours. This was due to the high burden of disease and the pressure on acute and chronic beds. Patients making use of this palliative facility typically have end-stage cardiac failure, metastatic cancer, chronic renal failure ineligible for the transplant program and less frequently progressive neurological conditions (Gwyther et al. 2018). ALS patients almost never get admitted to this facility because of the continued psychosocial support delivered to them in the community by the MND Association and the Hospice Palliative Care Associations.

A few district hospitals (less than ten country-wide) now have palliative care services which implement a plan for each referral with a terminal illness, or for those who are admitted two or more times in a four-week period (Gwyther et al. 2018). The South African Department of Health has adopted a policy document which aims to offer a support system to individuals to help them live as actively as possible until death and to have a team approach to support patients and their families. However, in practice the service remains fragmented. For example, care for palliative patients in the Cape Town community should include transport as required such as Dial-a-Ride to improve access to the ALS clinic, but this service is unreliable in many areas. State-funded home-based community care is also available in a few centers for those who are severely disabled (confined to a bed or chair over 50 percent of the waking day), in which home-based carers visit the home three times per week to wash and provide some care relief to the family.

However, despite these noble efforts to provide basic palliative care for South Africans in need, the poorest individuals living in informal housing continue to suffer substantial indignity while battling with ALS. The toilets in these areas comprise mobile communal facilities, often in unpaved surroundings and completely unsuitable for wheelchairs. It is heart-breaking to hear how patients who have become chair- or bed-bound must be carried to toilets to relieve themselves during all kinds of weather (personal observations).

The needs of ALS patients in the developing world are therefore very different to those in well-resourced areas. Despite these limitations, the state does provide certain items to improve patient comfort for those with ALS. The occupational health team supplies solid support (adjustable wooden structures) for patients to put on their beds to assist with turning in bed for those with flail arms or breathing for those with orthopnea (see later in the text). However, non-invasive ventilation equipment is not provided by the state, and patients are reliant on the availability of limited stock on loan from the MND Association.

Non-governmental Organization Support Structures in South Africa

The MND Association is a registered non-profit organization and a member of the MND/ALS International Alliance. It was founded in 1990 in the Western Cape province. Within four years, it became affiliated to the Hospice Palliative Care Association (HPCA) of South Africa and expanded to the northern and eastern regions of the country. Although there are presently 140 hospice facilities affiliated to the HPCA that are independently run across South Africa, ten had to close in 2018 due to financial constraints. These hospices are mostly reliant on international donations as they only receive 10 percent of their funding from the government (Gwyther, personal communication; www.timeslive.co.za/news/southafrica/2018-08-07).

The MND Association relies almost solely on donations and bequests, and fundraising is increasingly difficult due to an economically constrained environment. It is managed from a one-person office with branches in a few of the larger cities spanning South Africa. The patient/family advisors mainly have nursing or palliative care backgrounds. In Cape Town, the advisors attend the monthly ALS clinics to interact with families at the two Cape Town academic hospitals, and they maintain regular contact with their patients through home visits and phone calls. While the Association provides support for all sufferers of ALS and advice on care and counseling, they also facilitate the loan of medical equipment from their stocks to those who have been identified by the ALS clinics to need equipment, such as non-invasive ventilation machines.

CURRENT SERVICES AND MEASURES TO STRENGTHEN PALLIATIVE CARE

The Department of Health has identified the need to expand the delivery of palliative care to other provinces in South Africa, increase the number of health care workers trained in palliative care, improve the availability of morphine and increase the number of palliative care beds at all district levels. By 2022, it hopes to have achieved these goals, with 60 percent coverage of all national districts. Few patients in South Africa have health care insurance. Specialist multidisciplinary ALS clinics are available at three main teaching hospitals: Groote Schuur Hospital (University of Cape Town), Tygerberg Hospital (Stellenbosch University) in Cape Town and the Chris Hani Baragwanath Hospital in Soweto (University of Witwatersrand). Here, patients will receive comprehensive care from the neurology team for symptomatic therapies, speech therapy to assess and discuss the option of placing a percutaneous endoscopic gastrostomy (PEG) tube, dieticians for supplemental feeds, occupational therapists and physiotherapists. As stated earlier, the MND/ALS Association has numerous non-invasive ventilation devices for loan at no cost, but patients often need to wait due to limited availability. The request and provision of tracheostomies and invasive home-based ventilation is not an option in this resource-limited setting. By contrast, ALS sufferers living outside the major population centers have very limited access to a multidisciplinary team.

Home-based nurse care teams can provide basic nursing assessment and support, but legislation does not allow them to dispense drugs such as liquid morphine. These drugs are available only at the ALS clinics, at tertiary hospitals and at select community-based clinics within the coverage area of the few district hospitals offering palliative care. Given the shortage of doctors on the continent, Uganda has led the way in decentralizing the administration of palliation medicine by allowing nurses to dispense liquid morphine to their home-based terminal patients for pain relief in terminal cancer (Lohman; www.health-e.org.za/2013/09/19; accessed 2 Feb 2019).

A neglected area is the need to recognize the burden of the caregivers of those reaching the end of their independent life. The state provides a small caregivers grant (less than $30 per month), but caregivers frequently sacrifice their own livelihood, education and resources to look after their loved ones. In Kenya, Grant et al. (2003) reported that caregivers often do not discuss their difficulties within the family for fear of becoming vulnerable to "evil forces."

CULTURAL ISSUES: PROCESSES REQUIRED FOR HAVING A "GOOD DEATH" IN SOUTH AFRICA

In Africa, most people consult both Western biomedicine practitioners and traditional healers. However, many people, more so in the rural and semi-urban areas, consult with traditional healers as their preferred source for culturally appropriate spiritual advice (Graham et al. 2013). In a study conducted in South Africa, interviews with isiXhosa-speaking traditional healers about death and dying revealed that, during the dying process, the spiritual aspects of suffering were considered more important than the physical ones (Graham et al. 2013). Despite this, traditional healers felt that Western biomedicine and the dying person's family were the principal role players in palliative care.

A study conducted at Soweto's Chris Hani Baragwanath Hospital palliative care center, in which people with advanced cancer were interviewed, found that most patients did not want to acknowledge that they were terminally ill, that they did not want to know their prognosis and similarly that they had not had a conversation about end-of-life preferences with their doctor (Shen et al. 2018). Nevertheless, 80 percent of 221 patients indicated that, as they approach the end of life, their wishes would be to focus on comfort care rather than having aggressive life-extending measures implemented by their physicians (Shen et al. 2018).

In Xhosa culture, death is viewed as a collective family affair. This aligns with the African philosophy of *ubuntu* in which a person is only a person through his interaction with other people (in Graham et al. 2013). The spoken word and end-of-life conversations are considered important for comforting the dying person, to allow the dying person to express their "after-life" wishes and to allow for the opportunity to restore relationships. Following the last wishes of a dying person will allow the person to have a "good death" and therefore an easier passage to the spiritual world where they will continue to occupy an important role as an ancestor and guardian of the happiness of the remaining family and community. The sense of connectedness to family roots and the ancestors often determines the strong motivation to die not in institutions but close to the ancestral home (Graham et al. 2013). Graham et al. (2013) emphasize the importance of awareness among health care providers practicing in multicultural environments and that different communities may have different psychosocial needs for an end-of-life palliative care service.

Interestingly, part of having a good death in many African cultures is to receive a proper, public funeral (Gysels et al. 2011). Indeed, even poor South Africans without health or life insurance will have a funeral plan (Shen et al. 2018).

LEGALIZING PHYSICIAN-ASSISTED SUICIDE IN SOUTH AFRICA

Suicide and attempted suicide are legal in South Africa. While assisted suicide is generally considered unlawful, the Appellate Division (now the Supreme Court of Appeal) in a seminal case on the issue avoided a definitive determination of whether this will always be the case (Burchell 2016). The cessation or withdrawal of life-sustaining medical treatment is lawful and regulated by the Health Professions Council of South Africa (South African Law Commission 1998; www.hpcsa.co.za). While voluntary active euthanasia is unlawful, sentences handed down by the courts tend to be lenient. A case in point is that of Professor Sean Davison, who is not a clinician but an active advocate for assisted suicide and who received a short, partially suspended sentence of house arrest following a conviction on three counts of premeditated murder for assisting several individuals in dying (Nombembe 2019). Thus, there is little policy governing the process of assisted dying. This is concerning, since there are already instances in which doctors assist terminally ill patients in dying with dignity, but this happens behind closed doors to avoid criminal sanction (http://saflii. org/za/cases/ZAGPJHC/2010/129.html, 2010).

There have been some developments in South Africa around this issue. In 2015, a High Court judgment granted a man suffering from terminal cancer permission to be assisted in ending his life. While this was subsequently overturned by the Supreme Court of Appeal, the Court did note that a development of the law with respect to assisted dying was imminent, particularly given developments in foreign jurisdictions. Furthermore, in 2019, the National Health Amendment Bill, which aims to give legal recognition to advance directives and living wills (which are currently not legally binding in South Africa), was introduced to Parliament. However, lawmakers appear reluctant to address this sensitive and controversial issue as there has been no parliamentary response to the South African Law Commission's comprehensive *Report on Euthanasia and the Artificial Preservation of Life*, which was published in 1998.

Nevertheless, South Africa does appear to be following the global trend and slowly moving toward accepting patient autonomy regarding the end-of-life decisions (Jacobs 2018; Jacobs and Henricks 2018). DignitySA is a prominent non-profit organization which advocates "for the right of the individual to self-autonomy in end-of-life decisions" by challenging existing laws and educating South Africans on their rights (https://dignity-southafrica.org/). This is largely based on the rights to dignity and bodily integrity contained in the Bill of Rights in the South African Constitution.

Proposed Priorities for South African Policy Makers to Support ALS/MND

1. Recognition of the important work being performed by non-governmental organizations such as the MND/ALS Association and hospices.
2. Expansion of the training and support for community nurses/care-givers to provide palliative care for ALS outside of the metropolitan areas.
3. Accessibility of low-cost symptomatic therapies, such as oral morphine for dyspnea-associated anxiety or the availability of atropine eye drops to be used off-label for excessive drooling of saliva, in primary and secondary hospitals and clinics away from the centers.
4. Expansion and support for ancillary medical services, such as speech therapy, and dietetics, occupational therapy and physiotherapy to train family members to perform basic chest physiotherapy for clearing secretions.
5. Development of national policies to provide culturally appropriate implementation of palliative services at all levels of society (Ddungu 2011).
6. Awareness of and provision for the support and needs of caregivers.

Proposed Research Priorities in South Africa for ALS

Although research on ALS in Africa has until very recently been largely neglected, in South Africa there is a definite shift to change this, largely due to the establishment of research partnerships with international collaborators. The ALS Association is funding a project at the University of Cape Town, in which currently used ALS cognitive screening and assessment batteries are being adjusted to be more linguistically and culturally appropriate for use in South African ALS patients, namely, South African English, Afrikaans and isiXhosa speakers (Albertyn, in progress). This will allow the accurate phenotyping of cognition and behavior in African ALS patients. The isiXhosa version can easily be adapted to other Nguni languages, such as isiZulu.

The ALS Association is also funding an international project that includes two sites in South Africa in which resource materials and policies are being developed specifically for younger caregivers, that is, the children/adolescents of family members affected by ALS (Kavanaugh, forthcoming). In addition, the University of Cape Town is participating in the Rare Diseases- and NIH-funded CReATe ALS phenotype, genotype and biomarker discovery program led by Michael Benatar at the University of Miami. This is the first time that an African site is participating in an international ALS genomic study.

Concluding Thoughts

In a developing country such as South Africa, the media shows interest in ALS when a public figure (such as a sports star) develops the disease, but this interest quickly fades when the person dies. There is a great need for ongoing appeals to buy equipment and support for non-governmental organizations such as the MND Association. Legal development with respect to assisted dying requires that the public put pressure on lawmakers to address and draft clear policy in response to this issue (Jacobs 2018).

Presently, only symptomatic therapies are offered to most patients with ALS in South Africa. Furthermore, few patients are offered genetic testing outside of a research environment, and most patients will never have access to electronic communication devices. Therefore, in a resource-constrained environment such as ours, the ongoing support from the global ALS research community and patient advocacy groups is vital. Being part of the broader community makes everyone feel that they are fighting ALS in some meaningful way. This extends to recognizing an alternate pricing structure for potential participants from lower- and lower-middle-income countries to attend international ALS meetings so their voices may be heard. There is much to do, and Africa wants to—and should be—part of the solution.

Acknowledgments The authors wish to thank Drs Roger Cummins and Clint Cupido for their helpful comments.

References

Burchell, J. (2016). *Principles of Criminal Law*, 5th ed. Cape Town: Juta & Co Ltd.

Centner, C.M., K.J. Bateman and J.M. Heckmann (2013). Manifestations of HIV infection in the peripheral nervous system. *Lancet Neurology* 12 (3): 295–309. https://doi.org/10.1016/S1474-4422(13)70002-4.

Ddungu, H. (2011). Palliative care: what approaches are suitable in developing countries? *British Journal of Haematology* 154 (6): 728–35. https://doi.org/10.1111/j.1365-2141.2011.08764.x.

Dekker, M. C. J., S.J. Urasa, M.B. Aerts and W.P. Howlett (2018). Motor neuron disease in sub-Saharan Africa: case series from a Tanzanian referral hospital. *Journal of Neurology, Neurosurgery and Psychiatry* 89 (12): 1349–50. https://doi.org/10.1136/jnnp-2017-317858.

Graham, N., L. Gwyther, T. Tiso and R. Harding (2013). Traditional healers' views of the required processes for a "good death" among Xhosa patients pre- and post-death. *Journal of Pain Symptom Management* 46 (3): 386–94. https://doi.org/10.1016/j.jpainsymman.2012.08.005.

Grant, E., S.A. Murray, A. Grant and J. Brown (2003). A good death in rural Kenya? Listening to Meru patients and their families talk about care needs at the end of life. *Journal of Palliative Care* 19 (3): 159–67. https://www.ncbi.nlm.nih.gov/pubmed/14606327.

Gwyther, L., R. Krause, C. Cupido, J. Stanford et al. (2018). The development of hospital-based palliative care services in public hospitals in the Western Cape, South Africa. *South African Medical Journal* 108 (2): 86–89.

Gysels, M., C. Pell, L. Straus and R. Pool (2011). End of life care in sub-Saharan Africa: a systematic review of the qualitative literature. *BMC Palliative Care* 10: 6. https://doi.org/10.1186/1472-684X-10-6.

Henry, K.A., J. Fagliano, H.M. Jordan, L. Rechtman and W.E. Kaye (2015). Geographic Variation of Amyotrophic Lateral Sclerosis Incidence in New Jersey, 2009–2011. *American Journal of Epidemiology* 182 (6): 512–19.

Jacobs, R.K. (2018). Legalising physician-assisted suicide in South Africa: should it even be considered. *South African Journal of Bioethics Law* 11 (2): 66–69.

Jacobs, R.K. and M. Hendricks (2018). Medical students' perspectives on euthanasia and physician-assisted suicide and their views on legalising these practices in South Africa. *South African Medical Journal* 108 (6): 484–89.

Logroscino, G., B.J. Traynor, O. Hardiman, A. Chio et al. (2010). Incidence of amyotrophic lateral sclerosis in Europe. *J Neurol Neurosurg Psychiatry* 81 (4): 385–90.

Mehta, P., W. Kaye, J. Raymond et al. (2018). Prevalence of Amyotrophic Lateral Sclerosis—United States, 2014. *MMWR Morb Mortal Wkly* Rep 67: 216–18.

Mombaur, B. and J.M. Heckmann (2015). Myasthenia gravis is a rare but treatable disease. *South African Medical Journal* 105 (8): 619. Retrieved from.

Nel, M., G.M. Agenbag, F. Henning, H.M. Cross, A. Esterhuizen and J.M. Heckmann (2019). C9orf72 repeat expansions in South Africans with amyotrophic lateral sclerosis. *Journal of Neurological Sciences* 401: 51–54.

Nombembe, P. (2019, June 19). Right-to-die activist Sean Davison gets three years' house arrest for murders. *Times LIVE* https://www.timeslive.co.za/news/south-africa/2019-06-19-right-to-die-activist-sean-davison-gets-three-years-house-arrest-for-murders/ (accessed 28 July 2019).

Shen, M.J., H.G. Prigerson and M. Ratshikana-Moloko (2018). Illness understanding and end-of-life care communication and preferences for patients with advanced cancer in South Africa. *Journal of Global Oncology* 4: 1–9. https://doi.org/10.1200/JGO.17.00160.

South African Law Commission. (1998). *Report on Euthanasia and the Artificial Preservation of Life*. Project 86; 79–80.

Weru, J. (2017). Most people in Africa don't have access to palliative care. This needs to change. https://theconversation.com/africa.

WEBSITES

www.westerncape.gov.za.

www.statssa.gov.za.

https://www.brandsouthafrica.com/south-africa-fast-facts/health-facts/health-care-in-south-africa. last accessed 2 Feb 2019.

https://hpca.co.za.

www.timeslive.co.za/news/southafrica/2018-08-07.

www.health-e.org.za/2013/09/19; accessed 2 Feb 2019.

https://www.hpcsa.co.za/Uploads/editor/UserFiles/downloads/conduct_ethics/Booklet%207.pdf.

http://saflii.org/za/cases/ZAGPJHC/2010/129.html at para 14.

https://dignitysouthafrica.org/.

CHAPTER 19

Public Policy in ALS Care: South Korea

Seung Hyun Kim, Kiwook Oh, and Bugyeong Son

Abstract Amyotrophic lateral sclerosis (ALS) in South Korea is designated as a rare disease. Therefore, medical expenses for the affected patients and finances related to essential medical facilities are supported by the government under the Rare Disease Management Act. The Act on Welfare of Persons with Disabilities provides additional assistance for disabled patients. The Korean ALS Association, Seungil Hope Foundation and Lou Gehrig's Network are three main patient advocacy groups supporting patients and families, raising awareness of ALS throughout the community and influencing policy change. National Health Insurance covers the entire Korean population. Therefore, all basic medical benefits are provided to all citizens regardless of their income. However, the

S. H. Kim (✉)
Department of Neurology, Hanyang University Medical Center,
Seoul, Republic of Korea
e-mail: kimsh1@hanyang.ac.kr

K. Oh
College of Medicine, Hanyang University, Seoul, Republic of Korea
e-mail: kiwook-oh@hanyang.ac.kr

B. Son
Hanyang University Medical Center, Seoul, Republic of Korea
e-mail: sonbugyeong@hanyang.ac.kr

© The Author(s) 2021
R. H. Blank et al. (eds.), *Public Policy in ALS/MND Care*,
https://doi.org/10.1007/978-981-15-5840-5_19

247

payments for uninsured services, which include alternative treatments and precision medicine, require out-of-pocket payment, which financially challenges patients. Increasing support for caregivers and providing equal medical access across the nation are problems to be resolved.

Keywords ALS • Rare Disease Management Act • Korean ALS Association • Seungil Hope Foundation • Palliative care

INCIDENCE AND PREVALENCE OF ALS

The Republic of Korea (ROK) has a population of 51 million. The mean annual incidence for amyotrophic lateral sclerosis (ALS) is 1.20/100,000, the prevalence rate is 3.43/100,000 and the mean age of diagnosis is 61.4. The gender ratio (male: female) is 1.60. When including other types of motor neuron diseases (G12.2~G12.28), the incidence and prevalence is increased twofold. Sporadic ALS (G12.21)-diagnosed individuals across all motor neuron disease (MND) cases (G12.20~G12.28) are approximately 50 percent. Of those with MND, familial ALS (G12.20, KCD-6) represents about 2 percent of the full MND spectrum. Across the MND spectrum, the combined proportion of G12.22 (primary lateral sclerosis), G12.23 (progressive bulbar palsy) and G12.24 (progressive muscular atrophy) is less than 10 percent (Jun et al. 2018).

RARE DISEASE MANAGEMENT ACT

The Korean Ministry of Health and Welfare (MOHW) has designated ALS/MND as a rare disease. In Korea, the Rare Disease Management Act defined rare disease as a disease affecting fewer than 20,000 patients or for which the prevalence is unknown because of its rarity or difficulty in diagnosis. Under the MND category, familial and sporadic ALS, primary lateral sclerosis, progressive bulbar palsy, progressive muscular atrophy and X-linked spinobulbar muscular atrophy are designated as rare diseases (Ministry of Health and Welfare 2019).

The purpose of the Rare Disease Management Act is to reduce individual and social burdens caused by rare diseases and to contribute to improving people's health and welfare by setting and implementing comprehensive policies on the prevention, treatment and research of rare diseases.

State and local governments have implemented education and publicity projects concerning rare disease management. Projects extend from public government level to each patient. May 23 of each year is designated as Rare Disease Day in order to enhance understanding of rare diseases among the public and encourage the will to prevent, treat and manage rare diseases. MOHW formulates a comprehensive rare disease management plan every five years and established the Management Committee and Rare Disease Support Center.

The designation of regional rare disease hub centers has also been expanded. There were four hub centers in 2018, which was extended to eleven in 2019. Regional hub centers support diagnosis through a diagnosis-management network and enhance professional consultation and education for patients and family. In addition, the central hub also supports the development of networks among the regional hub centers, in this way constructing networks across the regional hub centers. By doing so, MOHW plans to eliminate uneven treatment between the metropolitan and rural areas by allowing residents in less populated districts to receive continuous disease management.

Most importantly, since July 2007, once diagnosed with ALS, the patient pays 10 percent of their medical expenditure and the government covers the rest, including the purchase of assistive technologies, the expenses of providing care, ventilator rent and cough-assist machines. With the revision in September 2018, the approach to the treatment of rare diseases is being strengthened and medical expenses are alleviated. MOHW introduced a post-facto approval system, so that the medicines and treatment for rare diseases would be accessed quickly for actual treatment.

Based on patients' economic capabilities to bear expenses, the state and local governments may provide supplementary financial support for necessary expenses for the diagnosis and treatment of rare diseases. When patients are diagnosed with ALS, they can also apply for additional economic support under the Act regarding Support for Catastrophic Health Expenditures. The purpose of this Act is to promote social security and help protect the national health by increasing healthcare access through partially subsidizing costs for citizens who suffer economic difficulties arising from excessive healthcare expenses relative to their income. For instance, MOWH and the Korean National Health Insurance Service (NIHS) subsidize out-of-pocket payment charged for diagnostic examinations. The eligibility criteria are set based upon the characteristics of the disease, household conditions and necessity of support. The amount of aid is provided up to 50 percent of the total medical expense, or 20,000 USD.

FIGHTING THE DISEASE

Riluzole is approved and widely used in Korea. When the patient is diagnosed as clinically definite or probable ALS by El-Escorial Criteria, NHIS covers 90 percent of the cost which results in patients paying approximately 1 USD per pill. Edaravone (Radicut) was approved in 2015 and is available nationwide. The cost is not covered by the NIHS but can be reimbursed by the patient's private health insurance. Additionally, under Medicine Law, any procedure that includes an intravenous injection must be performed in a medical institution by medical personnel; thus, patients must commute or be admitted to a hospital to receive an edaravone injection.

Stem cell therapy (Neuronata-R, Lenzumestrocel) was developed in Korea and designated as an orphan drug by the Korean Ministry of Health and Drug Safety (MFDS) in 2014, as well as the U.S. FDA and EMA in 2018. The treatment strategy is based on stem cells' own functions including stimulating intrinsic neurogenesis, releasing diverse neurotrophic factors and modulating the immune-inflammatory processes. Since its commercialization in 2015, over 250 patients have received the treatment. There are a growing number of tourist patients from overseas that receive stem cell treatment in Korea.

Nuedexta became accessible by way of revisions to the Enforcement Decree of the Narcotics Control Act in 2018. With a doctor's recommendation letter and medical reports which demonstrate the possible benefit from Nuedexta, a patient can obtain an Approval for Handling Narcotic Drugs for Personal use from the MFDS and start the importing process through the Korean Orphan and Essential Drug Center (KODC).

CLINICAL TRIALS AND INNOVATIVE RESEARCH

Research in ALS is supported by the Rare Disease Management Act. The government supports necessary expenses in performing research projects, diagnosis and treatment of the disease, and education and training of professionals. State and local governments may give additional administrative and financial support to persons who produce or sell medications for the diagnosis and treatment of rare diseases, including tax support as prescribed by the Restriction of Special Taxation Act. Hence, greater support is available from the public sector as compared to the private. There are three major funding resources in the field of medical research.

1. National Research Foundation (NRF), https://www.nrf.re.kr/eng/index

   The NRF was established in 2009 by the Ministry of Science & ICT for the purpose of setting the direction of the nation's basic and applied research across all academic disciplines. NRF is the nation's largest funder of science research. In 2019, the total budget was 5.23 billion USD. Academic research and university funding amounted to 1.64 billion USD (31.3%) and National Strategic R&D Programs funding amounted to 1.67 billion USD (31.9%).

2. Korea Health Industry Development Institute (KHIDI), www.khidi.or.kr

   The KHIDI was established in 1999. It is a government-affiliated institution which performs professional and systematic support to develop the national health industry and enhance health services. In 2019, the total budget was 2.91 billion USD.

3. Korean Drug Development Fund (KDDF), http://eng.kddf.org/

   The KDDF was established in 2011 for the purpose of supporting novel drug developments. The total project budget was 890 million USD (445 million USD from the government and 445 million USD from the private sector) between 2011 and 2020.

Reports on the implementation of national R & D projects have been registered in the National Digital Science Library (NDSL, http://www.ndsl.kr). As of September 2019, 58 ALS national R & D reports have been registered.

Use of Clinical Drugs for Therapeutic Purpose

The Korea National Enterprise for Clinical Trials (KoNECT) analyzed the U.S. National Institutes of Health registered clinical trial protocol world-wide data and announced that Korea ranked sixth (3.5%) in the share of clinical trial protocols, exceeded only by the US (24.5%), Germany (5.3%), UK (5.0%), Canada (3.9%) and China (3.7%). A growing number of rare disease clinical trials was also reported (Yoo 2018).

The authorization of new drug takes a long time because it requires a thorough review process by the Minister of Food and Drug Safety (MFDS). Waiting for this authorization process of new drug can be viewed as cruel for patients with rare and intractable diseases that currently have no treatment. Therefore, providing new treatment opportunities before their authorization can be argued from a humanitarian perspective. However, patients are not permitted to pay for research drugs. According to Article 34 of the Pharmaceutical Affairs Act, pre-authorized use of clinical trial drugs is described as follows:

> No drugs manufactured or imported after being manufactured for the purpose of clinical trials shall be used for any purpose other than for clinical trials. Provided that where the Minister of Food and Drug Safety has granted approval, the drugs for medical treatment of any of the following persons can be used for any purpose other than for clinical trials as prescribed by Ordinance of the Prime Minister: 1. A patient with a serious life-threatening disease, such as terminal cancer or AIDS; 2. An emergency patient prescribed by Ordinance of the Prime Minister, such as a patient whose life is threatened and a patient without alternative means of treatment.

Article 34, then, partially allows the use of pre-licensed, clinical trial drugs. If the doctor decides to use pre-licensed clinical trial drugs for patients who meet the description in the Article, the doctor may apply for the "use of clinical drugs for therapeutic purposes" (Ministry of Food and Drugs Safety 2018). The application would proceed through the MFDS and the Institutional Review Board (IRB) review. In this process, informed consent by the patient as well as a Letter of Intent to Provide from the manufacturer of clinical trial drugs are required. Most of the expenses are covered by the research fund or the study drug manufacturer.

STATUS OF MULTIDISCIPLINARY TEAM CARE AND CLINICS

There is only one multidisciplinary ALS clinic in Korea registered by the World Federation of Neurology Research Group on Motor Neuron Diseases—Amyotrophic Lateral Sclerosis (WFNALS), the Hanyang ALS Clinic. However, there are 42 tertiary hospitals which have twenty or more specialized departments and have medical specialists exclusively dedicated to each department. Patients can easily have consultations with multiple specialists in one hospital.

THE ENFORCEMENT DECREE OF THE ACT ON WELFARE OF PERSONS WITH DISABILITIES

The MOHW supports ALS patients' daily activities with a disability policy enacted under the enforcement decree of the Act on Welfare of Persons with Disabilities (Act No 14892). The disability policy has five categories:

- Reorganization of welfare and health support system
- Education, culture, sports and opportunities guarantee
- Strengthening of economic independence
- Enhancement of rights and security
- Activation of social participation

Patients with physical difficulties, despite the diagnosis, can apply for a disability certificate with their local government. The government officials review his/her medical report and visit the household in person to examine and determine the severity of the disability. Then, the patient may consult the official and apply for various support programs to the appropriate extent according to the disability. The following are key programs from which most ALS patients receive help:

1. Disability Activity Assistance: Persons with severe disabilities and difficulty in performing daily and social activities alone may receive vouchers, depending on their activity assistance eligibility assessment and living conditions. The vouchers are issued to provide home-visit bathing and nursing care, housework and physical and social activity support. Depending on the severity and household income, patients pay up to 15 percent of the expense.
2. Disability Pension: Persons aged over 18 with severe disabilities whose income, including that of their spouse, is equal to or less than the eligibility threshold can be provided a disability pension of up to 250 USD/month.
3. Assistive Device Support: State and local governments support the expense for buying or renting assistive devices. Patients pay up to 10 percent of the total expense but can only apply for each device once a limited time period depending on the devices. There are 88 devices listed, including a wheelchair (electronic, automatic, light weight, reclining, tilted, etc.), air mattress, posture support tools and ankle support braces.

THE MOST ACTIVE ALS ASSOCIATIONS AND ADVOCACY GROUPS

The Korean ALS Association (KALSA) was founded in 2000 and currently has more than 2000 members. It communicates with patients, families, doctors and researchers to share information on new treatments and care methods, induce policy changes and stimulate social awareness. Through an annual academic conference and regular meetings, it opens a forum for communication and education among its members. Furthermore, KALSA supports patients' out-of-pocket medical expenses, funds research and provides feeding formulas for patients on a quarterly basis. Patients may also apply for medical supplies such as gauze, suction catheters, sterilized gloves and Ambu bags. KALSA supports self-help groups in each region where patients and families exchange information on fighting the disease and share tips for daily activities (Korean ALS Association 2019).

Another active group is the Seungil Hope Foundation. Seongil Park, an ALS patient, a former basketball player and the youngest professional basketball coach, established a foundation for ALS patients. He published a book written with his eyeball tracking mouse titled "Write Hope with the Eye." He has worked actively in various communities and contributed greatly in informing the public about the seriousness of the disease and giving hope to patients. The Foundation is currently working toward three goals: building an ALS specialized hospital, providing practical support for patients and families and creating an enjoyable donation culture. In addition, the Foundation supports the purchase of medical equipment and supplies for patients, supports tuition for patients' children and provides emergency medical expenses for gastrostomy and tracheostomy.

Finally, the Lou Gehrig's Disease Network is the most active online community for sharing information about ALS. There are 6000 members including patients, families, friends, doctors and researchers, and around 500–600 members visit its website in a day. It is free and extremely easy to use, providing means to socialize, seek and offer support and learn about the illness.

Currently there are no cohort or nation-wide surveys regarding ALS caregivers. However, it was found that 92.1 percent of ALS patients are at home, 6.6 percent in general hospitals and 1.3 percent in tertiary hospitals. However, because of how the disease progresses, most of the patients end up receiving breathing assistance through a tracheostomy and nutritional assistance through gastrostomy, which result in being completely dependent on the help of others. Such characteristics put a large burden on caregivers. However, patients who require respiratory assistance are not often admitted to long-term care facilities because of the high needs of professional care, or because medical costs may exceed affordable levels.

In all, 56.8 percent of home-residing ALS patients are provided care by family members and 42.3 percent of the patients hire a formal caregiver. Among them, 22.6 percent of patients received government subsidies based on disability policies, 10.9 percent from long-term care insurance systems for the elderly and 8.8 percent from hired private caregivers.

There is a shortage of medical care facilities with personnel who have a good understanding of the disease and take care of ALS patients. Especially due to the difficulty in assistance with tube feeding, ambulatory support, managing medical devices such as BiPAP, preparing for emergency care and care for the patient's psychological burdens, ALS patients are not always welcome in general nursing homes for an extended time. Based within the Seungil Hope Foundation, there is currently a movement to build a systematic care structure through the construction of a medical care hospital which specializes in care for ALS patients, helping patients and their families rehabilitate and providing a shared facility in cooperation with local communities.

GENETIC TESTING OF PATIENTS WITH ALS

Genetic testing for several common genes such as *SOD1, FUS, SMN1, ATXN2, PABPN1, SPAST, SPG11* is available within the coverage of NHI, with the patient paying 10 to 50 percent of the cost. Genetic tests such as NGS, WES or WGS can be performed for research purposes at no additional cost to the patient. Genetic counseling is usually provided by a physician with the help of clinical genetics departments. The Personal Information Protection Act and Bioethics and Safety Act are main statutes designed to regulate the protection of patients' privacy and information. Under these acts, patient's genetic information cannot be given to others without their consent. Furthermore, presenting a distinct distribution of genetic variants, Korean ALS patients may have a different genetic background from other ethnic groups. Mutations of common genes found in the European population, including *C9orf72, TARDp* and *OPTN* have not been found in Korean ALS patients.

KOREAN ORIENTAL MEDICINE

Korean oriental medicine is a distinctive feature whose practice originated and developed in Korea. Under the Korean Medicine Law, "medical personnel" refers to a physician, a dentist, an oriental medical doctor, a midwife or a nurse who holds a license granted by the MOHW. They administer oriental medical treatment including acupuncture, prescribe herbal drugs and provide guidance for health promotion based on a systematic oriental medicine perspective. Acupuncture and herb medication are easily accessible in local oriental medical clinics and people consider them beneficial for pain management. The cost is partly covered under the NIH except liquid form herbal medicine.

END-OF-LIFE CARE

Home Healthcare Nurses

A home healthcare certified nurse provides care under the Medicine Law. A doctor writes a request letter to the hospital in the patient's district and the hospital sends a health-care specialized nuse to the patient's home. The service includes taking blood and urine samples for examination, administering medication prescribed by a doctor, consulting or educating the patient and their caregivers, exchanging tracheostomy and gastrostomy tubes and taking care of pressure sores. In Korea 120 hospitals provide home healthcare nurses, and ALS patients pay only 10 percent of the cost.

Hospice and Palliative Care

No types of euthanasia are allowed in Korea. The Act on Hospice and Palliative Care and Decisions on Life-sustaining Treatment for Patients at the End of Life came into effect in 2018. The Act was enacted to protect the dignity and value of human beings by ensuring the best interests of the patients and by respecting their self-determination of life-sustaining treatment. Key sections include:

1. Determination to terminate life-sustaining treatment: Patients undergoing end-of-life care can decide to withhold life-sustaining treatment or to terminate it. At least two doctors must verify the details of the patient's advance statement to implement such a determination.
2. Advance statement on life-sustaining treatment: Korean citizens over 19 years old can provide a written statement regarding their own determination to terminate life-sustaining treatment and hospice care. The MOHW has designated 300 regional healthcare institutions, hospitals, a non-profit organization and public institutions for one-to-one consultation and registration.
3. Hospice care: The MOHW implements hospice projects with following aims to develop and disseminate guidelines for controlling

symptoms, including appropriate pain management for terminal patients; establish and operate hospitals, counseling and home hospices; research and develop projects for hospice care; foster institutions specialized in hospice care and training of human resources; develop hospice education programs for terminal patients and families; and support medical expenses to minimize economic burden of patients. However, diseases which warrant patients eligible for hospice care are limited to cancer, AIDS, chronic obstructive pulmonary disease (COPD), chronic liver cirrhosis or any other disease by ordinance of the MOHW, but currently do not include ALS.

Since its implementation in 2018, the number of cases which have carried out a patient's will to end treatment has been constantly growing. In January 2019, a total of 35,994 patients followed through with their end-of-life decision, and by August the number grew to 62,546 (National Agency for Management of Life-Sustaining Treatment 2019). The policy is still in its early phase, and the Ministry is cautious with regards to giving the patients' desire to end treatment top priority. Furthermore, considering the Korean culture in which the family decision is as important as the patient's, the frequent revision of the policy will likely continue.

OVERVIEW OF KOREAN MEDICAL POLICY

Healthcare Financing

The MOHW plays the central role in health policy at the national level. As a compulsory social insurance, the Korean Health Insurance (NHI) covers the entire population. The Ministry makes NHI policy and the National Health Insurance Service (NHIS) manages the NHI as a single insurer. The NHI provides service benefits (healthcare benefits, health check-ups) or cash benefits (care expense, co-payment ceiling system, compensation for excessive co-payment, appliance expenses for the disabled, pregnancy and childbirth examination expenses). The Health Insurance Review and Assessment Service (HIRA) is responsible for claim reviews, assessment of the appropriateness of healthcare, technical support to benefit packages and the design of the provider payment system.

Persons who receive healthcare pay certain portions of the healthcare costs as co-payments. Most people have a co-payment rate of 20 percent for inpatient care, 30–60 percent for outpatient care and 30–50 percent for pharmacy copayments (NHI 2019). The co-payment ratio varies according to the level and type of medical care institution. NHIS distinguishes citizens between workplace subscribers and local subscribers. Workplace subscribers are employees and users of a company, government employees and faculty and their dependents. The remainder are local subscribers. In 2018, 70.4 percent were workplace subscribers, 26.8 percent local subscribers and 2.8 percent got medical benefits for public aid under the National Basic Living Security Act. Employees pay 3 to 6 percent of their total salary to NIH, depending on their income, district and family situation.

In addition, there is private insurance to cover out-of-pocket expenses. According to the Insurance Report 2018, 60 percent of Korean citizens pay into at least one private insurance to cover out-of-pocket expenses of major diseases such as cancer, stroke and cardiovascular disease, and 28.6 percent have indemnity medical insurance.

Healthcare Delivery System

The Korean healthcare delivery system was introduced in 1989 to promote convenience for its citizens, efficiency of medical resources, balanced healthcare development across the country, efficient and effective use of national medical resources and fiscal stability.

Medical institutions are divided into three categories: community clinics, general hospitals (medium-sized hospitals) and tertiary hospitals (superior general hospitals). Community clinics provide primary care services in which the principal goal is to maintain health and disease control for local residents. General hospitals act as community hospitals, which meet hospitalization demands in most communities or serve as specialized hospitals in a local area. Superior general hospitals treat severely ill patients, educate about health and medical personnel and perform medical research. Patients can go to any doctor or any medical institution depending on their preference, except tertiary hospitals. If the patient wants to go to a secondary or tertiary hospital, or if the doctor recommends the patient visit larger hospitals, a referral letter issued by the doctor is required.

Long-Term Care Insurance Systems for the Elderly

Korea has a social insurance policy that provides support to elderly citizens who have mobility problems due to old age or disease to improve old age health and stable living while decreasing the burden on family. All Korean citizens over 65, or patients with dementia or Parkinson's disease of any age, may apply. The benefits range from aged care facilities to in-home services (home visit care, home visit nursing, home visit bathing, day and night care) and cash benefits. ALS patients pay 15 percent of the service expense.

Under the National Basic Living Security Act, all Korean citizens have a right to a minimum level of living and the government must help by furnishing them with the following benefits: livelihood benefits, housing benefits, medical benefits, education benefits, childbirth benefits, funeral benefits and self-sufficiency benefits. The recipients of each type of benefit will be determined by the MOHW or by the heads of the central administrative agencies with consideration of age, size of a household, area of residence and living conditions.

Medical benefits consist of various tests and treatments necessary for assisting a healthy life. When the medical benefit recipient has received treatment in relation to disease, injury or childbirth, the head of the local government shall pay the equivalent amount. The benefit includes the doctor's consultant, medication, medical supplies, treatment fee, operation fee and administration fee. Even though the recipient must pay out of pocket, they are able to get 50 percent of it reimbursed if the cost is over 20 USD.

DISCUSSION

Thanks to the Ice Bucket challenge and other continuing education efforts, ALS awareness has recently escalated and donations have expanded leading to stronger support and innovative research.

Korea has universal health coverage with ALS being designated as a rare disease. Although the Korean government is actively trying to alleviate the burden placed upon patients and their caregivers as a result of such illnesses, there are a few points that still need to change in order to improve care.

First, despite universal health coverage for the population, out-of-pocket payments remain high. ALS patients spend 7902 USD per month, which increases with disease progression. The direct medical costs amount to 3436 USD, with 44.8 percent of the expense borne by the patient and the rest paid by the government. Even though the NHI has reduced the cost of ALS with the Rare Disease Act, ALS patients still face economic burdens. The cost of new drugs worsens this load, especially since a patient must bear the full cost of orphan drugs which is one of the main obstacles for starting treatment. Despite discussions to expand NIHS support for certain orphan drugs, efforts to add edaravone and stem cell treatment for ALS have to date failed.

The second key area that needs improvement is that of support for caregivers. Family caregivers spend, on average, 95.6 hours per week and professional caregivers spend about 25 hours per week tending to those affected by ALS (Oh et al. 2015). This burden, and the accompanying caregiver costs, increases with disease progression. Moreover, many family members of ALS patients quit their jobs to provide care for the patients. Policies must be implemented to ensure that government-supported professional caregivers, who can provide a high quality of care, are available to care for ALS patients for a longer time. Introducing programs to support the psychological well-being for the caregivers should also be considered.

Lastly, the gap between the metropolitan areas and the rural areas should be diminished. South Korea is approximately 99,720 sq. km., with travel from the North to the South by train taking about three hours. However, patients in rural areas have poorer access to hospitals and healthcare services. Also, among 42 tertiary hospitals which provide high-quality multidisciplinary care, 13 are in Seoul and 8 are in Gyeonggi Province surrounding Seoul. The freedom in selecting a hospital offers advantages, but at the same time, patients prefer tertiary hospitals which often results in long waiting times for treatment. The number of doctors and nurses has been increasing, but the numbers are still below the OECD average with most of them serving metropolitan areas (Kwon et al. 2015). Due to this difference, rural areas must receive more support from the government by way of better-quality hospitals and health delivery systems, to serve as an enhancement to patients being referred from tertiary hospitals to community clinics for continuum of care.

REFERENCES

Jun, K.Y., J. Park, K.-W. Oh et al. (2018). Epidemiology of ALS in Korea using nationwide big data. *Journal of Neurology, Neurosurgery and Psychiatry*, https://doi.org/10.1136/jnnp-2018-318974.

Korean Amyotrophic Lateral Sclerosis Association (2019). http://www.kalsa.org/.

Kwon, S., T.-J. Lee and C.-Y. Kim (2015). Republic of Korea Health System Review, Health Systems in Transition, 5 (4), https://iris.wpro.who.int/bitstream/handle/10665.1/11358/9789290617105_eng.pdf.

Ministry of Food and Drugs Safety (2018). Guideline for use of clinical trial drugs for therapeutic purpose. Seoul, South Korea.

Ministry of Health and Welfare (2019). https://www.socialservice.or.kr:444/user/htmlEditor/view2.do?p_sn=6.

National Agency for Management of Life-Sustaining Treatment (2019). https://www.lst.go.kr

National Health Insurance (2019). http://www.bokjiro.go.kr/welInfo/retrieve WelInfoDetail.do?welInfSno=344.

Oh, J., J.W. An, S.I. Oh, K. Oh et al. (2015). Socioeconomic costs of amyotrophic lateral sclerosis according to staging system. *Amyotrophic Lateral Sclerosis and Frontotemporal Degeneration* 16 (3–4): 202–08.

J. Yoo (2018). KoNECT.

CHAPTER 20

Amyotrophic Lateral Sclerosis Care in Tunisia

Imen Kacem, Ikram Sghaier, Amina Nasri,
and Riadh Gouider

Abstract Amyotrophic lateral sclerosis (ALS) is rare in Tunisia, where access to new etiopathogenic treatment is still limited. In this review, we examine the existing model of care for ALS patients in Tunisia, the law that governs ALS care and how multidisciplinary care is delivered. We also shed light on the clinical particularity of Tunisian ALS patients. We believe that funding challenges for ALS care, improvement of ALS awareness and increased knowledge for ALS management are required. The current challenges of ALS in Tunisia are to ensure coordinated interprofessional care and establish an interdisciplinary model care for people with ALS and their family caregivers as key stakeholders and decision markers.

I. Kacem • A. Nasri • R. Gouider (✉)
Faculty of Medicine of Tunis, University of Tunis El Manar, Tunis, Tunisia
e-mail: drkacemimen@yahoo.fr; dr.nasri.amina@gmail.com;
riadh.gouider@gnet.tn

Department of Neurology, Razi Hospital, La Manouba, Tunis, Tunisia

I. Sghaier
Department of Neurology, Razi Hospital, La Manouba, Tunis, Tunisia
e-mail: sghaiere.ikram@gmail.com

© The Author(s) 2021
R. H. Blank et al. (eds.), *Public Policy in ALS/MND Care*,
https://doi.org/10.1007/978-981-15-5840-5_20

Keywords Amyotrophic lateral sclerosis • Tunisia • Phenotype • Care coordination • Interdisciplinary • Management • Quality of life • Ethics

INCIDENCE, PREVALENCE AND DEATHS OF ALS PATIENTS IN TUNISIA

Through the 1980s, the Tunisian ALS incidence was reported equal to 0.45/100,000, which is lower than what was reported worldwide (Ben Hamida 1990; Beghi 2006; Logroscino 2018). There are several explanations to the incidence variability. First is the sample size of the source population, which was only 102 patients (Ben Hamida 1990). Second is heterogeneity across countries, differences in diagnostic criteria and the inclusion or exclusion of the disease variants. A consistent finding in studies is that there is a slight excess of males affected with ALS. Similarly, our Tunisian data suggest the predominance of male patients with sex ratio of 2.75:1 (Ben Hamida 1990). More recently, data suggest that the gender ratio may be approaching equality as it is the case in our Tunisian population, with sex ratio decrease to 2.0 in our 2019 study (Kacem et al. 2019).

Although there is no specific mortality rate of ALS patients in Tunisia, it was estimated to be 19/million (15–29) motor neuron disease (MND)-related death, with age-standardized mortality rates of MND increased by 15.6 percent (95%UI-22.2 to 54.7) from 1999 to 2016 (Logroscino 2018). Our recent study in the Neurology Department of Razi Hospital, which included 210 patients diagnosed with ALS from 2003 to 2019, reports longer progression among Tunisian population (Kacem et al. 2019). In fact, the median survival time from onset to death was five years. About 8 percent of cases in our cohort have survived more than ten years. The longest survival time was 27 years, with the patient still alive at the end of the study. The overall 1- 2- 3- and 4-year survival rates were 86.7, 74.3, 66.6 and 53.1 percent, respectively.

The longer survival rate reported in the Tunisian population could be explained by younger age of onset (juvenile form), which is more frequent than what is reported in European studies. Additionally, patients were diagnosed early; thus, the disease courses were longer with a slower degenerative process (Luna 2019). Hence, a combination of environmental and genetic factors could orchestrate the clinical phenotype of Tunisian ALS patients. The epidemiological research conducted in Africa (Ben Hamida 1990; Marin 2012; Luna 2019) remains inconclusive, and more efforts are needed to improve the knowledge about the true disease burden in these countries. The efforts that substantially reduce the uncertainty, such as our recent descriptive study (Kacem et al. 2019), will be a major advance toward this goal.

With increasing limitations on resources for healthcare in Tunisia, the priority in this sector is the collection of comprehensive, comparative and global information about the impact of ALS and the risk factors on population health. This priority will be aided by the establishment of a national register which will lead to more useful monitoring national health priorities and ensuring the right time and manner for disease management. Consequently, more effort is needed to obtain data sets on the health of populations in all cities of Tunisia.

Major Governmental Agencies Involved in ALS Care

To date, there has been no government action, reports or committees on ALS in Tunisia. Like other low- and middle-income countries (LMICs), disparities in access to timely ALS care for patients constitute a significant barrier in providing quality healthcare in Tunisia (Peters 2008; Alkire 2015). Adequate health coverage and efficient health systems are necessary to provide access to ALS screening, timely diagnosis and treatment (Jennum 2013). Unfavorable socioeconomic conditions such as high unemployment and low education and income levels are related to higher odds of later ALS diagnosis in advanced stages, leading to rapid death (Jennum 2013). A few studies have reported on the access to ALS care and treatment worldwide, showing significant differences in delays of ALS care by type of healthcare coverage (Mitsumoto 2007; Zoccolella 2007; Hogden 2015), but none has included Tunisia.

The health system in Tunisia is comprised of three main providers: the public health system, social security health insurance and private health insurance. The public healthcare system, financed from the state and the national budgets, ensures universal coverage including access to public hospitals and primary care facilities. Since independence in 1956, Tunisia has established free healthcare for all individuals through a government-funded system, and in 1960, it implemented the social protection system and health insurance.

In order to improve coverage and accessibility to health system care, Tunisia implemented the large-scale reform in 1996 (Achour 2011). Numerous insurance plans covering different professional groups were merged under the Social Security Fund, and it was extended to include the private sector. Furthermore, an optional supplementary health insurance managed by mutual health insurance companies was introduced. In 2004, the Tunisia's National Health Insurance (Caisse Nationale d'Assurance

Maladie (CNAM)) was implemented which provides universal health coverage for those affiliated with the national insurance (Caisse Nationale de Sécurité Sociale (CNSS) and Caisse Nationale de Retraite et de Prévoyance Sociale (CNRPS)). In 2007, CNAM introduced a reimbursement scheme under which beneficiaries can use either public or private providers with payment required first and then reimbursed from CNAM after a request from the affiliated provider (Makhloufi 2015). CNAM is funded by a compulsory payment from the employees and employers. There is also private health insurance which can provide medical care in private hospitals to their beneficiaries.

In summary, all ALS patients have full access to examination by a specialized neurologist. Moreover, the public healthcare system ensures coverage for riluzole for all patients who are members in the social security health insurance. Patients not covered by CNAM, however, are responsible for paying the entire cost. Meanwhile, vitamin therapy, speech therapy and motor rehabilitation treatment are accessible for all Tunisian ALS patients without charge in public institutions. However, while CNAM partially covers the ALS health expenses, it does not cover all costs, especially indirect ones. Moreover, no public or private association or care agencies are involved in managing the cost-effectiveness of treatment for ALS Tunisian patients.

Currently, there is no governmental organization or association for ALS in Tunisia, and neurodegenerative diseases are poorly known. However, in the recent years there has been increased awareness of Alzheimer's disease and the implementation of a governmental organization dedicated to treat and spread the knowledge of it. Hopefully, ALS will receive the same attention in the coming years.

The exponential growth of the science system, the rising costs of conducting health research and financial pressures on governmental budgets have impacted on the funding of health science. Many countries, including Tunisia, have gone through changes in the funding of their universities and the research fields with one of the main trends being creating a balance between the recurrent funding which is provided annually by the university and the external funding of projects. Moreover, classifying ALS as a rare disease poses challenges to investigators and researchers. Consequently, this requires the creation of multi-institutional and international collaborations to conduct clinical investigations in ALS.

PUBLIC FUNDING FOR RESEARCH

Tunisia has relatively low research and development (R&D) intensity. In fact, the gross domestic expenditure on research and development (GERD) accounted for only 0.63 percent of gross domestic product (GDP) in 2015. This represents a continuing downward trend since 2011, bringing the current share of GDP invested in R&D down to the levels of 2003 (UNESCO Institute for Statistics 2018). However, Tunisia still has a higher level of R&D intensity than the average for North Africa and the Arab States and the countries categorized by the World Bank as lower-middle-income economies. In fact, the Science Report of the UNESCO of 2015 points out that a GERD/GDP ratio of around 0.7 percent is close to the average for upper-middle-income economies (Makhloufi 2015). Despite the low proportion of the government sector accounted in GERD, which is equal to 50 percent in Tunisia, the Tunisian GERD/GDP ratio continues to increase. It is noteworthy that R&D activities are constantly increasing; thus, R&D funding needs to be proportionally adjusted.

One of the principal characteristics of the Tunisian research system is the high level of institutional density. Hence, the large number of Tunisian research institutions causes fragmentation in financial and administrative resources as well as problems for knowledge management. The funding by the Ministry of Higher Education and Scientific Research (MESR) suggests a modest share of the overall national budget for higher education and research dedicated to steering the research effort to specific research programs or structures. The institutional funding for research is allocated predominantly by the MESR. The MESR allocates 60 percent of its research budget as institutional funding for the research labs and research units based on five-year contracts. The regular accreditation of each research institution is based on many performance indictors related to scientific production, the openness of the institution to external environment and collaborations and the human resources.

Other ministries especially Health and Agriculture provide additional institutional funding in their areas of responsibility. For instance, the Ministry of Health allocates R&D funding to research projects based on the main objectives of the quality of health services, training, employment and excellence in the public healthcare system. The strategic priorities of the Ministry of Health in funding research laboratories are assessed against performance related to these priorities. A key focus is also in funding clinical trials as there are four clinical investigation centers (CIC) in Tunisia.

Public and Media Perceptions of ALS

Despite the recent improvement in the understanding of neurodegenerative diseases in Tunisia and the appearance of associations and publicity for Alzheimer's disease, ALS is still viewed as a rare disease. Unlike some countries, in Tunisia ALS is less known, and there is no media or association that promotes the knowledge of the early symptoms. However, patients with ALS require a large amount of community support and may be a priority over other slowly progressive neurological diseases by neurologists and individuals with specialized disease knowledge.

Care of ALS Patients

Although Tunisia does have institutions for long-term care, it is mostly for aged people. At present, there is no public or private institution specialized in ALS disease management; thus, virtually all ALS patients reside in their own home. In Tunisia, most caregivers are the children of the patients, patient's partners and/or a stepdaughter. This limited scope of caregivers reflects the general lack of ALS knowledge and the limited specialized formal training for ALS patient management and care. Nevertheless, it is possible to get treated by specialized medical personal or by paid caregivers hired by families who can afford the costs.

As discussed in Chapter 1, ALS is characterized by the progressive loss of voluntary motor activity and the ability to perform activities of daily life. Consequently, there is a negative impact on quality of life for both patients and their families (Gauthier 2007; Ozanne 2011; Santaniello 2018). Because ALS remains an incurable disease, its management must focus on improving the daily life of patients (Bali and Miller 2013; Scott 2017). The economic burden of ALS to patients and families can be large. The expenses associated with the disease management can be divided into direct and indirect costs (Steen 2009). The direct costs include medications, equipment for ALS patients to improve their daily activities, medical devices and services, home adaptations and mobility of patients and families. The indirect costs include the loss of income due to the patient's illness related to absence from work.

In our Tunisian cohort, the inequality of age and sex frequency distributions in early ($\leq$45 years) and late ALS onset ($\geq$75 years) were found. We report 19.5 percent of Tunisian patients with early ALS onset, and among them 11.5 percent were men and 8 percent women. Hence, being affected with ALS disease in such critical ages would influence the normal income of patients and their families. Unfortunately, until now, there has been no published study on estimation of the direct and indirect costs for ALS patients and their families in Tunisia and no government assistance program for informal caregivers.

Access to Assistive Technologies

Patients with ALS frequently and increasingly face difficulties in performing daily functional tasks due to the progression of muscle weakness. The assistive technologies to facilitate ALS patients' mobility are necessary in order to optimize indoor and outdoor mobility, communication, body postures, dressing and bathing. The CNAM provides limited coverage for direct patient's needs.

STATUS OF MULTIDISCIPLINARY TEAM CARE AND CLINICS

It is well established that the multidisciplinary care for ALS patients can achieve an optimal care for both patients and their families. In Tunisia, given the multitude of areas impacted by ALS (physical issues, psychosocial problems, etc.), the multidisciplinary care team should include medical practitioners in neurology, respiratory, gastroenterology, pharmacology, rehabilitation and palliative care; allied healthcare professionals in physiotherapy, occupational therapy, speech therapy and nutrition; as well as professionals in nursing, genetics and psychology including neuropsychology. Decision-making barriers are found in three major factors: the patient's acceptance of the final diagnosis of ALS, the patient–carer relationship and the absence of dynamic collaboration among practitioners in different fields.

Our multidisciplinary team in the Neurology Department in Razi Hospital was built with the aim to guide the patient and the caregiver through ongoing decisions regarding the patient's situation. This is conducted in a timely manner by providing the patient and family with evidence-based information on the available choices and the appropriate options to be taken. An inter-professional approach to address the needs of ALS patients is represented in many models of care (Mayadev 2008; Güell 2013; Hogden 2015; Dharmadasa 2016; Hogden 2017). Our model recognizes that patients and their family members are key stakeholders and must all have active roles in the decision-making process.

Table 20.1 Multidisciplinary team disease management in Tunisia

Problems	Intervention	Healthcare involved
Announcing the diagnosis	Counseling Support the patients and families	– Neurologist – Neuropsychologist
ALS progression	Riluzole	– Neurologist – Pharmacologist
Breathing issues	Ventilation	– Pneumologist – Intensive care specialist – Nurse
Eating issues	Gastrostomy	– Gastroenterologist – Dietitian – Nursing – Speech pathologist
Mobility	Equipment for ensuring the facility of patient mobility	– Physiotherapist
Cognitive issues	Counseling	– Neuropsychologist
Care issues	Counseling	– Neuropsychologist – Family's patient
Communications issues	Proposing other means of communication	– Speech pathologist

Consequently, the process of ALS management is conducted through regular discussions consistent with the patient's projected healthcare needs. Due to the increasing deterioration of the patient, the multidisciplinary team collaborates to facilitate his/her decisions to match the inevitable changes in health and lifestyle and hence the engagement with a variety of healthcare disciplines (Table 20.1).

TUNISIAN CARE MODEL

<u>Initial consultation:</u> A patient with suspected ALS undergoes electroneuromyography tests (ENMG), MRI brain imaging and laboratory testing. Following the diagnosis of ALS, the neurologist provides the medications available to slow its progression. The only FDA-approved drug for ALS patients is riluzole.

<u>Breaking the bad news:</u> Breaking the bad news of the ALS diagnosis has always been a burden for specialists, especially when dealing with diagnosis of a fatal disease (Buckman 1984). Under our disease management strategy, the neurologist has the responsibility of revealing the diagnosis and explaining the details of ALS progression to the patient and his family. However, the expectation that the patient has the right to know the truth,

and the real diagnosis, has not been the norm and still is not in Tunisia even though the issue of nondisclosure has been debated worldwide. Cultural diversity means that not all our patients and families relate to/or accept the idea of individual autonomous decision-making. Rather, the family makes the medical decisions when one of the members is sick.

In Tunisia, the diagnostic announcement should be made according to a 1993 law which declares that: "A serious or fatal prognosis can be concealed from the patient. It cannot be revealed to him with the greatest circumspection, but it can be generally to the close family, unless the patient has previously prohibited this revelation or appointed third parties to which it must be made" (Article 36 of the Tunisian Code of Medical Ethics (Decree No. 93–1155 of May 17, 1993, on the code of medical ethics, J.O.R.T No. 40 of May 28 and June 1, 1993 page 764).

Genetic screening for personalized medicine: The geographical position of Tunisia at the crossroads of Africa, Asia and Europe made it a unique place where the genetic background of the population reflects the heritage of many ethnicities. A strong tradition of consanguineous marriage gave the Tunisian population some particular characteristics where the pioneering studies of Mongi Ben Hamida and the subsequent studies allowed participating in advances in neurosciences and identification of new several clinical phenotypes of ALS by describing for the first time the juvenile ALS form (Ben Hamida 1990; Ben Hamida and Hentati 1984) and the associated gene *ALS2* (alsin) (Hentati 1994).

In the Department of Neurology of Razi Hospital, we initiated the first step for studying the genetic side of ALS disease in Tunisia. The first genetic research on ALS disease is conducted by exploring mutation in *SOD1, TARDBP (TDP-43)* and *FUS* gene via Sanger sequencing for the gene's exome. A two-step protocol was followed for the detection of the GGGCC hexanucleotide in the chromosome 9 open reading frame 72 (C9orf72) gene: first by performing fragment length analysis, and then by repeat-primed PCR (unpublished data). The Department bears the total cost of genetic exploration; thus, there are no costs for patients.

Implementation of the strategy of disease management: Once the diagnosis of ALS has been confirmed, the neurologist establishes the strategy of disease management according to patient's situation followed by the evaluation of disease progression during a daily care consultation. For this, the neurologist works collaboratively with a neuropsychologist, speech pathologist and occupational therapist to evaluate the degree and/or the stage of the disease in order to adapt the treatment.

Respiratory, speech, rehabilitation and nutritional/dietitian assessment: The pneumologist makes the initial respiratory interventions based on medical tests, the physical examination, chest radiography and a lung function study which includes spirometry, lung volumes, peak respiratory pressures, arterial blood gases and cough peak flow. The rehabilitation physician assesses the patient's walking ability and manipulation of objects and evaluates the technical aids needed to sustain quality of life and maintain the highest degree of independence.

The speech therapist provides the strategies and advice to ALS patients and their families for ensuring the optimum normality of the daily actions such as swallowing, talking and monitoring the saliva. Meanwhile the dietitian and/or the nutritionist participate in monitoring good nutrition. The nutritionist assesses the eating habits and swallowing, and then carries out an initial diagnostic nutritional evaluation and calculates the energy-nutritional requirement for spontaneous ingestion. Consequently, the nutritionist and the dietitian will establish a strategy to optimize the qualitative and quantitative composition of the patient's food (Brooks et al. 1994). In this context, in our department at Razi Hospital, we have established a nutrition guide designed specifically for ALS patients.

Gastroenterologists and resuscitation assessments: When complications such as malnutrition and the necessity of weight-loss stabilization arise in a patient, the gastroenterologist assesses gastrostomy tube placement by endoscopic (PEG) and multiple radiologic (RIG) methods. While G-tubes provide an alternative route for delivering nutrition and have been shown to stabilize weight loss, most ALS patients in Tunisia refuse gastrostomy even after explanation by the neurologist that the consequences of such decision could be harmful. Resuscitation for ALS patients appears in the final stage of the disease where the patients are completely incapable for monitoring the vital actions.

RIGHT TO TRY AND PARTICIPATION IN CLINICAL TRIALS

Tunisian legislation enables ALS patients to participate in therapeutic clinical trials specific to their disease and to be treated with drugs that have not yet been approved (according to Decree No. 2014–3657 of October 03, 2014, on the code of medical ethics). In Tunisia, to participate in a clinical trial, ALS patients and/or the patients' caregivers must provide a written informed consent. After the agreement of the Committee for the Protection of Persons (CPP) and the authorization of the Ministry of Health, the trials can be conducted.

In 2016, the clinical investigation centers (CIC) were created to develop and facilitate clinical trials and translational research studies that may lead to new drugs, devices, procedures and treatments for the benefit of patients. This mission is ensured by providing scientific expertise, facilities, technical staff and overall study coordination. Most clinical trials in Tunisia are in phases II and III, and the conduct of them is closely governed by specifications relating to the medical or scientific experimentation of medicinal products intended for human medicine (Order of the Minister of Health of 1 June 2015). However, to date, there have been no clinical trials for ALS in Tunisia.

GENETIC TESTING FOR ALS

The genetic testing for patients with ALS has not, so far, been approved for routine use in Tunisia. Hence, any genetic screening for ALS patients or their family members is not reimbursed by the government. Consequently, it is considered as a research activity and funded from the R&D budget.

Ethically, genetic testing in Tunisia is approved first by an institutional ethics committee (if one exists), and second by CPP. Genetic testing requires informed consent from all participants. Both committees must follow Helsinki Declaration for institutional medical research involving human subjects, including research on human material and identifiable data. In fact, the process followed by both committees is to examine after a request for authorization of all the candidates, their protocols, objectives and methodologies. The committees must identify the risks associated with the research, determine that these risks will be minimized to every extent possible, identify the benefits that this research would bring, determine that the risks are reasonable in relation to beneficial effects on subjects as well as the importance of gaining knowledge and ensure that potential subjects will be accurately informed about the risks or discomfort and the expected benefits of this research.

Additionally, the International Declaration on Human Genetic Data (Knoppers 2006) concerning the conservation and use of biological samples and genetic data has been adopted in the Tunisian institutions and is well executed among the Tunisian research community. Importantly, this declaration emphasizes the vulnerability of developing countries to genetic data and the need to strengthen international collaboration. Indeed, this international declaration ensures the capacity of Tunisian institutions to retain their genetic data rights in the context of international collaborations.

THE LEGAL CONTEXT OF END-OF-LIFE DECISION-MAKING FOR ALS PATIENTS

Although the exact numbers are not available due to the scarcity of information about ALS in Tunisia, according to our observation, most patients die at home since there are no specialized structures and/or institutions for palliative care and reanimation for ALS patients. However, in case of respiratory failure, ALS patients can be hospitalized in intensive care.

Advance directives (ADs) are a vital part in care planning which requires the communication with the patient, patient's family and healthcare providers. ADs in Tunisia are not yet governed by law nor by legislation. Hence, in Tunisia, it is taken informally the patient decision by setting out what treatment/intervention is being refused and under what circumstances. In emergency cases the absolute authority of an AD must be followed by the caring doctors.

In case of respiratory failure when a patient refuses a tracheotomy, the doctor can choose continuous deep palliative sedation (PS) to relieve the suffering, but not shortening of life. In emergency situations, PS may have to be initiated immediately according to doctor's judgment after discussion with patient's family. Continuous deep PS is recommended in cases of advanced ALS where death is expected within hours or few days.

Due to religious objections, euthanasia or PAS are prohibited by Tunisian law. Despite this, the caring neurologist can discuss the possibilities of disease worsening with the patients and/or their families, specifically the respiratory complications expected at a very advanced ALS stage. Moreover, the doctor can describe to the patient the existing therapeutic choices accompanied by an explanation of the benefits and/or the limitations of each one according to patient's case with details of the interventions that will be applied (ventilation) when patient becomes unconscious. It is worthy to note, that according to our observations, most patients with ALS choose to not go through any resuscitation and/or tracheotomy.

CRITICAL FACTORS UNIQUE TO TUNISIA FOR UNDERSTANDING ALS POLICY

Cultural differences in Tunisia affect the view of truth-telling where it is the responsibility of the family to protect the patients from bad news. Hence, the neurologist informs the family about the disease details rather than the patient. Consequently, the family frequently receives the ALS diagnosis and clinical plan before the patient leading to situations where the family has the primary decision-making responsibility. This is unlike the European experience where a patient has the decision responsibility and might block his/her family from knowing the real diagnosis. The question whether the non-disclosure or telling the truth of diagnosis and prognosis is in the best interest of the patients is ongoing and reflects the cultural diversity across the world.

RECOMMENDED CHANGES IN ALS POLICY

The costly management of ALS patients and the burden on the patient as well as the caregivers pose a considerable challenge given the limited financial resources of the Tunisian health system and the underestimation of this fatal disease. Unfortunately, no study has been conducted to estimate the economic burden of ALS in Tunisia. Hence, measuring the costs of ALS management is needed to help decision-makers in healthcare establish a clear and common strategy for ALS management.

The main goal of this strategy once implemented is prioritizing healthcare interventions to reduce the economic burden of ALS for patients and their families. Additionally, enhancing the knowledge about ALS in Tunisia is needed to ensure stable and sustainable funding for medical and social benefits. Since the health insurances do not cover the full expenses of ALS or support certain specific treatments and the coverage remains insufficient, ALS patients' families presently bear the biggest portion of ALS costs.

While the research and development on rare diseases such as ALS may be considered to an extent the best topic for basic research, R&D in Tunisia faces challenges. Drug development for rare diseases presents an expensive process that R&D cannot support.

Indeed, while the big pharmaceutical companies show greater interest in ALS drug regulation and tend to take the R&D results to later development stages, the clinical particularity of ALS patients in Tunisia could create an attractive environment to productive long-term research. A more comprehensive scientific and medical strategy is needed, along with more funding opportunities for ALS. In order to build a fruitful research environment able to attract scientists, pharmaceutical companies need more investment for ALS in Tunisia. Overall, it is crucial that the budget for R&D into ALS be substantially increased in the coming years in Tunisia. This requires that the public sector be involved in a partnership with the private sector such as stakeholders and industry.

Acknowledgments The authors would like to express their thanks to multidisciplinary ALS Tunisian team: Prof. Dziri Catherine (Head of Department of Medicine Physical and Functional Rehabilitation of the National Institute of Orthopaedics "M.T. Kassab," Tunisia), Prof. Trabelsi Samah (Head of National Pharmacovigilance Center, Tunisia), Prof. Brahmi Nozha (Head of Department of Intensive Care and Toxicology, Montfleury, Tunisia) and Prof. Kallel Lamia (Head of Gastroenterology Department, Mahmoud El Matri Hospital, Tunisia) for their excellent assistance.

REFERENCES

Achour, N. (2011). Le systeme de sante tunisien: Etat des lieux et defis. http://www.unfpa-tunisie.org. (Article in French).

Alkire, B.C. (2015). Global access to surgical care: A modelling study. *The Lancet Global Health* 3 (6): e316–e323.

Ben Hamida, M. (1990). Hereditary motor system diseases (chronic juvenile amyotrophic lateral sclerosis). Conditions combining a bilateral pyramidal syndrome with limb and bulbar amyotrophy. *Brain* 113: 347–63.

Ben Hamida, M. and F. Hentati (1984). Maladie de Charcot et sclérose latérale amyotrophique juvénile. *Revue Neurologique* (Paris) 140 (3): 202–206.

Beghi, E. (2006). The epidemiology of ALS and the role of population-based registries. *Biochimica et Biophysica Acta (BBA)-Molecular Basis of Disease* 1762 (11–12): 1150–57.

Bali, T. and T.M. Miller (2013). Management of amyotrophic lateral sclerosis. *Missouri Medicine* 110 (5): 417–21.

Brooks, B., D. Lewis and J. Rawling (1994). The natural history of amyotrophic lateral sclerosis. Motor Neuron Disease, A.C. Williams, ed. London: Chapman & Hall Medical, 131–69.

Buckman, R. (1984). Breaking bad news: why is it still so difficult? *British Medical Journal (Clinical research ed.)* 288 (6430): 1597–99.

Dharmadasa, T. (2016). Treatment approaches in motor neurone disease. *Current Opinion in Neurology* 29 (5): 581–91.

Gauthier, A. (2007). A longitudinal study on quality of life and depression in ALS patient–caregiver couples. *Neurology* 68 (12): 923–26.

Güell, M.R. (2013). Comprehensive care of amyotrophic lateral sclerosis patients: A care model. *Archivos de Bronconeumología (English Edition)* 49 (12): 529–33.

Hentati, A. (1994). Linkage of recessive familial amyotrophic lateral sclerosis to chromosome 2q33–q35. *Nature Genetics* 7 (3): 425–28.

Hogden, A. (2015). Development of a model to guide decision making in amyotrophic lateral sclerosis multidisciplinary care. *Health Expectations* 18 (5): 1769–82.

Hogden, A. (2017). Amyotrophic lateral sclerosis: Improving care with a multidisciplinary approach. *Journal of Multidisciplinary Healthcare* 10: 205–15.

Jennum, P. (2013). Mortality, health, social and economic consequences of amyotrophic lateral sclerosis: A controlled national study. *Journal of Neurology* 260 (3): 785–93.

Kacem, I., I. Sghaier, S. Bougatef, A. Nasri et al. (2019). Epidemiological and clinical features of amyotrophic lateral sclerosis in a Tunisian cohort. *Amyotrophic Lateral Sclerosis and Frontotemporal Degeneration:* https://doi.org/10.108 0/21678421.2019.1704012.

Knoppers, B.M. (2006). The emergence of an ethical duty to disclose genetic research results: International perspectives. *European Journal of Human Genetics* 14 (11): 1170–78.

Logroscino, G. (2018). Global, regional, and national burden of motor neuron diseases 1990–2016: A systematic analysis for the Global Burden of Disease Study 2016. *The Lancet Neurology* 17 (12): 1083–97.

Luna, J. (2019). Clinical features and prognosis of amyotrophic lateral sclerosis in Africa: The TROPALS study. *Journal of Neurology, Neurosurgery and Psychiatry* 90 (1): 20–29.

Mayadev, A.S. (2008). The amyotrophic lateral sclerosis center: A model of multidisciplinary management. *Physical Medicine and Rehabilitation Clinics of North America* 19 (3): 619–31.

Marin, B. (2012). Juvenile and adult-onset ALS/MND among Africans: Incidence, phenotype, survival: a review. *Amyotrophic Lateral Sclerosis* 13 (3): 276–83.

Mitsumoto, H. (2007). A strategy to develop effective ALS therapy. *Brain and Nerve= Shinkeikenkyu no shinpo* 59 (4): 383–91.

Makhloufi, K. (2015). Have health insurance reforms in Tunisia attained their intended objectives? *International Journal of Health Economics and Management* 15 (1): 29–51.

Ozanne, A.G.O. (2011). Quality of life, anxiety and depression in ALS patients and their next of kin. *Journal of Clinical Nursing* 20 (1–2): 283–91.

Peters, D.H. (2008). Poverty and access to health care in developing countries. *Annals of the New York Academy of Sciences* 1136 (1): 161–71.

Santaniello, B. (2018). ALS managed care considerations. *The American Journal of Managed Care* 24 (15 Suppl): S336–S341.

Scott, A. (2017). Drug therapy: On the treatment trail for ALS. *Nature* 550 (7676): S120.

Steen, I.V.D. (2009). The costs of amyotrophic lateral sclerosis, according to type of care. *Amyotrophic Lateral Sclerosis* 10 (1): 27–34.

UNESCO Institute for Statistics (2018). http://uis.unesco.org/

Zoccolella, S. (2007). Riluzole and amyotrophic lateral sclerosis survival: A population-based study in southern Italy. *European Journal of Neurology* 14 (3): 262–68.

CHAPTER 21

Public Policy in MND Care: The United Kingdom

David Oliver and Christopher McDermott

Abstract There are over 4700 people living with MND in the United Kingdom and 1350 are diagnosed annually. Health care is provided within the universal National Health Service provision but social care, such as personal care, some equipment and respite care, is provided through local councils and is variable. Most people with MND are cared for at home, but MND Care and Research Centres across the United Kingdom provide specialist multidisciplinary team care. Palliative care is widely available, and under the NICE Guidelines there should be palliative care representation on the Multidisciplinary Team (MDT) from diagnosis. There is strong advocacy for people with MND from the MND Association of England and Wales and MND Scotland. The future of MND care in the United Kingdom will be based on the implementation of the NICE Guidelines and the development of increased skills to provide multidisciplinary care for patients and families.

D. Oliver (✉)
University of Kent, Canterbury, UK
e-mail: drdjoliver@gmail.com

C. McDermott
University of Sheffield, Sheffield, UK
e-mail: C.J.McDermott@sheffield.ac.uk

R. H. Blank et al. (eds.), *Public Policy in ALS/MND Care*,
https://doi.org/10.1007/978-981-15-5840-5_21

There is a challenge to continue to develop these services and to provide social care, within financial restraints.

Keywords Motor neurone disease • Multidisciplinary team care • Guidelines • Research strategy • Palliative care • Social care

INCIDENCE AND PREVALENCE OF MND

The United Kingdom has a population of 66.5 million—England 55.6 million, Wales 3.12 million, Scotland 5.42 million and Northern Ireland 1.9 million. The number of people with MND in England is stated to be 3962 with an incidence of 1132, and extrapolation for the whole of United Kingdom gives a prevalence of 4738 and an incidence of 1353 (Neurological Alliance 2019). These figures are similar to those extrapolated, using a prevalence of 7/100,000 the figure for the United Kingdom would be 4655, and with an incidence of 2/100,000, the incidence would be 1330.

GOVERNMENTAL REPORTS AND ACTIONS ON MND

The care of people with MND in the United Kingdom is within the National Health Service (NHS) and the support of social care from local councils. Health care in the United Kingdom is provided free of charge at the point of delivery—including care at home by a general practitioner (GP), outpatient appointments, hospitalization, investigations and rehabilitation services. However, these services vary across the country and are locally commissioned by bodies that have some local representation but are mainly dependent on funding from central government. Over the last 25 years these bodies have been under continual change. Medication is provided free of charge to children, people over 60 years old and those with certain long-term conditions, such as cancer, diabetes and thyroid issues. People with MND are usually able to claim for free medication, although they may need to confirm their disability. This does vary across the various countries within the United Kingdom—for instance, in Scotland all medication is free. Riluzole was not provided by the NHS in all areas until the NICE recommended its use in 2001 (NICE 2001).

Social care such as personal care and residential home care is provided by local councils and is not provided free for all people, but they may be expected to pay for some, or all, of the care, depending on their income and savings. There are also discrepancies across the country, depending on the funding provided by the local council. Some people with MND may receive NHS Continuing Care funding, covering all care costs, if they are very severely disabled or close to the end-of-life.

The main development in England and Wales has been the decision by the NICE to undertake Guidelines on MND in 2013 following discussion with the Motor Neurone Disease Association. A Guideline Development Group was established with Dr. David Oliver as the Chair. The Group included neurologists, a general practitioner, therapists and people with MND and carers. For each question a literature review was undertaken, and the evidence was assessed using the Grading of Recommendations, Assessment, Development and Evaluation (GRADE) methodology. The guidelines were produced using the best available evidence, but where this was not available, recommendations were made by consensus of the group. The areas considered were:

- Recognition of symptoms and referral to neurology
- Information and support at diagnosis by a neurologist who is knowledgeable and manages MND
- Organization of care—multidisciplinary team approach (MDT)
- Social care—integrating care at home and ensuring care is constant and coordinated
- Provision of equipment to aid activities of daily living—provided appropriately and speedily
- Nutrition—assessment of nutritional needs and coping with swallowing issues
- Communication—enabling communication face to face and by web-based systems
- Muscle problems—enabling mobility and reducing stiffness
- Saliva management—reducing and coping with drooling of saliva
- Cough effectiveness—enabling people to cough, if necessary
- Respiratory function—assessment, commencement and monitoring of respiratory function and the use of NIV
- Cognitive assessment—recognition of frontal lobe changes and frontotemporal dementia
- Prognostic factors—specific factors that are related to poor prognosis

- Planning for end-of-life care—facilitating palliative care and advance care planning, supporting patients and families at the end of life and in bereavement (NICE 2016a)

These guidelines aimed to improve care for people with MND and their families. It was found that the use of a multidisciplinary team did not only improve care and quality of life of patients but also led to an extension of life. Evaluation of the cost effectiveness showed that MDT is cost effective, with an incremental cost-effectiveness ratio (ICER) of £26,672 per quality of life year (QALY) gained (NICE 2016a).

As part of the guidelines, NICE produced Pathways and Quality Standards, which are "a concise set of prioritised statements designed to drive measurable improvements in the three dimensions of quality—safety, experience and effectiveness of care—for a particular area of health or care" (NICE 2016b). These aim to provide the priorities for those commissioning or providing services with the aim of improving care. The five quality standards are:

1. Adults diagnosed with MND are give information by a consultant neurologist with expertise in MND.
2. People with respiratory impairment are offered non-invasive ventilation based on regular assessment of respiratory function and symptoms.
3. Equipment and adaptations are tailored to people's needs and provided without delay.
4. Personal care is provided by a consistent team of workers who are familiar with the person's needs.
5. People with MND are given opportunities to discuss their preferences and concerns about end-of-life care at diagnosis and key stages of disease progression.

The guidelines and these quality standards should be implemented over time with an improvement in care for people with MND. However, they are considered "guidelines" and there is no compulsion on commissioners or providers to meet all these recommendations. The MND Association has started to audit the Standards and the Guideline recommendations, and this may encourage all involved in the care of people with MND to consider and implement the changes needed.

The NHS recently stated that the care for people with neurological conditions is not ideal, with a 39 percent increase in neurological deaths compared to a 6 percent decrease in deaths from all causes and evidence that people with neurological conditions have the lowest health-related quality of life of any long-term condition (NHS England 2019a). There is a new five-year plan for the NHS and active consideration of the needs for neurological conditions, including MND, with commissioners being encouraged to deliver new models of care (NHS Thames Valley Strategic Clinical Network 2019).

Major Governmental Agencies Involved in MND Care

Most care for people with MND occurs within the National Health Service. The neurology services within most hospitals are commissioned by local Commissioning Groups, which set contracts and monitor the care provided. However, the care of people with MND is commissioned as a "specialist service" by NHS England on a national basis. This does allow regional centers such as the MND Care Centres to be funded but does affect the provision of local services for patients who live far from the main population centers and the care centers.

Social care—personal care, equipment, adaptations to housing—is primarily provided by local council social services. The funding is often very limited since the care of the elderly and disabled must compete with education, childcare, local amenities and other community services. There is some funding from the national government with other monies raised locally from Council Tax, a tax based on your housing and not necessarily related to one's financial circumstances. Social care is also subject to assessment of the person's ability to pay from their salary and savings, and thus many people may have to pay a large proportion, or even all, of the cost of social care. There are often great variations according to the place of residence since councils may allocate funding differently due to different priorities.

The Most Active Private MND Organizations and Associations

Within England and Wales, the MND Association provides a great deal of support for people with MND, their families and the professionals involved in their care.

- MND Care Centres. Since 1990 the MND Association has helped to develop 22 MND Care Centres, often providing the initial funding, which is then continued by the NHS. The centres provide dedicated MND clinics with multidisciplinary teams within Regional Neuroscience Centres, a single point of contact for people with MND and a location for clinical drug trials.
- Area Support Coordinators (ASC) who are specialists available from the MND Association to provide information and support to people with MND, their families and the professionals involved.
- Local Association Visitors are volunteers who have been carefully selected and have undergone a thorough training program to provide support. They also liaise with the ASC and local branch.
- Many areas have a local branch, which may provide support with Association Visitors and/or regular support with information groups for people with MND and their families.
- A helpline—MND Connect is available during the week and some evenings. An online forum is also available.
- Advice on benefits.
- A loan service with limited range of equipment where it is not readily available from statutory sources.
- Financial support is available, including funding some equipment and services and funding for children and young people living with someone with MND, non-paid carers supporting someone living with MND and provision of any other ways to improve the quality of life for a person with MND.
- Information and leaflets on MND and its management for people with MND and families, carers and professionals who are caring for someone with MND.
- Educational sessions are available for professionals, including regular conferences and the annual International Symposium on MND/ALS, which has become the major meeting where new developments in research, management and care are discussed.
- Research—the MND Association funds research on MND—basic research, trials and management/care.

In Scotland, MND Scotland provides similar support for people with MND and their families and carers. However, they have advocated for MND clinical specialists, who are funded by the Scottish Health Boards and work closely with MND Scotland. They also provide specific services for people with MND, including advocacy workers to provide support and help reduce delays and disputes about care; loan for equipment including chairs and beds; financial support, including grants, such as "time out grants" for carers and families to have a break or holiday; financial advice from Welfare and Benefits Officers; loans for communication aids, including laptops, desktop computers, iPads with text to speech apps and eye-gaze equipment; local physiotherapy services; complementary therapies; support groups; information and education for health and social care professionals; and research on MND. There is also a Scottish MND register of people with MND.

There are other charities which provide support and care for people with MND and advocate for the improvement and development of care for people with neurological diseases. The Neurological Alliance represents 80 organizations involved in neurological care. It aims to increase awareness and understanding of neurological conditions and ensure access to high-quality services and information from first symptoms throughout life. Sue Ryder provides palliative and neurological support from specialist centers across the United Kingdom, day services, supported living and specialist Sue Ryder nurses in people's homes. They have also campaigned for improved care systems.

CONTRIBUTIONS FROM PRIVATE AND PUBLIC SECTORS FOR MND RESEARCH AND CARE

MND research in the United Kingdom is funded from a broad range of sources, including government, research councils, industry, charity, philanthropy and venture capitalists. Established in 1987, the Association of Medical Research Charities (AMRC) is the United Kingdom's national membership organization for health and medical research charities. The AMRC brings together and supports health and medical charities to produce high-quality research. In 2016 AMRC members funded 45 percent of publicly funded medical research and 29 percent of non-commercial research in the NHS (AMRC 2017).

The Charity Research Support Fund (CRSF) underpins charity investment in university research across England (similar funds are provided in the devolved nations). The fund means that universities can effectively leverage research funding from charities and enables researchers who receive charitable funding to recover the full economic costs that charities do not pay, such as shared IT and administration overheads. The CRSF is an element of government funding administered to universities as part of quality-related (QR) research funding. In England, it was allocated by Higher Education Funding Council for England (HEFCE) before April 2018, and through Research England under UK Research and Innovation (UKRI) after April 2018. It was introduced in 2006 at £135.5 million and in 2018/19 the CSRF was set at £204 million per annum.

Key MND charities include MND Association, MND Scotland, My Name'5 Doddie Foundation and Marie Curie. The MND Association is one of the largest charity funders of MND research. In 2017, £4.5 million (24% of its expenditure) supported MND research (MNDA 2018).

The National Institute for Health Research (NIHR) was established in 2006 under the government's health research strategy Best Research for Best Health. Today, the NIHR is the nation's largest funder of health and care research with £227 million of funding awarded to research projects in 2017–2018 (NIHR 2018). In addition to funding specific projects, the NIHR funds infrastructure and a clinical research network in England, which supported 1375 studies in 82 percent of NHS Trusts in 2017–2018. Although the NIHR is centered on England, it works closely with the devolved administrations in Scotland, Wales and Northern Ireland which co-fund many of its programs.

The UK Motor Neurone Disease Clinical Studies Group (UK MND CSG) represents a central component of the framework for MND research in the United Kingdom, providing the primary, but not sole, route through which MND studies can be monitored and supported, and through which new ideas for clinical research studies are developed. The group meets monthly and has representation from all major population centers in the United Kingdom (http://www.mndcsg.org.uk). In 2016–2017 the recruitment was 7719 into 21 studies in England; of these, five studies were commercial and recruited 31 participants.

PUBLIC AND MEDIA PERCEPTIONS OF MND

The perceptions of MND in the press and media vary and are often tied to celebrities who have the diagnosis or die from MND. The main areas are:

- Human-interest stories of the person with MND "fighting" the disease or facing deterioration. For instance, Stephen Hawking was viewed as a person who continued to work and publish despite his diagnosis of MND and he featured widely in the press and media when new books were published. His death in 2018 was widely covered.

- New treatments becoming available—some are reports of early, unsubstantiated trials or of treatments with very unsure provenance or applicability. For instance, "remarkable new drug can slow down the disease by 70%" in the discussion in the newspaper of CuATSM in Australia (Daily Mail 6.4.19).
- Fundraising events organized by the MND Association and MND Scotland. In 2014 this focused on the Ice Bucket challenge, although as the origin was in the United States, there was confusion with the use of ALS, as this term is rarely used in the United Kingdom.
- MND is often used within the debates of changing the law on assisted dying. The organizations pressing for change, such as Dignity in Dying, use examples of people with MND in their literature, talking of their fear of a distressing death when making the case for assisted dying. For instance, in 2018 Noel Conway asked for the right for an assisted death when he was maintained on non-invasive ventilation and feared his only options were to "effectively suffocate" if he removed a mask or to travel to Dignitas in Switzerland for assisted dying. His application was turned down by the courts (Dignity in Dying 2019a).

People with MND have also featured in the discussions when new legislation allowing assisted dying was debated in Parliament. This has again often focused on the fears of a distressing death.

Although the press coverage on MND has often been about the fears of distress at the end of life, there has been more positive coverage in the human-interest stories. Moreover, there has usually been the opportunity for the MND Association or MND Scotland to provide accurate information on MND.

PROPORTION OF PEOPLE WITH MND AT HOME AND INSTITUTIONAL CARE

It is very difficult to elucidate where people with MND are cared for in the United Kingdom. Admissions to hospital are not common, with only 1887 inpatient admissions for MND and spinal muscular atrophy recorded in 2015–2016 in England: 10 percent of these were for less than one day and the mean length of stay was 15.75 days (Public Health England 2017). Thus, although hospital is the place of death for about 40 percent of patients, the majority are cared for at home. Some patients may be in care homes for the elderly or residential settings for people with neurological disease, but they represent only 17 percent of deaths (Public Health England 2018). Although about 13 percent of patients die in hospices, this again is usually after a short end-of-life admission. Most people with MND remain at home. The aim of developments within the NHS is to increase choice for people, and since home is the predominant choice for place of care (Ali et al. 2019), this is likely to continue at the same level or increase.

COMPOSITION OF CAREGIVERS: INFORMAL AND FORMAL OR PAID

Caregivers of a person with MND at home are primarily the family, usually a spouse or child. When paid carers are involved, they are either paid directly by funding from the local council social services or from the patient with monies obtained from benefits or their own funding. A small number of people have control of their own budget for care through direct payment. After their needs are assessed, they are helped in obtaining the care they wish, but they employ those who provide the care.

Governmental Aid for Caregivers

Allowances are available from the government to help with personal care for people with MND. These are not means tested and can be provided quickly if a doctor or other experienced professional completes a specific statement that person may die in the next six months ("special rules"). This can be a problem as some professionals do not wish to make this assertion and the MND Association are pressing for all people with MND to receive the allowance quickly as a result of the diagnosis rather than prognosis. There are also benefits if the person is not able to work or has a low income. If there are complex medical needs, the NHS provides funding through NHS Continuing Healthcare. It provides care for the person's needs, but a high level of disability must be demonstrated for it to apply.

Carers themselves may be able to receive benefits as well. A carers' allowance is available if care is provided for over 35 hours per week, or if the person with MND is already receiving other allowances. All carers should receive an assessment of their own needs from social services, although this may not lead to any additional support or funding. The benefits system is complex and often affected by the person's own financial state. Many are means tested and are only available for people with low income or low level of savings. Respite care may be supported by social services or may be possible within a specialist palliative care unit/hospice on occasions.

ACCESS TO ASSISTIVE TECHNOLOGIES

People with MND have multiple functional problems and have complex equipment needs that change as their disease progresses. Regular assessment by the MND multidisciplinary team can ensure that the provision of equipment and adaptations is responsive to a person's changing needs. Providing equipment and adaptations without delay maximizes the impact on the person's quality of life, allowing them to continue with usual activities and reduce the likelihood of harm from adverse events such as falls. Funding and routes of availability varies depending on the type of equipment and location.

In England, funding for communication aids for individuals with complicated needs falls under NHS England Specialised Commissioning. This means that if any individual meets the criteria for complex Augmentative and Alternative Communication (AAC) assessment, their assessment and provision will be funded by NHS England through a specialist AAC service. There are 15 NHS England specialist AAC services for the assessment and provision of complex AAC. If a person does not meet the criteria for a specialist AAC service assessment, their needs can be met by their local speech and language therapist and community team that is expected to provide more basic, low-tech equipment. Any equipment the person needs would have to be funded by the local Clinical Commissioning Group (CCG). In Wales a similar hub and spoke system operates. In Scotland as of March 2018, it is now a legal obligation for Health Boards to provide a communications device to one who needs it. This is a result of MND Scotland's successful "Let Me Speak" campaign and the subsequent legislation passing in the Scottish Parliament in March 2016.

The situation regarding wheelchair provision is more complicated. Patients need to be referred to one of over 150 wheelchair services in England. There is great variation in how services are run and the type of wheelchairs that are provided. In April 2017, NHS England introduced personal wheelchair budgets to improve choice for patients either through the NHS or third-party organizations or by using top-up private funding to purchase wheelchairs that would fall outside of normal statutory provision. As a result of the geographical variations in the provision of equipment and adaptations, the major charities MND Association and MND Scotland offer equipment loans and/or financial help.

STATUS OF MULTIDISCIPLINARY TEAM CARE AND CLINICS

In England, MND services are commissioned centrally by NHS England as a "specialised service" as opposed to regional commissioning, which takes place for non-specialist services by clinical commissioning groups (CCGs). The specialist services commissioned by NHS England are grouped into six National Programmes of Care (NPoC) and MND sits within the neuroscience specialized neurology CRG of the Trauma NpoC, which outlines the service specification (NHS England 2013). MND services are generally located in large regional neuroscience or neurology centers. A care center model has evolved in many areas with a central MND clinic acting as a specialist hub and providing specialist care. A new network model has also been developed in more geographically sparse regions such as the South West Peninsular and in Wales. Often these centers and networks are supported by the MND Association.

In Scotland, responsibility for NHS services is devolved to the Scottish government, which sets national objectives and priorities with 14 regional NHS boards and 7 national or special NHS boards. In January 2015, the Scottish Government invested £2.5 million to enhance the provision of nursing and care for its residents. This doubled the number of MND nurses in Scotland and for the first time ensured all were funded directly by NHS Scotland.

"RIGHT TO TRY" LEGISLATION FOR MND PATIENTS

In the United Kingdom, a drug that has been proven to be safe and shown to have a beneficial effect is licensed either directly through the Medicines and Healthcare Regulatory Authority (MHRA) or via a central European agency, the European Medicines Agency (EMA), where licenses are then adopted by the MHRA. Licensing a drug does not take into account the cost of the drug, its economic impact or when or how it should be made available. These are taken into consideration by other organizations such as the NICE in England and Wales, or the Scottish Medicines Consortium (SMC) in Scotland.

The EMA licenses drugs for the EU, and the licensing decision is valid across all member states. They can give a drug either a full license or a conditional license if a drug is at an earlier stage of development, is being developed for a condition where there are no drugs currently available, or the current treatments have a limited effect. This lasts for a year and has conditions or limitations in so much as the company must commit to finishing the studies required for full approval.

In the United Kingdom, the MHRA adopts decisions made by the EMA, but can also grant licenses on its own. The MHRA can issue either a full license or an approval within the Early Access to Medicines Scheme (EAMS). The EAMS scheme was introduced to make it possible for promising unlicensed drugs or treatments to be made available to patients faster. These medicines may be part of ongoing research, thus there is a chance the medication could have some unknown adverse side effects. Also, the full results from the phase II or III trials of the medicine may not be known. The scheme requires drug companies with promising compounds to undergo a two-stage evaluation process: (1) application for designation as a "Promising Innovative Medicine" and (2) the EAMS "Scientific Opinion" of available data (MHPRA 2019).

In addition to the formal early-access schemes described above, people in the United Kingdom can also ask their doctor to request a drug specifically for them, this is sometimes known as a "special." However, getting approval for a "special" is a lengthy and complex process involving numerous steps at different levels. The costs may be borne by the drug company, the local NHS Trust or local commissioners. In some circumstances a patient may seek to fund the costs themselves, although local NHS permission will still be necessary.

NICE is an independent body with an aim to improve outcomes for people using the NHS, and it assesses the clinical and cost effectiveness of approved health technologies, including new drugs. This is to ensure that all NHS patients have equitable access to the most clinically and cost-effective treatments, and, therefore, NICE recommendations can impact the availability of a drug once it has been given market approval by

MHRA. Guidance and assessments from NICE are directly applicable in England and are also routinely adopted in Scotland, Wales and Northern Ireland.

GENETIC TESTING OF PATIENTS WITH MND

Genetic testing is usually possible within the NHS at no cost to the patient. This is usually organized within an MND Care Centre or Clinical Genetics Departments, where well-informed genetic counseling is provided. Genetic testing may also be undertaken in research laboratories, but these are not accredited to provide feedback or reports for patients. Pre-symptomatic testing of family members is also possible for people over 18 years of age. This is provided by Clinical Genetics Services, across the country, or at specialized MND clinics. Genetic counseling is provided during a series of appointments over several months before blood is taken for testing. Further counseling is given when the results are given to the patients over a series of follow-up appointments, if a mutation is detected. All testing is completely confidential, and the person being tested will decide who should be informed. If appropriate, and with consent, counseling and predictive gene testing can be offered to other at-risk family members. In some areas, testing may be available for payment, but the same counseling should be provided, and the centers providing testing should be fully accredited and work under the auspices of the UK Genetic Testing Network.

PLACE OF DEATH

Within England the place of death in 2012 to 2104 for people with MND and spinal muscular atrophy were: hospital, 39 percent; home, 29 percent; care home, 17 percent; hospice, 13 percent; and other, 1 percent (Public Health England 2018). Corresponding figures for the rest of the United Kingdom are difficult to obtain, but it would be expected that they are not unlike those in England.

ACCESS TO PALLIATIVE CARE

Palliative care is widely available across the United Kingdom and is provided by specialist palliative care units/teams and/or hospices. Hospices are inpatient units, which may be funded wholly or partly by the NHS, with support from charitable donations. Care is provided without any charge. Specialist palliative care may be provided in several ways:

- Inpatient care within a hospice—there are 220 hospices in the United Kingdom caring for over 200,000 or 38 percent of all deaths per year. Although 95 percent of patients receiving care have cancer, people with MND represent one of the largest non-cancer groups.
- Day care—with patients attending for the day for assessment, psychosocial support and providing respite for families and carers. Twenty-five percent of all patients attending day care have a non-malignant diagnosis and many are people with MND.
- Hospital care—with hospital palliative care teams providing advice and support for patient, families and professionals. People with MND are less likely to be seen by these teams as hospital admission is unusual.
- Home care—specialist teams supporting patient and families at home in collaboration with the primary care service, including the GP.

Surveys in the past have shown that many hospices do provide care for people with MND. In 1999, a survey of 170 hospices showed that of these hospices 100 percent provided inpatient care, 76 percent day hospice care, 61 percent home care and 28 percent hospital care (Oliver and Webb 2000). However, 48 percent of these hospices only provided care in the terminal stages and only 39 percent from diagnosis or within six months. A later survey in 2003 showed only 8 percent of services saw patients at diagnosis, 36 percent restricted the number of patients with MND they saw at any one time and 32 percent felt that MND patients were a greater strain on resources than cancer patients (Oliver et al. 2003).

There has been no survey in recent years, but there are anecdotal reports that hospices are restricting their involvement for MND patients and only seeing them toward the end of the disease progression. This may reflect improved care from specialized MND multidisciplinary teams, who provide palliative care within their regular assessments and support, and the increased pressures on hospices to care for patients from all disease groups, regardless of diagnosis.

LEGAL STATUS OF ADVANCE DIRECTIVES

Within the United Kingdom there are differences in the legal situation and nomenclature of advance care planning in England and Wales compared to Scotland. In England and Wales, the Mental Capacity Act (2005) addresses the assessment of capacity and future decision making:

- Capacity assessment—everyone is assumed to have capacity, but if they have an impairment of mind or brain, which would restrict their ability to make the specific decision, it is necessary to assess capacity before any decision making.
- An Advance Statement can be completed by anyone—this may cover their wishes and preferences in relation to their care and treatment, such as how they wish to be cared for, their values and beliefs, relationships and aspects of care and treatment. Such a statement gives information to those making decisions if the person loses capacity, but is not legally binding.
- An Advance Decision to Refuse Treatment (ADRT) can be completed by a person with capacity, stating the treatments that they do not wish to receive and the circumstances when this would apply. There is a need to be more specific than an Advance Statement—for instance, a person with MND receiving non-invasive ventilation may state that they do not wish this to continue when they can no longer communicate. If the refusal relates to a treatment that is potentially life-sustaining, the ADRT should be in writing, witnessed and include a declaration that the decision applies even if the person's life would be at risk. An ADRT is legally binding and should be adhered to.
- Proxy decision making can be used, with a Lasting Power of Attorney (POA). This may relate to either health care matters or financial matters. The person, when they have capacity, appoints someone else to make decisions on their behalf if they lose capacity. There is a specific form and a fee is charged to register it with the Office of the Public Guardian. As with an ADRT, it only becomes operative when the person loses capacity.
- If a person has lost capacity to make an informed decision and there is no clear statement of their wishes, then a "best interests" decision may be necessary. The "decision maker" will normally be a professional responsible for the day-to-day care, usually the doctor, or it

could be a nurse or social worker. The carers, family and wider multidisciplinary team should be consulted but the decision stays with the "decision maker."

- If there are conflicts within a family or team about a decision, the Court of Protection can be involved, which will make the decision independently after having heard all the information from all involved.

In Scotland the overall structure is very similar but with some differences:

- The Adults with Incapacity (Scotland) Act 2000 has established Continuing Powers of Attorney and Welfare Powers of Attorney. There are three versions of Power of Attorney—financial, welfare and combined. The other implications of a POA are like those in the United Kingdom.
- An advance directive is used to express wishes about future care. It is not legally enforceable under the Act, but one of the general principles of the Act states that the wishes of an adult should be taken into consideration when acting or making a decision on their behalf. Thus, it is generally agreed that a medical practitioner should not ignore an advance directive if the treatment which is to be refused applies to the specific circumstances of the person.

Thus, in the United Kingdom advance care planning is possible, and if specific actions are taken, the wishes of the person should be respected. Both ADRTs and POAs are legally binding.

WITHHOLDING AND WITHDRAWAL OF TREATMENT

The withholding and withdrawal of treatment has a legal basis in the United Kingdom. It is understood that the primary goal of any medical treatment is to benefit the patient by restoring or maintaining health, and maximizing benefit and minimizing harm, and that the treatment that does not provide net benefit to the patient may, ethically and legally, be withheld or withdrawn and the goal should shift to the palliation of symptoms.

If a person has capacity, they may refuse treatment and their decision should be respected and complied with, even if complying with this refusal could lead to significant harm or even death. To continue a treatment which the patient does not wish to have or continue could constitute a criminal offense of battery. Moreover, treatment may be withdrawn using a valid and specific ADRT, or at the request of an attorney and where this is seen by a team review to meet the "best interests" criteria. When the "best interests" of the patient has been determined to allow withdrawal, then this withdrawal of treatment is legal and is not considered euthanasia (Faull 2015).

Ethically and legally, in the United Kingdom the withholding and withdrawing of treatment are seen in the same way, with the same deliberations and discussions with the patient, if possible, the family and carers and the wider multidisciplinary team. Decisions to withhold or withdraw treatment should be made by the clinician in overall charge of a patient's care following discussion with the health care team and, where appropriate, patient and/or those close to the patient (GMC 2010).

Legal Status of Assisted Dying and Palliative Sedation

At present there is no legal basis for assisted dying, either euthanasia or physician-assisted suicide. There have been several attempts to legalize it over the last ten years, but these have failed. There are continuing campaigns to introduce assisted dying, but at present there is no support to make a change in legislation in Parliament, although surveys of the general population have shown that 84 percent of the public supports the choice of assisted dying for the terminally ill (Dignity in Dying 2019b).

Palliative sedation is a complex area. A recent review (Twycross 2019) has suggested the term Continuous Sedation until Death (CDS) and that in the United Kingdom the aim is the management of symptoms with proportionately titrated doses of medication, maintaining awareness if possible—as defined by the EAPC: "Therapeutic/palliative sedation in the context of palliative medicine is the monitored use of medications intended to induce a state of decreased or absent awareness (unconsciousness) in order to relieve the burden of otherwise intractable suffering in a manner that is ethically acceptable to the patient, family and health-care providers" (Cherny and Radbruch 2009). In the United Kingdom medication may be used at the end of life to relieve symptoms, including physical distress and psychosocial distress, knowing that such medication may lead to death (Twycross 2019). However, the use of CDS, with the aim of ensuring death without any distress, is not common in the United Kingdom.

Factors Unique to UK Culture in Decision Making

The United Kingdom is increasingly a multicultural society with many varied cultures, religious affiliations and social and spiritual outlooks. However, under the law, and for the vast proportion of the population, there is an emphasis on patient decision making and the role of the health professionals in facilitating these decisions with careful discussion and relevant wider discussion with family and the multidisciplinary team. There can, on occasions, be conflicts with some families, who may consider that they should have greater involvement in the decision making, even at the exclusion of the patient. However, the law is clear and there are legal ways to reduce conflict, including, if necessary, involvement of the Court of Protection or other courts. This can be a lengthy and difficult process but can allow a decision to be made.

Policy Changes to Improve Care of MND Patients and Advance MND Research

In many ways the policies and guidelines are present that would lead to the improvement in care for people with MND and their families. In particular, the NICE Guidelines, if fully implemented and funded, would lead to major changes in the care provided with an increase in multidisciplinary care, integrated and supportive social care and improved access to care and interventions (NICE 2016). This would require a change in the funding available for MND care as part of an improved care system for all neurological disease.

Social care remains an important issue. At present this varies across the country depending on the local council and funding. There has been increasing discussion of the provision of social care, including provision free of charge and the removal of means testing. This would require a move by all political parties and an agreement to make these changes over a longer period than the life of a single Parliamentary period. This may remain an elusive aim, but to improve care for people with MND, and all people with disability and age-related issues, the change is necessary.

Research into MND, whether basic research on the disease process or the development of treatment or the assessment of care approaches and symptom management has been primarily stimulated by the MND Associations. There has been increasing involvement of the national research organizations allowing an increase in studies and patient involvement. MND care, and neurological care, increasingly has been on the agenda of palliative care organizations and the James Lind Alliance setting priorities for research. Of the top ten priorities, two mention MND directly and most would help to improve MND care at the end of life and earlier in the disease progression (James Lind Alliance).

Acknowledgments The authors acknowledge the advice on genetic testing from Professor Chris Shaw, Professor of Neurology and Neurogenetics, Director of the Maurice Wohl Clinical Neuroscience Institute and Associate Director of the UK Dementia Research Institute at the Institute of Psychiatry, Psychology and Neuroscience at King's College, London and King's Health Partners.

REFERENCES

Ali, M., M. Capel, G. Jones and T. Gazi (2019). The importance of identifying preferred place of death. *BMJ Supportive and Palliative Care* 9: 84–91.

Association of Medical Research Charities (2017). Unlocking the investment power of medical research charities. How the Charity Research Support Fund enables the unique contributions of charities to health and well-being. November.

Cherny N.I. and L. Radbruch (2009). European Association for Palliative Care (EAPC) recommended framework for the use of sedation in palliative care. *Palliative Medicine* 23: 581–93.

Dignity in Dying. The facts. https://www.dignityindying.org.uk/why-we-need-change/the-facts/.

Dignity in Dying (2019a). The facts. https://www.dignityindying.org.uk/why-we-need-change/personal-stories/

Dignity in Dying (2019b). The facts. https://dignityindying.org.uk/why-we-need-change/the-facts/

Faull C. (2015). Withdrawal of ventilation at the request of a patient with motor neurone disease: guidance for professionals. *Association for Palliative Medicine of Great Britain and Ireland*, https://apmonline.org/wp-content/uploads/2015/02/APM-Guidance-on-Withdrawal-of-Assisted-Ventilation-Consultation-1st-May-2015.pdf.

General Medical Council (2010). Treatment and care towards the end of life: good practice in decision making, https://www.gmc-uk.org/-/media/documents/treatment-and-care-towards-the-end-of-life%2D%2D-english-1015_pdf-48902105.pdf.

James Lind Alliance. Palliative and end of life care Top 10, http://www.jla.nihr.ac.uk/priority-setting-partnerships/palliative-and-end-of-life-care/top-10-priorities/.

Medicines and Healthcare Products Regulatory Agency (2019). Guidance: Apply for the early access to medicines scheme (EAMS), https://www.gov.uk/guidance/apply-for-the-early-access-to-medicines-scheme-eams.

Motor Neurone Disease Association (2018). Annual Report and Consolidated Financial Statements.

National Institute for Health and Care Excellence (2001). Guidance on the use of Riluzole (Rilutek) for the treatment of Motor Neurone Disease, https://www.nice.org.uk/guidance/ta20.

National Institute for Health and Care Excellence (2016a). Guideline 42 Motor neurone disease: assessment and management, https://www.nice.org.uk/guidance/ng42.

National Institute for Health and Care Excellence (2016b). Motor Neurone Disease Quality Standards, https://www.nice.org.uk/guidance/qs126/chapter/Introduction.

National Institute for Health and Care Excellence (2016c). Motor Neurone Disease Endorsed resource—Transforming MND care audit tool, https://www.nice.org.uk/guidance/ng42/resources/endorsed-resource-transforming-mnd-care-audit-tool-4664620189.

National Institute for Health Research (2018). Annual Report Neurological Alliance 2019, https://www.neural.org.uk/assets/pdfs/neuro-numbers-2019.pdf.

Neurological Alliance. Neuro Numbers. Neurological Alliance 2019, https://www.neural.org.uk/wp-content/uploads/2019/07/neuro-numbers-2019.pdf.

NHS England (2019a). Neurological Conditions, https://www.england.nhs.uk/ourwork/clinical-policy/ltc/our-work-on-long-term-conditions/neurological/.

NHS England (2019b). National Programmes of Care and Clinical Reference Groups, https://www.england.nhs.uk/commissioning/spec-services/npc-crg/.

NHS England (2013). NHS Standard contract for neurosciences: specialised neurology (adult), https://www.england.nhs.uk/wp-content/uploads/2013/06/d04-neurosci-spec-neuro.pdf.

NHS Thames Valley Strategic Clinical Network (2019). Transforming community neurology, http://tvscn.nhs.uk/wp-content/uploads/2016/06/Transforming-Community-Neurology-Part-A-Transformation-Guide-version-1.pdf.

Oliver, D. and S. Webb (2000). The involvement of specialist palliative care in the care of people with motor neurone disease. *Palliative Medicine* 14: 47–48.

Oliver, D., S. Webb, R. Sloan, N. Sykes and J. Smithy (2003). Survey of specialist palliative care involvement in the care of people with MND/ALS. Poster at 14th international Symposium on ALS/MND. Milan.

Public Health England (2017). Hospital aactivity compendium:England. www.gov.uk/government/publications/neurology-services-hospital-activity-data

Public Health England (2018). Deaths associated with neurological conditions in England 2001–2014. Deaths associated with neurological conditions datasheet. https://www.gov.uk/government/publications/deaths-associated-with-neurological-conditions.

Twycross R. (2019). Reflections on palliative sedation. *Palliative Care: Research and Treatment* 1–16, https://doi.org/10.1177/1178224218823511.

CHAPTER 22

ALS Public Policy in the United States

Benjamin Rix Brooks and Jerome E. Kurent

Abstract The burden of amyotrophic lateral sclerosis (ALS) in the United States continues to grow as the aging population increases. Access to high-quality care varies depending on a patient's medical insurance, geographical location and socioeconomic status. The National ALS Registry was established in 2010 and is a vital resource of epidemiology including the identification of possible environmental risk factors. The federal insurance program Medicare provides clinical care for most patients with ALS. More recently, identification of military service as a risk factor for developing ALS has resulted in significant medical and financial support provided through the Department of Veterans Affairs (VA). The estimated annual costs of providing clinical care for patients with ALS in the United States ranges from $1.05 to 2.25 billion. The National Institute of Neurological Diseases and Stroke under the National Institutes of Health (NIH)

B. R. Brooks
Atrium Health Neurosciences Institute, University of North Carolina School of Medicine, Charlotte, NC, USA
e-mail: benjamin.brooks@atriumhealth.org

J. E. Kurent (✉)
Medical University of South Carolina, Charleston, SC, USA
e-mail: kurentje@musc.edu

© The Author(s) 2021
R. H. Blank et al. (eds.), *Public Policy in ALS/MND Care*,
https://doi.org/10.1007/978-981-15-5840-5_22

provides most public ALS research funding, but non-governmental and philanthropic ALS organizations contribute substantially to research support.

Keywords Amyotrophic lateral sclerosis • Motor neuron disease • Public policy • Palliative care • Hospice • Multidisciplinary clinic • Genetic testing • ALS association • CDC ALS registry

BACKGROUND AND EPIDEMIOLOGY OF ALS IN THE UNITED STATES

In the United States amyotrophic lateral sclerosis (ALS) is most familiar to the American public as *Lou Gehrig's disease*. Lou Gehrig was a legendary baseball player, nicknamed the *Iron Horse*, who died of ALS in 1941 (Innes and Chudley 1999). On the other hand, the term *motor neuron disease*, or MND, would not be a term familiar to most Americans although it is used in many other parts of the world to designate ALS.

As an instrument of public policy, the congressionally mandated *National ALS Registry* collects vital epidemiological data including possible environmental risk factors. The National ALS Registry was established at the Center for Disease Control and Prevention (CDC) through a concerted effort of patient advocacy groups working with Congress to enact the ALS Registry Act in 2008. The legislation provided the Agency for Toxic Substances and Disease Registry (ATSDR), a branch of the CDC, with the authorization and guidance necessary to create the National ALS Registry (Kaye et al. 2014; Kaye et al. 2018). The National ALS Registry acquires data from administrative databases including Medicare, commercial Medicare Advantage and other sources (Wagner et al. 2015). In addition, there is a web-based portal accessible by patients who can provide basic demographic information. Patients followed in ALS multidisciplinary clinics (MDCs) are routinely provided contact information for the ALS Registry and are encouraged to enroll because the National ALS Registry also serves as a recruitment tool for research (Malek et al. 2014).

The National ALS Registry has geocoded all patients with ALS by city using geographic information system (GIS) software and includes the locations of all 72 ALS MDCs. The estimated prevalence of ALS cases in 2015 as reported in 2018 was 5.2 per 100,000 (Mehta et al. 2018). A total of 16,583 cases were identified with an estimated lifetime risk of developing ALS in the United States as 1 in 325 males and 1 in 450 females. In 1996 there was one hospital admission for every two to three living ALS patients, with 15 percent in-hospital deaths mostly related to respiratory failure and related complications (Dubinsky et al. 2006; Lechtzin et al. 2001).

Significant variation in the incidence of ALS by race and ethnicity occurs in the United States and has been well documented (Rechtman et al. 2015). In the United States, most ALS decedents during 2011–2014 were Caucasian (91%) and were men (56%) (Larson et al. 2018). Mortality rate ratios by race were 2.64 for Caucasians and 1.48 for African-American patients. States in more northern latitudes have statistically significant greater age-adjusted ALS mortality rates than states at more southern latitudes (Noonan et al. 2005; Wagner et al. 2015). The association between northern latitudes and increased ALS mortality rates among Caucasians may possibly be related to confounding factors such as geographic patterns of European immigrant settlement in the United States (Gunnarsson and Bodin 2018; Mehta et al. 2018; Raymond et al. 2019). In the USA, prevalence varies by state and even regions within states. ALS prevalence also correlates with socioeconomic factors. The higher ALS prevalence in the Midwest and Northeast likely reflects the higher proportion of whites in those regions, compared with that in the South and West. The lowest prevalence in the West Census region is most likely related to the population diversity in states such as California. Payer type is also important for the National ALS Registry because it relies on federal administrative data sets and a self-registration web portal. Over one-third of all ALS cases listed no federal payer (Medicare, Medicaid or VA) and might not be captured in the federal data sets. The self-pay payer type was highest among Asians followed by African-American/Blacks and then Whites (Jordan et al. 2015; Rechtman et al. 2015).

Other factors including genetic predisposition along with environmental exposures cannot be ruled out at this time and need further investigation (Mehta et al. 2018, Raymond et al. 2019). In contrast to the rest of the country, ALS is now a reportable disease in the state of Massachusetts. Based on data from newly diagnosed patients in Massachusetts, the prevalence of ALS in that state rose steadily from 5.1 per 100,000 to 5.9 per 100,000 between 2007 and 2011 (Massachusetts Department of Public Health 2016). Continued surveillance will indicate whether prevalence will continue to increase as a result of better treatment, and if there is potential to further understand the role of underlying or mitigating risk factors leading to this observation.

The potential relationship between environmental exposures and the development of ALS was raised following Gulf War I when there appeared to be an increased prevalence of ALS in returning Veterans. Subsequent epidemiological studies suggested that Veterans from conflicts prior to Iraq including Viet Nam, Korea and World War II also had an increased risk of developing ALS (Horner et al. 2008; Barth et al. 2009; Kasarskis et al. 2009). Thus far, no specific risk factors have been identified for ALS among these diverse military populations (Weisskopf et al. 2005; Allen et al. 2008; Bove et al. 2014; Beard et al. 2017; Sagiraju et al. 2019). Although one of the strongest risk factors for the development of ALS is military service, tobacco smoking, occupational and other environmental exposures are also considered important (Spencer et al. 2019; Gunnarsson and Bodin 2018).

PUBLIC POLICY AND MAJOR GOVERNMENTAL AGENCIES SUPPORTING PATIENT CARE

Medicare is a federally funded insurance program and is administered by the Center for Medicare and Medicaid Services (CMS). It was enacted in 1965 as Health Insurance for the Aged (under Title XVIII) of the Social Security Act. Medicare insurance initially covered only individuals aged 65 years and older. In 1972 Medicare eligibility was subsequently extended to individuals under age 65 having certain long-term disabilities, and in 2001, Congress passed a landmark legislation which added ALS as a qualifying condition for automatic Medicare coverage (HR 353 Amyotrophic Lateral Sclerosis (ALS) 2000; Williams et al. 2013). The 24-month waiting period typically required to obtain benefits was eliminated for ALS patients. Medicare coverage is not automatic for ALS patients. People must first apply for Social Security Disability Insurance. Once this is granted, ALS patients under the age of 65 are provided with Medicare coverage.

Medicare Part A medical insurance covers inpatient care provided in a hospital or skilled nursing facility and applies to patients with ALS. Home health care services are also covered by Medicare Part A, and include skilled nursing care, physical therapy, occupational therapy and speech-language pathology assistance. Hospice care benefits are also provided under Part A for patients with ALS who are expected to live six months or less (Krivickas et al. 1997; McCluskey and Houseman 2004). Medicare coverage typically requires a deductible and co-payment, which may be supplemented by private insurance. Medicare Part B medical insurance helps cover outpatient care. Medicaid is a joint federal-state insurance program active in 37 of 50 states and District of Columbia for patients qualifying based on very low income and poverty levels.

The estimated total annual cost for ALS care for an estimated prevalent 15,000 patients ranges from $1,050,000,000 to $2,250,000,000 USD (Larkindale et al. 2014; Obermann and Lyon 2014; Meng et al. 2018). Currently 4000 patients in the United States are receiving edaravone, which increases the annual cost by an estimated $600,000,000.

The Americans with Disabilities Act, The Family Medical Leave Act of 1993 and the Social Security Administration can provide varying degrees of social and financial support for patients with ALS and their family caregivers depending on individual needs and the availability of resources.

PUBLIC POLICY RELATED TO VETERANS WITH ALS AND SERVICE-CONNECTED DISABILITY

The Institute of Medicine (IOM) report, *Amyotrophic Lateral Sclerosis in Veterans: Review of the Scientific Literature*, was released on November 10, 2006 (Institute of Medicine 2006). Evidence supported a 1.5 to 2 times increased incidence of ALS in association with military service. ALS was subsequently declared a 100 percent service-connected disability (Beard et al. 2017). An average of 1520 Veterans with ALS across the United States are evaluated and managed by the Veterans Health Administration (VHA) each year. There is an estimated prevalence of 4220 Veteran patients living with ALS. The VHA Handbook 1101.07 (2011) describes the necessary structural, procedural and educational components required for the comprehensive care of Veterans with ALS and will be discussed later in this chapter. The ALS Association's ALS in the Military White Paper: Defense Health Research (www.alsa.org/Military) and website (https://www.als.org/navigating-als/military-veterans) are excellent resources summarizing this topic.

PUBLIC POLICY AND GOVERNMENT-SUPPORTED ALS RESEARCH

The National Institute of Neurological Diseases and Stroke under the National Institutes of Health (NIH) maintains an intramural research program supporting research at its main campus. The NIH also provides extramural funding for researchers across the country via competitive grants for basic science and preclinical drug studies, which typically take

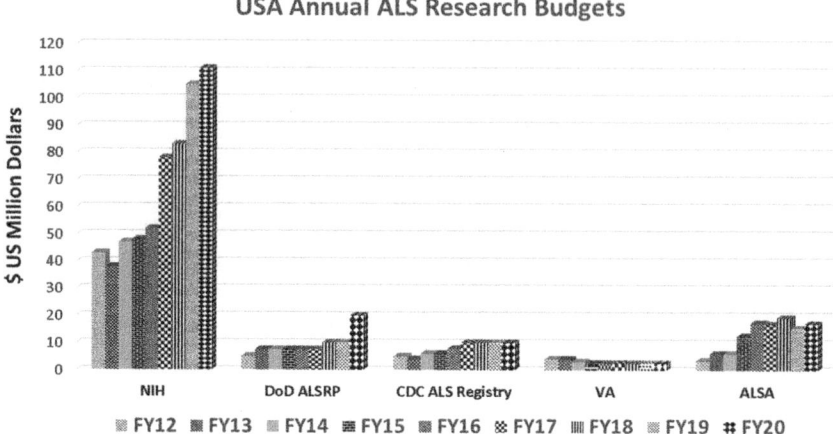

Fig. 22.1 USA Annual ALS Research Budgets 2012–2020. Annual ALS Research Budgets for Fiscal Years 2012–2020 for National Institutes of Health (NIH), Department of Defense ALS Research Program (DoD ALSRP), Center for Disease Control and Prevention—Agency for Toxic Substances Disease Registry National Amyotrophic Lateral Sclerosis Registry (CDC ALS Registry), Department of Veterans Affairs (VA) and Amyotrophic Lateral Sclerosis Association (ALSA). Original source material available at NIH = https://report.nih.gov/categorical_spending.aspx; DoD ALSRP = http://cdmrp.army.mil/about/funding-history; CDC ALS Registry = https://www.atsdr.cdc.gov/features/alsregistryanniversary/index.html; VA = https://cdmrp.army.mil/alsrp/pdfs/ALSRP%20Strategic%20Plan.pdf; ALSA = http://www.alsa.org/about-us/financial-information.html

place at academic medical centers. Federally funded basic science and clinical research supported by the NIH budget is distributed through individual Institutes, as noted in Fig. 22.1. This includes the National Institute of Neurological Diseases and Stroke, National Institute on Aging, National Institute of Environmental Health Sciences and the National Institute of General Medical Sciences. The NIH was expected to allocate $110 million to ALS research in 2020. Figure 22.1 also indicates support from other governmental entities as well as the ALS Association. The development of

Table 22.1   ALS deaths per year with location of death

Location	2005	2006	2007	2008	2009	2010	Total
Acute care	1739 (27%)	1656 (25%)	1716 (26%)	1698 (25%)	1709 (24%)	1726 (24%)	10,244
Home or hospice	3018 (46%)	3210 (49%)	3350 (50%)	3455 (50%)	3449 (49%)	3839 (49%)	20,321
Nursing home	1406 (22%)	1401 (21%)	1308 (19%)	1293 (19%)	1307 (19%)	1294 (19%)	8009
Other	337 (5%)	312 (5%)	344 (5%)	436 (6%)	539 (8%)	369 (8%)	2337
Total ALS deaths	6500	6579	6718	6882	7004	7228	40,911

possible new treatments for ALS typically takes place in basic science laboratories within academic medical centers and is often sponsored by the pharmaceutical industry or other private commercial entities.

Non-governmental and Community-Based ALS Organizations and Resources

The face of ALS in the United States was transformed by the Ice Bucket Challenge, which resulted in an estimated $222 million USD generated across the globe for ALS research. It should be noted that Pete Frates, a professional baseball player who only recently died from ALS, is credited with catalyzing the Ice Bucket Challenge following his diagnosis (https://petefrates.com/).

The ALS Association (ALSA) is the only national organization dedicated solely to ALS and serves numerous vital functions. These include research funding obtained through private contributions, ALS Walk events, as well as providing a support mechanism for ALSA multidisciplinary clinics (Boylan et al. 2015). The Muscular Dystrophy Association (MDA) provides support to patients with more than 100 different neuromuscular conditions including ALS. MDA also provides financial support for MDA Care Center ALS multidisciplinary clinics (Ward et al. 2010; Young et al. 2011).

There are also numerous other non-federal community-based philanthropic initiatives and organizations which have been developed to overcome knowledge gaps and empower ALS patients with useful internet resources. These include ALS Untangled, Patients Like Me, ALS Worldwide, Answer ALS and Target ALS, among others. Many local ALS organizations directly affiliated with MDCs have also been established, such as the Les Turner Foundation at Northwestern University and Joe Martin ALS Foundation at Atrium Health ALS Clinics.

Providing Care to the Patient with ALS

The patient typically experiences a delay from onset of symptoms to diagnosis of ALS which averages nearly one year (Brooks et al. 1994; Williams et al. 2013). Patients experience multiple diagnostic encounters over the course of several months often beginning with the primary care provider, followed by an evaluation by a consulting neurologist. The patient is then usually referred to a tertiary medical care center for a confirmatory diagnosis of ALS by a neurologist with neuromuscular diseases expertise (Boylan et al. 2015; Goutman et al. 2014). It is not unusual for an ALS mimic to be identified by the ALS specialist which results in a non-ALS diagnosis that therefore may not be life-limiting (please see Chapter 1, Table 1.1, Conditions that can Mimic ALS/MND). Several excellent comprehensive books are available to help guide the care and support patients with ALS (Bedlack and Mitsumoto 2012; Mitsumoto 2009; Oliver 2006).

Guidelines for coordination of care for ALS patients have been developed over the past three decades. These include the American Academy of Neurology (AAN) evidence-based ALS Quality Measures in 2013 (Miller et al. 2013) used to benchmark clinical care. The Northeast ALS Consortium (NEALS) Bulbar Speech and Swallowing Committee has also published consensus guidelines for the diagnosis and management of bulbar dysfunction in ALS (Pattee et al. 2019). The NEALS consortium has recently developed an ALS *Clinical Trials Platform* to more efficiently evaluate multiple ongoing clinical trials and is expected to provide significant acceleration in drug development (Paganoni et al. 2019a).

Status of ALS Multidisciplinary Clinics

Most patients will be followed on a regular basis at an ALS Multidisciplinary Clinic (MDC), which is usually located at an academic medical center. ALS MDCs typically function under the auspices of the ALS Association (http://www.alsa.org/community/centers-clinics/) or the Muscular Dystrophy Association (https://www.mda.org/care/care-center-list). Some degree of financial support is typically provided for clinic operations

(Ward et al. 2010). In addition, the vital role of committed individuals serving in a voluntary capacity as liaisons between ALS organizations and the community cannot be overstated. In-person patient clinic encounters are increasingly supplemented with ALS telemedicine, especially for patients encumbered by severe physical disability or long-distance travel. ALS telemedicine is in the process of being established in conjunction with ALS MDCs across the country and appears to be highly successful (Pulley et al. 2018; Geronimo et al. 2017), along with associated cost savings (Paganoni et al. 2019b). Patients are interviewed in their homes by ALS clinic staff using computer-based technology, typically with a family member facilitating the interview for the patient. ALS telemedicine sessions can be arranged at intervals of one to three months. Palliative care telemedicine is also available in some regions of the country and is coordinated with ALS clinic staff. During the current COVID-19 pandemic ALS telemedicine is proving to be an invaluable resource in assisting patients with ALS and their families.

There are 170 Veterans Administration Medical Centers (VAMC) in the United States. The VA National Task Force has established the need for comprehensive, multidisciplinary services for Veterans with ALS, which is described in its Strategic Plan. At least one ALS multidisciplinary clinic was to be established for each of the 19 geographic regions across the United States called Veterans Integrated Service Networks (VISNs).

Veterans with ALS are typically provided care at a VAMC ALS multidisciplinary clinic, but they have the option of receiving care at a non-VA facility if closer to the patient's residence. Goals of care include maximizing quality of life by providing state-of-the-art patient-centered care while providing education for the Veteran and family caregivers. Additional VA benefits include a Homemaker Home Health Aid program, which provides professional caregiver services at the patient's home for basic self-care needs such as bathing. Adaptive housing grants provide home renovations such as to accommodate wheelchairs by widening doorways in order to access showers. VA grants assist with purchase of vans or other transportation needs for the Veteran with ALS. Respite care for the family caregiver may be provided on an as-needed basis. Veterans may also be eligible for nursing home placement along with comprehensive care if the family is no longer able to provide for the patient at home. The Paralyzed Veterans of America (PVA) is the only congressionally chartered veterans service organization dedicated solely for the benefit and representation of veterans with spinal cord injury or disease that interacts closely with

Veterans diagnosed with ALS. PVA representatives facilitate access to service-connected benefits noted above. Opportunities for Veterans to participate in Institutional Review Board (IRB)-approved research projects are offered when available.

CAREGIVER SUPPORT

There is a need for enhanced federal and state policy to provide support for family caregivers of patients with chronic disease. This is particularly urgent for families of patients with ALS. The patient and family have the major responsibility of paying for chronic care of a patient with ALS. Public disability benefits are offered through the Social Security Administration. Social Security Disability Income (SSDI) provides certain working individuals who are no longer able to work monthly income based primarily on work history. Dependent children, spouses and disabled adult children may also qualify for payments depending on the patient's work history. In addition, following death of the disabled individual, certain survivorship benefits may also apply. Veterans with ALS are provided financial support that increases with progressive disability of the patient. Home modification allowances, assistance with purchasing a modified vehicle for transportation as well as outpatient care and care at the veteran's residence are also provided.

ACCESS TO DRUG TREATMENTS FOR ALS

There are currently three FDA-approved, disease-modifying treatments for ALS: riluzole as tablets or suspension can extend the natural history of ALS by 2–3 months in clinical trials and 6–19 months in clinic-based observational studies (Andrews et al. 2020); dextromethorphan-quinidine was approved for the symptomatic treatment of pseudobulbar affect (PBA) common in ALS and other neurological conditions; and edaravone was approved with studies currently underway to further define its efficacy. Although the American Academy of Neurology (AAN) ALS Practice Parameters in 1999 and 2009 as well as the ALS Quality Measures 2013 recommended that riluzole treatment be discussed with each patient, based on data from medical insurance plans utilization of this drug has been low in the United States compared with Europe (Miller et al. 1999b, 2013). Analyses of ALS patient populations during 1998–2017 covered by different insurance plans also revealed variable rates of utilization of riluzole based on the type of insurance. Patients followed in ALS MDCs have higher rates of riluzole use than those not in MDCs. Medicare and commercial insurance will pay for some portion of the cost of riluzole and edaravone but will often require a patient to pay a deductible and co-pay to offset the total expense of this drug (ALS Association 2016; U.S. Army Medical Research and Materiel Command. Congressionally Directed Medical Research Programs. Department of Defense. Amyotrophic Lateral Sclerosis Research Program 2018; U.S. Department of Health and Human Services, Food and Drug Administration 2018).

The Federal Drug Administration (FDA) is responsible for evaluating the safety and efficacy of ALS treatments including drugs and devices. Public policy interventions have led to Orphan Product drug designations, as well as fast-track evaluations for certain interventions earmarked for ALS. In 2017, there were 73 preclinical research projects, 6 phase 1 clinical trials, 12 phase 2 clinical trials, and 4 phase 3 clinical trials involving 105 ALS-related interventions (Long Analysis Group 2017). The development of possible new treatments for ALS typically takes place in basic science laboratories within academic medical centers and are often sponsored by private commercial entities, including the pharmaceutical industry.

ALS Practice Parameter Treatment Guidelines supported by the American Academy of Neurology (AAN) were first formulated by academic medical centers in 1999 and subsequently updated (Miller et al. 1999b, 2009). ALS Quality Measures for Medicare Provided Care were developed by the AAN and submitted to Medicare in 2013 with the palliative care and falls assessment measures being accepted but the other meaures returned for further development that recommenced with the activities of the AAN ALS Quality Measures Update Working Group in early 2020 (Miller et al. 2013). The Airlie House Consensus Symposium on Clinical Trials in ALS in 2016 supported by many governmental and non-governmental organizations summarized standard guidelines for the design and implementation of ALS clinical trials. This was forged by academic centers and patient groups in collaboration with regulatory agencies to include advances in promising gene therapies and bioengineering options provided by stem cells to accelerate development of ALS treatments (ALS Association 2016; van den Berg et al. 2019).

ACCESS TO ASSISTIVE TECHNOLOGIES
AND NON-PHARMACOLOGICAL TREATMENTS

Respiratory treatment interventions including noninvasive ventilation (NIV), cough assist devices, secretion oscillation treatment devices and nebulization are of great benefit to patients with ALS. These interventions are widely available, and the utilization of these interventions has increased dramatically throughout the United States, as documented in several Medicare and commercial insurance database analyses. Although their value has been documented by randomized control trials and survey (Bourke et al. 2012; Heiman-Patterson et al. 2018), there are significant variations in the use of respiratory devices. Patients followed at ALS MDCs are more likely to have access to these interventions compared to patients not followed at an MDC.

The Centers for Medicare and Medicaid Services (CMS) has provided guidelines for the utilization of respiratory devices in patients with acute and chronic neuromuscular respiratory failure. The guidelines are under review by numerous academic organizations as well as other entities which provide this equipment. Noninvasive ventilation was underutilized prior to 2006 but its use appears to have increased since then. ALS MDCs have the highest rates of noninvasive ventilation use. Patient advocate groups, voluntary ALS associations and clinicians as well as patients are trying to develop more rigorous guidelines to promote the appropriate utilization of noninvasive ventilation. The increased use of noninvasive ventilation may have modulated the use of tracheostomy invasive ventilation for the treatment of ALS.

Durable medical equipment including power wheelchairs have been a source of public policy concern with respect to payment mechanisms, but they have recently been liberalized. Speech-language pathology interventions have recently led to specific congressional actions to improve Medicare reimbursement. The influence of individuals with ALS on influencing policy is illustrated by Steve Gleason who was a professional football player diagnosed with ALS and helped bring major attention to the need for communication devices reimbursement (https://teamgleason.org/).

"RIGHT TO TRY" LEGISLATION

Although riluzole and edaravone are presently licensed as disease-modifying drugs for the treatment of ALS, many patients are interested in pursuing possible treatments not approved by the FDA and are willing to accept the risks of doing so. The "Right to Try" legislation provides a mechanism for patients with ALS to receive treatments not approved by the FDA, but it remains a challenging and controversial option (Joffe and Lynch 2018). It would be necessary for the patient with ALS to obtain the collaboration of the treating neurologist to administer the unlicensed intervention. The participating neurologist must be willing to monitor the patient's clinical status, as well as to help obtain treatment for any potential complications. At this point in time even though physician liability is waived, it appears that most neurologists in the United States would be hesitant to accept this responsibility. In addition, the patient would be responsible for paying for the drug since it is expected that most insurance carriers would not be willing to reimburse for the costs of medications not officially approved for the treatment of ALS.

Although it is possible that a drug development company might be willing to pay for the cost of the drug, there is no requirement that the sponsor provide the drug to the patient. The Right to Try Act states that the sponsor or manufacturer has no liability for actions under the Right to Try provisions. The no-liability provision also applies to a prescriber, dispenser or other individual entity unless there is "reckless or willful misconduct, gross negligence, or an intentional tort." Participation in Right to Try requires that the drug must be in clinical study development and has also completed Phase 1 testing. It does not require FDA approval or IRB oversight. The FDA also has the option of providing the special designation of "compassionate use" or "expanded access" (https://www.fda.gov/news-events/public-health-focus/expanded-access) for interventions not fully licensed, but still considered to have potential value.

GENETIC TESTING OF PATIENTS WITH ALS

In the United States most patients with sporadic ALS (sALS) are usually not offered genetic testing except in specific research settings (Klepek et al. 2019). Patients with familial ALS (fALS) are generally advised to have genetic testing. However, insurance company approval for genetic testing has been variable, sometimes denying approval claiming that results would have no practical implications for treatment. There is a clear need for policy which would guarantee insurance approval for genetic testing in patients already affected with fALS. There is also a need for policy which would provide payment for genetic testing of pre-symptomatic individuals in families known to carry a specific ALS gene. This would be accomplished with appropriate genetic counseling both prior to and after test results are known.

Intense study of patients with known genetic defects is presently ongoing and offers hope that meaningful therapies will be developed for specific subsets of fALS patients. For example, clinical trials using antisense oligonucleotides (ASOs) are presently underway for patients having the mutant *SOD1* and *C9orf72* genes (Ly and Miller 2018; Miller et al. 2020), as well as *SOD1* suppression with adeno-associated virus and microRNA (Mueller et al. 2020).

A US federal law in 2008 entitled the Genetics Information Nondiscrimination Act (GINA) is designed to protect people from discrimination based on genetic risk. In the past health insurance and employment could be denied to individuals known to be at risk for developing a genetic disorder. This could certainly apply to individuals at risk of developing an inherited form of ALS.

ACCESS TO PALLIATIVE CARE AND HOSPICE

Palliative care in the United States has experienced major development and recognition over the past 20 years (Carver and Foley 2001; Morrison and Meyer 2004; Kurent 2005). Certification for qualified health care professionals can be obtained through the American Board of Hospice and Palliative Medicine examination. There are numerous accredited palliative medicine fellowship training programs available to physicians who have completed their residency programs including Family Medicine, Internal Medicine and Neurology.

Most hospice care in the United States is provided through the Medicare Hospice program administered under the Health Care Financing Administration. Private insurance programs may also provide hospice care for patients who do not qualify for Medicare. Most multidisciplinary hospice care is provided at the private residence of the patient, and occasionally in skilled nursing facilities. Fewer than 10 percent of all hospice patients receive care at inpatient, free-standing hospice care facilities. Inpatient hospice care is usually reserved for the short-term management of patients who may experience severe symptoms that cannot be adequately addressed in the home setting.

An estimated 80 percent of patients with ALS will receive hospice care during the terminal phases of their illness, although precise statistics are difficult to obtain. Medicare hospice criteria for ALS include severely impaired respiratory function with forced vital capacity (FVC) of less than 30 percent; critical nutritional impairment usually associated with weight loss and rapidly progressive weakness; inability to swallow with the patient deciding not to implement a feeding tube unless one is already in place prior to hospice referral (Kirk and Mahon 2010). The need for more liberal Medicare hospice criteria for patients with ALS has been suggested (McCluskey and Houseman 2004).

Most hospice organizations in the United States are for-profit while relatively few are not-for-profit. These two different designations are governed by similar patient care and regulatory guidelines but have different tax-reporting requirements.

PLACE OF DEATH FOR PATIENTS WITH ALS

At least half of ALS patients die at home usually with support provided by Medicare hospice. However, analysis by the Centers for Disease Control and Prevention Multiple Cause Mortality Files from 2005 to 2010 indicated that approximately 25 percent of all ALS patients were admitted to a hospital and died in an acute care setting. It is expected that in the years ahead proportionately more patients will die at home with hospice care, and fewer patients will die in the acute care setting. Table 22.1 summarizes deaths per year for patients with ALS from 2005–2010.

PALLIATIVE SEDATION

Palliative sedation refers to the willful lowering of a patient's consciousness using medications such as benzodiazepines and morphine with the intent of reducing the terminally ill patient's awareness of intractable symptoms. Refractory pain, dyspnea and anxiety may be managed by palliative sedation, which is neither intended nor designed to end the life of the patient. It is considered an ethically and legally acceptable component of comprehensive palliative care and symptom management. The National Hospice and Palliative Care Organization (NHPCO) indicates that palliative sedation, or Sedation for the Imminently Dying, is a treatment option that may be considered by patients and their families as well as health care providers (Kirk and Mahon 2010). The US Supreme Court also supports the use of palliative sedation as a means of relieving intractable suffering not relieved by other available means, but it is considered to occur on only rare occasions.

Palliative sedation remains controversial since a patient receiving this intervention cannot eat or drink when heavily sedated. Palliative sedation has the potential to accelerate the time of death. The *Principle of Double Effect* is an analytical technique to justify the morality of a single act that has the potential of producing two morally opposite effects (Bernat 2008). It is necessary for the patient or surrogate decision-maker to provide informed consent for palliative sedation in collaboration with an experienced hospice or palliative care team. There are no data indicating the extent to which patients with ALS utilize palliative sedation in the United States.

The American Academy of Neurology Ethics Section membership was surveyed regarding the topic of Sedation for the Imminently Dying (Russell et al. 2010). Results of the survey suggested opportunities to further educate neurologists about this important potential intervention for patients with terminal neurological diseases. Palliative sedation has inherent ethical and moral dimensions which have been discussed in detail (Bernat 2008; National Ethics Committee VHA 2007; Cellarius 2008).

Legal Status of Advance Directives and Withholding/Withdrawing Care

Patients with ALS are encouraged to complete an advance directive (AD) prior to the onset of significant clinical decline. Several AD documents exist, including the Living Will and Durable Power of Attorney for Health Care (DPAHC). The DPAHC is the preferred document and patients should not be encouraged to complete both documents since they have the potential to conflict with each other. The term *durable* refers to the fact that such an appointment is not nullified by a patient's subsequent loss of decision-making capacity. Advance care planning should address the patient's understanding of the diagnosis, benefits and burdens of potential treatments (Fried et al. 2002).

The designation of a surrogate decision-maker by the patient as part of the AD would add much to ensure that the wishes of the patient be respected. In addition, the importance of effective physician-patient communication as a means of achieving the goals of an AD has been stressed (Messinger-Rappaport et al. 2009). It should also be noted although a Do Not Resuscitate (DNR) is a medical order, it can be included as a component of the AD. Only an estimated 15 percent of the US population has completed an AD, indicating a clear need to increase participation. Although physicians have been encouraged to have a conversation related to obtaining an AD, evidence suggests that most ADs are obtained by social workers, nurses and chaplains. ADs are considered legal documents which professional caregivers are bound to respect and to comply with the patient's expressed written wishes.

Many patients with different diagnoses may prefer not to provide written documentation of their avoidances, preferences and wishes for care at the end of life. This is due at least in part to difficulties confronting their own mortality and possibly mistrust of the medical establishment by members of some cultures. Many other patients are willing to have a discussion expressing their wishes for end-of-life care, but not in the form of a written document. However, patients with ALS in general are typically receptive to completing a written AD. It is important for the physician and the patient with ALS to discuss critical decision-making, such as implementation or avoidance of a feeding tube and invasive mechanical ventilation. The personal experience of this chapter's authors would indicate that the majority of patients with ALS have either a completed written AD, or at a minimum have had a discussion indicating their avoidance and preferences related to a feeding tube or tracheostomy with mechanical ventilation.

In the United States, there is no legal or ethical distinction between withholding and withdrawal of life-sustaining care. The Ethics Principle of Autonomy provides ALS patients with decision-making capacity to be the sole decision-maker regarding avoidances and preferences for care. This contrasts with many cultures around the world where critical health care decisions are often made by family consensus rather than based on the patient's preferences alone.

Most patients with ALS in the United States elect to not have tracheostomy and chronic ventilation. This is particularly true for patients older than 65 years. Probably fewer than 5 percent of all patients with ALS are managed with chronic ventilation. In addition to quality-of-life considerations, there are major economic and personal caregiver challenges associated with chronic ventilation. Most commercial medical insurance policies covering chronic care will be exhausted within one to two years. Such care requires around-the-clock attention to be shared by family members and paid professional caregivers. Most long-term ventilation care is provided in the home setting and occasionally in a chronic care facility. Long-term ventilation is very rarely provided in the acute care hospital.

It is not uncommon for a patient who has been maintained on chronic ventilation to express the desire to have the intervention withdrawn. This is an ethical and legal decision made by the patient which must be respected. Trained professional caregivers can schedule a time and place with the family for ventilator support to be withdrawn in a carefully moni-tored setting. This would include appropriate administration of medica-tions as needed during withdrawal of ventilation, which can take place in the patient's home or in the hospital, if the family prefers.

LEGAL STATUS OF PHYSICIAN-ASSISTED SUICIDE

Oregon was the first state to legalize physician-assisted suicide (PAS) in 1994 with the Death with Dignity Act (DWDA) (Ganzini et al. 2002; Oregon Department of Health and Human Services 2020). PAS has evolved as a very controversial issue with patient autonomy in conflict with the physician's Hippocratic oath to do no harm (Foley and Hendin 2002). Although polls indicate that the American public increasingly supports PAS, it remains an ethically and politically charged matter. In the United States, PAS is legal in nine states including California, Colorado, Hawaii, Maine, Montana, New Jersey, Oregon, Vermont and Washington, as well as the District of Columbia.

In 2006 patients with ALS represented the single most common diag-nostic category of patients requesting and completing PAS. ALS repre-sented 8 percent of all patients completing PAS. These statistics underscore the desperate circumstances experienced by patients suffering from ALS and their need for special support. Under the Act, ending one's life in accordance with the law does not constitute suicide, mercy killing or homicide. The DWDA and subsequent legislation in other states with legalized PAS specifically prohibit euthanasia. Euthanasia is not legal in any of the 50 US states or the District of Columbia.

To request a prescription for lethal medications, the DWDA requires that the patient must be a terminally ill adult with a life expectation of less than 6 months, 18 years of age or older, not pregnant and a legal resident of Oregon capable of making health care decisions. Patients meeting these requirements are eligible to request a prescription for lethal medication from a licensed Oregon physician willing to participate in the process. Similar policies are in place for other states where PAS is legal. In Oregon the patient must make two oral requests to his or her physician separated by at least 15 days. The patient must also provide a written request to the physician in the presence of two witnesses. The prescribing physician and a consulting physician must confirm the terminal diagnosis and prognosis while ascertaining that the patient has intact decision-making capacity. The prescribing physician must inform the patient of feasible alternatives to PAS such as comfort care provided by palliative care and hospice. The prescribing physician must request, but not require, the patient notify his or her next of kin of the prescription request.

FACTORS UNIQUE TO THE UNITED STATES: INCREASING ETHNIC AND CULTURAL DIVERSITY

The United States is a country of increasing ethnic and cultural diversity which should be considered when discussing critical decision-making during life-limiting illness such as ALS. The *Patient Self- Determination Act of 1990* gives each individual the right to indicate specific avoidances and preferences for medical care. However, shared decision-making is a more frequent dynamic which occurs among non-Caucasian patients and their families, including members of the African-American community (Crawley et al. 2000; Jenkins et al. 2005) and the growing and diverse Hispanic patient population. These are important factors to keep in mind when discussing decisions relating to the medical care of patients with ALS and especially during advanced illness.

In addition, Asians, Pacific Islanders, Muslims, Native Americans and Eskimo Natives each have their own needs and belief systems unique to their respective cultures. As health care providers, it is our goal to embrace these individual cultural needs as we provide care to our patients. More research is necessary in the area of cultural diversity and its relationship to decision-making during life-limiting diseases such as ALS. Effective communication between the patient and professional caregiver remains of paramount importance.

THE FUTURE

Rapid advances in understanding the underlying mechanisms of motor neuron cell injury as well as the genetics of ALS/MND have resulted in hope that more meaningful treatments and an ultimate cure will be possible. Public policy should continue to support research focused on drug development and other interventions, genetics and the possible role of environmental risk factors for ALS/MND. The economic, emotional and financial impact on family caregivers of patients with ALS is apparent. Further research and support in these vital areas are necessary.

Acknowledgments Many people, subjected to the challenges of ALS, and their committed caregivers, have worked diligently toward the development of public policy initiatives to sculpture an appropriate system of care and research in the USA. Their efforts, by participating in clinical studies and clinical trials to provide insights for novel future solutions to the burden of ALS, are gratefully acknowledged and appreciated. The authors also recognize the important observational clinical studies undertaken by the ALS Multidisciplinary Teams in the last quarter century that have educated this chapter.

We thank Calaneet Balas for her detailed review of this chapter and suggestions, and also thank the ALS Association Advocacy Team for being in the forefront of public policy while working to improve the lives of people living with ALS and their caregivers. The longstanding commitment and advocacy of Barbara Kurent-Byrum, NP, on behalf of patients with ALS and their families are gratefully appreciated. The authors also appreciate the thoughtful advice, support and proof-reading expertise provided by Patricia Warner Kurent, MBA.

REFERENCES

Allen, K.D., E.L. Kasarskis, R.S. Bedlack et al. (2008). The National Registry of veterans with amyotrophic lateral sclerosis. *Neuroepidemiology* 30 (3): 180–90.

ALS Association (2016). Guidance for Industry. Drug Development for Amyotrophic Lateral Sclerosis http://www.alsa.org/advocacy/fda/assets/als-drug-development-guidance-for-public-comment-5-2-16.pdf.

Andrews, J.A., C.E. Jackson C.E., T.D. Heiman-Patterson, et al. (2020). Real-world evidence of riluzole effectiveness in treating amyotrophic lateral sclerosis, Amyotrophic Lateral Sclerosis and Frontotemporal Degeneration, https://doi.org/10.1080/21678421.2020.1771734

Barth, S.K., H.K. Kang, T.A. Bullman and M.T. Wallin (2009). Neurological mortality among U.S. veterans of the Persian Gulf War: 13-year follow-up. *Am J Ind Med.* 52 (9): 663–70.

Beard, J.D., L.S. Engel, D.B. Richardson, M.D. Gammon et al. (2017). Military service, deployments, and exposures in relation to amyotrophic lateral sclerosis survival. *PLoS One.* 12 (10): e0185751. https://doi.org/10.1371/journal.pone.0185751.

Bedlack, R.S. and H. Mitsumoto (2012). *Amyotrophic Lateral Sclerosis: A Patient Care Guide for Clinicians.* New York: Demos Medical Publishing.

Bernat, J.L. (2008). *Ethical Issues in Neurology.* 3rd edition, American Academy of Neurology Press, Lippincott Williams & Wilkins, New York, London.

Bourke, S.C., C.L. O'Neill, T.L. Williams, E.T. Peel et al. (2012). The changing landscape of non-invasive ventilation in amyotrophic lateral sclerosis. *Journal of Neurology, Neurosurgery and Psychiatry* 83 (4): 368–69.

Bove, F.J., P.Z. Ruckart, M. Maslia and T.C. Larson (2014). Evaluation of mortality among marines and navy personnel exposed to contaminated drinking water at USMC base Camp Lejeune: A retrospective cohort study. *Environmental Health* 13 (1): 10, https://doi.org/10.1186/1476-069X-13-10.

Boylan, K., T. Levine, C. Lomen-Hoerth, M. Lyon et al. (2015). ALS Center Cost Evaluation W/Standards and Satisfaction (Access) Consortium. Prospective study of cost of care at multidisciplinary ALS centers adhering to American Academy of Neurology (AAN) ALS practice parameters. *Amyotrophic Lateral Sclerosis and Frontotemporal Degeneration* 17 (1–2): 119–27.

Brooks, B.R. (1994). El Escorial World Federation of Neurology criteria for the diagnosis of amyotrophic lateral sclerosis. Subcommittee on Motor /Neuron Diseases/Amyotrophic Lateral Sclerosis of the World Federation of Neurology Denmark Group on Neuromuscular Disease and the El Escorial: Clinical limits of amyotrophic lateral sclerosis" workshop contributors. *Journal of Neurological Sciences* 124: 96–107.

Carver, A.C. and K.F. Foley (2001). Palliative care in neurology. *Neurology Clinics* 194: 789–1044.

Cellarius, V. (2008). Terminal sedation and the "imminence condition." *Journal of Medical Ethics* 34: 69–72.

Crawley, L.V., R. Payne, J. Bolden, T. Payne et al. (2000). Palliative and end-of-life care in the African-American community. *JAMA* 284: 2518–21.

Dubinsky, R., J. Chen and S.M. Lai (2006). Trends in hospital utilization and outcome for patients with ALS: analysis of a large U.S. cohort. *Neurology* 67 (5): 777–80.

Foley K and H. Hendin. (2002). *The Case against Assisted Suicide: For the Right to End-of-life Care.* Baltimore: Johns Hopkins University Press.

Fried, T.R., E.H. Bradley, V.R. Towle and H. Allore (2002). Understanding the treatment preferences of seriously ill patients. *New England Journal of Medicine* 346: 1061–66.

Ganzini, L., M.J. Silveira and W.S. Johnston (2002). Predictors and correlates of interest in assisted suicide among patients with amyotrophic lateral sclerosis in Oregon and Washington. *Journal of Pain and Symptom Management* 3: 312–17.

Geronimo, A., C. Wright, A. Morris, S. Walsh et al. (2017). Incorporation of telehealth into a multidisciplinary ALS clinic: Feasibility and acceptability. *Amyotrophic Lateral Sclerosis and Frontotemporal Degeneration* 18: 555–61.

Goutman, S.A., D.G. Nowacek, J.F. Burke, K.A. Kerber et al. (2014). Minorities, men, and unmarried amyotrophic lateral sclerosis patients are more likely to die in an acute care facility. *Amyotrophic Lateral Sclerosis and Frontotemporal Degeneration* 15 (5–6): 440–43.

Gunnarsson, L.G. and L. Bodin (2018). Amyotrophic lateral sclerosis and occupational exposures: A systematic literature review and meta-analyses. *International Journal of Environmental Research and Public Health* 15 (11): E2371.

HR 353 titled the Amyotrophic Lateral Sclerosis (ALS). Treatment and Assistance Act of 1999; introduced in January of 1999; and, passed as part HR 5661, the Medicare, Medicaid, and SCHIP Benefits Improvement and Protection Act of 2000.

H.R.353 - Amyotrophic Lateral Sclerosis (ALS). Treatment and Assistance Act of 1999 106th Congress (1999–2000). https://www.congress.gov/106/bills/hr353/BILLS-106hr353ih.pdf.

Heiman-Patterson, T.D., M.E. Cudkowicz, M. De Carvalho, A. Genge et al. (2018). Understanding the use of NIV in ALS: Results of an international ALS specialist survey. *Amyotrophic Lateral Sclerosis and Frontotemporal Degeneration* 19 (5–6): 331–41.

Horton, D.K., S. Graham, R. Punjani, G. Wilt et al. (2018). A spatial analysis of amyotrophic lateral sclerosis (ALS) cases in the United States and their proximity to multidisciplinary ALS clinics, 2013. *Amyotrophic Lateral Sclerosis and Frontotemporal Degeneration* 19 (1–2): 126–33.

Horner, R.D., S.C. Grambow, C.J. Coffman, J.H. Lindquist et al. (2008). Amyotrophic lateral sclerosis among 1991 Gulf War veterans: Evidence for a time-limited outbreak. *Neuroepidemiology* 31 (1): 28–32.

Innes, A.M. and A.E. Chudley. (1999). Genetic landmarks through philately–Henry Louis 'Lou' Gehrig and amyotrophic lateral sclerosis. *Clinical Genetics* 56 (6): 425–27.

Institute of Medicine. (2006). *ALS in Veterans*. The National Academies of Sciences, Engineering and Medicine, Washington, DC.

Jenkins, C., N. Lapelle, J.G. Zapka and J.E. Kurent (2005). End-of-life care and the African-American community: Voices from the community. *Journal of Palliative Medicine* 8: 585–92.

Joffe, S. and H.F. Lynch (2018). Federal right-to-try legislation: Threatening the FDA's public health mission. *New England Journal of Medicine* 378: 695–97.

Jordan, H., J. Fagliano, L. Rechtman et al. (2015). Effects of demographic factors on survival time after a diagnosis of amyotrophic lateral sclerosis. *Neuroepidemiology* 44 (2): 114–20. doi: 10.1159/000380855.

Kasarskis, E.J., J.H. Lindquist, C.J. Coffman, S.C. Grambow et al. (2009). Clinical aspects of ALS in Gulf War veterans. *Amyotrophic Lateral Sclerosis* 10 (1): 35–41.

Kaye, W.E., M. Sanchez and J. Wu (2014). Feasibility of creating a National ALS Registry using administrative data in the United States. *Amyotrophic Lateral Sclerosis and Frontotemporal Degeneration* 15 (5–6): 433–39.

Kaye, W.E., L. Wagner, R. Wu and P. Mehta (2018). Evaluating the completeness of the national ALS registry, United States. *Amyotrophic Lateral Sclerosis and Frontotemporal Degeneration* 19 (1–2): 112–17.

Kirk, T.W. and M.M. Mahon. (2010). Palliative Sedation Task Force of the National Hospice and Palliative Care Organization (NHPCO) position statement and commentary on the use of palliative sedation in imminently dying terminally ill patients. *Journal of Pain and Symptom Management* 39: 914–23.

Klepek, H., H. Nagaraja, S.A. Goutman, A. Quick et al. (2019). Lack of consensus in ALS genetic testing practices and divergent views between ALS clinicians and patients. *Amyotrophic Lateral Sclerosis and Frontotemporal Degeneration* 20 (3–4): 216–21.

Krivickas, L.S., L. Shockley and H. Mitsumoto (1997). Home care of patients with amyotrophic lateral sclerosis (ALS). *Journal of the Neurological Sciences* 152 (Suppl 1): S82–9.

Kurent, J.E. (2005). Palliative care in specific neurological diseases. In *Continuum*, Vol 11, ed. by A.E. Miller. American Academy of Neurology Lippincott, Williams &Wilkins, Philadelphia.

Larkindale, J., W. Yang, P.F. Hogan, C.J. Simon et al. (2014). Cost of illness for neuromuscular diseases in the United States. *Muscle Nerve* 49 (3): 431–38.

Larson, T.C., W. Kaye, P. Mehta and D.K. Horton (2018). Amyotrophic lateral sclerosis mortality in the United States, 2011–2014. *Neuroepidemiology* 51 (1c2): 96–103.

Lechtzin, N., C.M. Wiener, L. Clawson, V. Chaudhry et al. (2001). Hospitalization in amyotrophic lateral sclerosis: Causes, costs, and outcomes. *Neurology* 56 (6): 753–57.

Long Analysis Group (2017). The biopharmaceutical pipeline: Innovative therapies in clinical development, https://www.phrma.org/report/the-biopharmaceutical-pipeline.

Malek, A.M, D.E. Stickler, V.C. Vinicius et al (2014). The National ALS Registry: a recruitment tool for research. *Muscle Nerve* 50 (5): 830–34.

Massachusetts Department of Public Health (2016). Data Brief: The Argeo Paul Cellucci Amyotrophic Lateral Sclerosis (ALS) Registry of Massachusetts https://www.mass.gov/doc/als-2007-2011-data-brief-0/download.

McCluskey, L. and G. Houseman. (2004). Medicare hospice referral criteria for patients with amytrophic lateral sclerosis: A need for improvement. *Journal of Palliative Medicine* 7: 47–53.

Mehta, P., W. Kaye, J. Raymond, R. Punjani et al. (2018). Prevalence of amyotrophic lateral sclerosis—United States, 2015. *MMWR Morbidity and Mortality Weekly Report* 67 (46): 1285–89.

Meng, L., A. Bian, S. Jordan, A. Wolff et al. (2018). Profile of medical care costs in patients with amyotrophic lateral sclerosis in the Medicare programme and under commercial insurance. *Amyotrophic Lateral Sclerosis and Frontotemporal Degeneration* 19 (1–2): 134–42.

Messinger-Rappaport, B.J., E.E. Baum and M.L. Smith (2009). Advance care planning: Beyond the living will. *Cleveland Clinical Journal of Medicine* 76: 277–85.

Miller, R.G., B.R. Brooks, R.J. Swain-Eng et al. (2013). Quality improvement in neurology: Amyotrophic lateral sclerosis quality measures: Report of the quality measurement and reporting subcommittee of the American Academy of Neurology. *Neurology* 81 (24): 2136–40.

Miller, R.G., C.E. Jackson, E.J. Kasarskis et al. (2009). Practice parameter update: The care of the patient with amyotrophic lateral sclerosis: Drug, nutritional, and respiratory therapies (an evidence-based review): Report of the Quality Standards Subcommittee of the American Academy of Neurology. *Neurology* 73 (15): 1218–26.

Miller, R.G., T.L. Munsat, M. Swash and B.R. Brooks (1999a). Consensus guidelines for the design and implementation of clinical trials in ALS. World Federation of Neurology committee on Research. *Journal of the Neurological Sciences* 169 (1–2): 2–12.

Miller, R.G., J.A. Rosenberg, D.F. Gelinas, H. Mitsumoto et al. (1999b). The care of the patient with amyotrophic lateral sclerosis (an evidence-based review): Report of the Quality Standards Subcommittee of the American Academy of Neurology: ALS Practice Parameters Task Force. *Neurology* 52 (7): 1311–23.

Miller, T., M. Cudkowicz, P.J. Shaw, et al. (2020). Phase 1-2 Trial of Antisense Oligonucleotide Tofersen for SOD1 ALS. *New England Journal of Medicine* 383 (2): 109–19.

Mitsumoto, H. ed. (2009). *Amyotrophic Lateral Sclerosis: A Guide for Patients and Families*. New York: Demos.

Mitsumoto, H., M. Bromberg, W. Johnston, R. Tandan et al. (2005). Promoting excellence in end-of-life care in ALS. *Amyotrophic Lateral Sclerosis and Other Motor Neuron Disorders* 6 (3): 145–54.

Mueller, C., J.D. Berry, D.M. McKenna-Yasek, et al. (2020). SOD1 Suppression with Adeno-Associated Virus and MicroRNA in Familial ALS. *New England Journal of Medicine* 383 (2): 151–58.

Morrison, R.S. and D.E. Meyer (2004). Palliative care. *New England Journal of Medicine* 350: 3582–90.

Muscular Dystrophy Association (2017). Highlights of the MDA U.S. Neuromuscular Disease Registry (2013–2016) https://www.mda.org/sites/default/files/MDA%20Registry%20Report%20Highlights_Digital_final.pdf.

National Ethics Committee Veterans Health Administration (2007). The ethics of palliative sedation as a therapy of last resort. *The American Journal of Hospice and Palliative Care* 54: 483–91.

Nelson, L.M., B. Topol, W. Kaye, D. Williamson et al. (2018). Estimation of the prevalence of amyotrophic lateral sclerosis in the United States using National Administrative Healthcare Data from 2002 to 2004 and Capture-Recapture Methodology. *Neuroepidemiology* 51 (3–4): 149–57.

Noonan, C.W., M.C. White, D. Thurman and L.Y. Wong (2005). Temporal and geographic variation in United States motor neuron disease mortality, 1969–1998. *Neurology* 64 (7): 1215–21.

Obermann, M. and M. Lyon (2014). Financial cost of amyotrophic lateral sclerosis: A case study. *Amyotrophic Lateral Sclerosis and Frontotemporal Degeneration* 16 (1–2): 54–57.

Oliver, D. ed. (2006). *Palliative Care in Amyotrophic Lateral Sclerosis: From Diagnosis to Bereavement*. Oxford: Oxford University Press.

Oregon Department of Health and Human Services. (2020). https://www.deathwithdignity.org.

Paganoni, S., B. Saville, J. Andrews and J. Shefner (2019a). Healey ALS Platform Trial, https://www.massgeneral.org/assets/MGH/pdf/neurology/als/healey-prize-presentation-2019.pdf.

Paganoni, S., M. van de Rijn, K. Drake, K. Burke et al. (2019b). Adjusted cost analysis of video televisits for the care of people with amyotrophic lateral sclerosis. *Muscle Nerve* 60 (2): 147–54.

Pattee, G.L., E.K. Plowman, K.L. Focht Garand et al. NEALS Bulbar Subcommittee (2019). Provisional best practices guidelines for the evaluation of bulbar dysfunction in amyotrophic lateral sclerosis. *Muscle Nerve* 59 (5): 531–36.

Pulley, M.T., R. Brittain, W. Hodges and C. Frazier (2018). Multidisciplinary amyotrophic lateral sclerosis telemedicine care: The store and forward method. *Muscle Nerve* 59: 34–39.

Qadri, S., C.D. Langefeld, C. Milligan, J.B. Caress et al. (2019). Racial differences in intervention rates in individuals with ALS: A case-control study. *Neurology* 92 (17): e1969–e1974.

Raymond, J., B. Oskarsson, P. Mehta and K. Horton (2019). Clinical characteristics of a large cohort of US participants enrolled in the National Amyotrophic Lateral Sclerosis (ALS) Registry, 2010–2015. *Amyotrophic Lateral Sclerosis and Frontotemporal Degeneration* 20 (5–6): 413–20.

Rechtman L., H. Jordan, L. Wagner, D.K. Horton et al. (2015). Racial and ethnic differences among amyotrophic lateral sclerosis cases in the United States. *Amyotrophic Lateral Sclerosis and Frontotemporal Degeneration* 16 (1–2): 65–71.

Russell, J.A., M.A. Williams and O. Dragan (2010). Sedation for the imminently dying. Survey results from the AAN ethics section. *Neurology* 74: 1303–09.

Sagiraju, H.K.R., S. Živković, A.C. VanCott, H. Patwa et al. (2019). Amyotrophic lateral sclerosis among veterans deployed in support of Post-9/11 U.S. conflicts. *Military Medicine* Oct 23. pii: usz350. https://doi.org/10.1093/milmed/usz350. [Epub ahead of print].

Selkirk, S.M., M.O. Washington, F. McClellan, B. Flynn et al. (2017). Delivering tertiary centre specialty care to ALS patients via telemedicine: A retrospective cohort analysis. *Amyotrophic Lateral Sclerosis and Frontotemporal Degeneration* 18 (5–6): 324–32.

U.S. Army Medical Research and Materiel Command. Congressionally Directed Medical Research Programs. Department of Defense. Amyotrophic Lateral Sclerosis Research Program (2018), https://cdmrp.army.mil/alsrp/pdfs/ALSRP%20Strategic%20Plan.pdf.

U.S. Department of Health and Human Services, Food and Drug Administration (2018). Amyotrophic lateral sclerosis: Developing drugs for treatment. Guidance for Industry. https://www.fda.gov/downloads/Drugs/Guidance ComplianceRegulatoryInformation/Guidances/UCM596718.pdf.

van den Berg, L.H., E. Sorenson, G. Gronseth, E.A. Macklin et al. (2019). Revised Airlie House consensus guidelines for design and implementation of ALS clinical trials. *Neurology* 92 (14): e1610–e1623.

Wagner, L., L. Rechtman, H. Jordan, M. Ritsick et al. (2015). State and metropolitan area-based amyotrophic lateral sclerosis (ALS) surveillance. *Amyotrophic Lateral Sclerosis and Frontotemporal Degeneration* 17 (1–2): 128–34.

Ward, A.L., M. Sanjak, K. Duffy, E. Bravver et al. (2010). Power wheelchair prescription, utilization, satisfaction, and cost for patients with amyotrophic lateral sclerosis: Preliminary data for evidence-based guidelines. *Archives of Physical Medicine and Rehabilitation* 91 (2): 268–72.

Williams, J.R., D. Fitzhenry, L. Grant, D. Martyn et al. (2013). Diagnosis pathway for patients with amyotrophic lateral sclerosis: Retrospective analysis of the US Medicare longitudinal claims database. *BMC Neurology* 4 (13): 160.

Weisskopf, M.G., E.J. O'Reilly, M.L. McCullough, E.E. Calle et al. (2005). Prospective study of military service and mortality from ALS. *Neurology* 64 (1): 32–37.

Young, J.L. (2011). A National Study of Amyotrophic Lateral Sclerosis Multidisciplinary Clinic Utilization. *PCOM Psychology Dissertations.* Paper 245. https://digitalcommons.pcom.edu/cgi/viewcontent.cgi?article=1244&context=psychology_dissertations.

CHAPTER 23

Conclusions: What We Can Learn from the Country Perspectives

Robert H. Blank, Jerome E. Kurent, and David Oliver

Abstract This chapter summarizes the wealth of information related to ALS/MND policy as presented in the preceding chapters written by experts from twenty-one diverse countries. An overview of findings related to ALS/MND policy issues is described and discussed. Major disparities between high- and low- and middle-income countries are noted, including differences within each wealth category regarding the activity and support of government and private organizations. Disparities are observed with research funding, diagnosis and care of patients, access to assistive technologies and palliative care, the availability of multidisciplinary care, support for caregivers and decision making at the end of life. This chapter

R. H. Blank (✉)
University of Canterbury, Christchurch, New Zealand
e-mail: rblank24601@hotmail.com

J. E. Kurent
Medical University of South Carolina, Charleston, SC, USA
e-mail: kurentje@musc.edu

D. Oliver
University of Kent, Canterbury, UK
e-mail: drdjoliver@gmail.com

© The Author(s) 2021
R. H. Blank et al. (eds.), *Public Policy in ALS/MND Care*,
https://doi.org/10.1007/978-981-15-5840-5_23

327

also stresses the importance of cultural and societal differences in understanding policy variation across countries while recognizing the need to take these into account when framing and implementing policy in any country.

Keywords ALS • MND • Cross-cultural analysis • Public policy • Multidisciplinary care • Palliative care

ALS/MND POLICY

All governments make decisions that set priorities regarding regulation and distribution of public goods. ALS/MND is no exception. Chapter 1 introduced a wide range of policy areas that are relevant to ALS/MND. Although some are more pertinent and encompassing than others, they include funding for research and care, long-term services and support for informal family caregivers, health promotion and prevention, and housing and community services, such as day care and respite centers. In addition, assistive technologies, workforce policy to meet the growing needs for formal caregivers and support for family carers, as well as policies designed to safeguard ALS/MND patients are very important. Also important are a wide range of policies surrounding end-stage disease and eventual death of patients with ALS/MND. These include the use of advance directives, withholding or withdrawing life-prolonging care and palliative sedation. Physician-assisted suicide (PAS), or medical aid in dying, and euthanasia remain highly controversial issues, even in countries where they have been implemented.

As will be clear from countries represented in this book, getting ALS/MND on the public agenda depends on the dedicated work of concerned professionals and advocacy groups, including patients and their families. Within the context of limited public resources, the ALS/MND community faces an uphill battle to secure necessary resources for both research and care because it is always in competition for public attention and funding with other areas. ALS/MND must frequently compete for limited resources often directed to increasing elderly populations around much of the globe, as well as the poor and under-served patient populations.

CROSS-NATIONAL LEARNING

Cross-country comparison is an appealing strategy for social enquiry and can provide a basis for identifying the variety of options that exist in ALS/MND policy. As such, comparison holds the promise of learning from other countries including their policy successes and failures. The examination of international experiences with ALS/MND can elucidate both the difficulties faced by, and the range of strategies available to, policy makers. They can also give us insights as to what works or does not work under an array of institutional and cultural contexts. The importance of *culture* and its potential influence on policy development cannot be overstated. Culture has been defined as a complex whole consisting of systems of beliefs, values, morals, law and communication that people share. Given the complexity of ALS/MND care, comparative studies can generate the evidence necessary to consider the full range of policy options and, therefore, strengthen policy making.

The preceding twenty-one country chapters provide a wealth of authoritative comparative information on numerous key facets of ALS/MND policy. Moreover, although there is a clear divide between high-income countries (HICs) and low- and middle-income countries (LMICs), even within each broad grouping there are significant differences in the scope and level of research and care activity, including considerable variation in end-of-life policies. This chapter attempts to summarize some of the major findings and provide an international context for developing ALS/MND policy across its many dimensions. Hopefully, this book will also contribute to a cross-cultural dialogue on ALS/MND policy that will be helpful in generating support across all countries, including those not represented in this book, and especially those that are finding it most difficult to do so at the present time.

EPIDEMIOLOGY OF ALS/MND

In only a few countries are there reliable, national figures on the incidence and prevalence of ALS. In many countries, data is very crude at best. On the other hand, Ireland has a national population-based registry that has tracked ALS/MND patients for the last 25 years and is linked to DNA samples. The Japanese Consortium for ALS (JaCALS) is a patient registry system with 33 institutes. The United States has a National ALS Registry administered by the Communicable Diseases Center (CDC). In most

Table 23.1 Incidence and prevalence of ALS/MND

	Incidence	Prevalence
Australia	3.14/100,000	8.7/100,000
Belgium	2.0/100,000	8–12/100,000
Brazil	1.49/100,000	3.92/100,000
Canada	2–3/100,000	8.1/100,000
China		1.23/100,000
Germany	2.0/100,000	6–8/100,000
India		4.0/100,000
Ireland	2.6/100,000	8.0/100,000
Israel	1.66/100,000	6.7/100,000
Italy	3.23/100,000	10.5/100,000
Japan	1.0/100,000	7–8/100,000
Mexico	0.4/100,000	1.44/100,000
Nigeria		15/100,000
Pakistan		1.44/100,000
Poland	2–3/100,000	5–7/100,000
Russia		0.7–1.25/100,000
South Africa	Caucasians like Europe, Africans much lower	
South Korea	1.20/100,000	3.43/100,000
Tunisia		0.45/100,000
United Kingdom	2.0/100,000	7.0/100,000
United States	3–5/100,000	5.9/100,000

countries, however, there is a need for more information concerning the incidence and prevalence of ALS. All countries should consider a national registry in order to obtain comparable data. Table 23.1 displays available data which demonstrate considerable variations in incidence and prevalence.

Timely diagnosis and communicating this to the patient are very important in the care and treatment of patients with ALS/MND and offer the opportunity for optimal care, as well as the potential for participation in clinical trials. As noted in Chapter 1, even under the best of circumstances, this can be a challenging process of excluding ALS/MND mimics. In many countries, diagnosis is haphazard at best. For instance, in India, Pakistan and Tunisia, extremely late diagnosis is commonplace. In South Africa, as in many African nations, the heavy burden of AIDS, tuberculosis and other common diseases means that ALS/MND is often underdiagnosed or only diagnosed very late in its progression. Similarly, the diagnostic delay for ALS in Brazil is much higher than in Europe. The most important problems relate to the lack of adequate funding and trained professionals. Most general practitioners and even general neurologists are often unfamiliar with this relatively rare disease.

FACING LIMITED RESOURCES

As noted in Chapter 1, the wealth of a country and the amount of funds available for health care are likely to be critical limiting factors in ALS/MND policy. The accounts provided in individual country chapters certainly bear this out. For instance, in Nigeria the health system is characterized by disparity in patients' location, financial inaccessibility, poverty, rapid turnover of people in key positions and a lack of continuity in policy. This is further complicated by impaired implementation of limited resources and poor management. Religious customs and cultural beliefs of "spiritual attack" are often considered to play a role in causing illness and represent additional complicating issues. These factors in Nigeria pose a tremendous challenge to the management and ongoing care for patients with ALS/MND.

Similarly, despite recent encouraging policy developments, including increased emphasis on multidisciplinary team care, the services available for people with ALS/MND and their caregivers in Russia are very limited. Pakistan is "poorly equipped to deal with ALS," while in South Africa the poor especially suffer without care. In India bad deaths seem to be the norm. These countries face many difficult issues including the unavailability of trained healthcare practitioners, inaccessibility to appropriate healthcare facilities, a high personal cost of care and a lack of governmental support for patient care and research.

In addition, geographic and regional inequalities in ALS/MND care are found across HICs and LMICs, usually between rural and urban settings. These disparities are most conspicuous in countries with large, dispersed populations but also can occur in smaller countries with a limited number of ALS/MND centers. For instance, while Brazil has many positive policies for ALS in place, they often are not implemented in many regions particularly due to the lack of qualified professionals in remote parts of the country. As a result, patients from different regions of the country have distinct standards of care leading to delayed diagnosis and suboptimal care.

In South Korea there is a significant gap between metropolitan areas and rural areas where patients have limited access to hospitals and health-care services. Superior hospitals which provide high-quality multidisciplinary care are located mostly in Seoul. South Africa has great inconsistencies in care across regions. Given its widely dispersed population, it is not surprising that Australia has difficulty providing care to patients with ALS/MND in remote rural areas and has large variations in support across states. Even in Israel which has two major ALS clinics operating within academic institutions, comprehensive ALS/MND multidisciplinary care is not widely available for many patients.

GOVERNMENT AND PRIVATE ORGANIZATION ACTIVITY IN ALS/MND

There are great variations in the involvement of governmental and private/charitable organizations in the care and support of people with ALS/MND. It is hoped that this book might be a stimulus for countries without access to multidisciplinary care for patients with ALS/MND to consider the development of comprehensive policies and guidelines to achieve this goal. This could be accomplished in close collaboration with private ALS/MND organizations. There are excellent examples of support provided by non-governmental ALS/MND organizations in Australia, Brazil, Canada, Germany, Israel, Italy, Japan, South Korea, the United Kingdom and the United States. Similarly, ALS Liga Belgium, GILA in Mexico and Dignitas Doletium in Poland are active associations committed to caring for persons with ALS/MND. Other countries have more limited involvement by private ALS/MND organizations, but many are working to develop similar ALS/MND advocacy/support groups and aiming to encourage governments to provide leadership and funding for patient care and family caregiver support.

PUBLIC AWARENESS AND MEDIA ATTENTION FOR ALS/MND

If ALS/MND is going to compete for its fair share of public resources, it must have increased public awareness and engender broad media attention. As a rare disease, this can be difficult, especially when competing for attention with diseases such as AIDS, Alzheimer's disease and cancer. The

Ice Bucket Challenge was credited with raising awareness around the world, including Belgium, Canada, China, Germany, Israel, Japan, South Korea, United Kingdom and the United States.

Another source of extensive media coverage in some countries including Italy, the United Kingdom and the United States has been that of athletes and other prominent persons with ALS/MND. In contrast, in most parts of the world including India, Mexico, Nigeria, Pakistan and Tunisia, there is little or no public awareness or media coverage of ALS/MND. This can be recognized as a major opportunity for private sectors to develop further.

FUNDING FOR ALS/MND RESEARCH

Dedicated, publicly funded research programs in ALS/MND are scarce in most countries. ALS/MND must compete with other diseases to secure funding primarily through a process of competitive grant programs. Virtually all country authors in this book have stressed the need for increased research funding, especially related to clinical trials. There are many notable examples of success. For instance, the Irish ALS/MND Research group, the Israel ALS Research Association and the active dedicated research in Canada, Germany, the United Kingdom and the United States.

Australia has been successful in funding MND research through a combination of public, private philanthropic and other non-government sources. These include the MND Research Institute Australia and FightMND. Since its inception in 2014, FightMND has raised over 28.5 million USD for research. Funding obtained from competitive research grants through the National Health and Medical Research Council (NHMRC), the Medical Research Future Fund (MRFF) and other Commonwealth agencies, as well as the federal government has helped fund research focused on clinical trial pathways.

ACCESS TO DRUGS TO TREAT ALS/MND PATIENTS

There are currently three drugs approved by the US Food and Drug Administration (FDA) for the treatment of ALS—riluzole, edaravone and quinidine/dextromethorphan. Riluzole and edaravone have been marketed as agents which can affect the natural history of ALS/MND. Quinidine/dextromethorphan is used primarily for the symptomatic treatment of emotional lability associated with pseudobulbar affect (PBA). Riluzole has been found to delay the onset of ventilator-dependence or tracheostomy and may increase survival by two to three months. Edaravone has been reported in one study to slow progression of disability for patients with ALS studied over a six-month period compared with patients not receiving this intravenous medication.

Riluzole is currently available in most countries represented in this book, but not all cover the cost of this medication. In Israel, riluzole is the only government-funded therapy for ALS/MND. However, edaravone is available for patients who can pay with their own resources. Both riluzole and edaravone are available in India if the patient has resources to pay for it. Brazil, China, Poland and Tunisia cover the full costs of riluzole. Belgium and South Korea public funding pays for 90 percent of the cost of the drug, while patients in Nigeria must pay the total cost. Neither riluzole nor edaravone are available in Russia. In the United States, Medicare or private insurance will pay for most if not all of the cost of this medication. The Veterans Administration pays for this medication for Veterans diagnosed with ALS.

RIGHT TO TRY

A "Right to Try" policy offers the potential for patients with incurable diseases to gain access to unlicensed drugs and other therapeutic interventions not presently available. It always involves a trade-off between concerns related to patient safety and the patient's right to exercise self-determination and take possible uncertain risks. Policy regarding right to try varies from country to country, and it is important to note that not all countries even recognize a patient's right to make independent decisions for themselves.

In many countries of Europe, laws are in place supporting the use of experimental drugs in a compassionate use or named patient format prior to registration. In Belgium, experimental drugs not considered unacceptably expensive can be prescribed by any physician even though not yet approved and not on the market. However, experimental drugs with a very high cost are problematic unless the company is willing to provide the drug without charge in an early access program. If this is not possible, most physicians and ethics committees could consider it unethical for the patient to have to cover the cost of the treatment.

CLINICAL TRIALS

Clinical trials are taking place across the world, but primarily led by North America, Europe and Australia. In contrast, patients with ALS/MND in LMICs may have severely reduced opportunities to be involved in a trial. For example, very few therapeutic trials come to Brazil primarily due to the bureaucracy involved with regulatory approvals. There is a need to update the regulatory framework for clinical research, particularly for rare diseases, which would greatly improve opportunities to develop ALS/MND-focused clinical trials

GENETIC TESTING

The availability of genetic testing for patients with ALS/MND varies greatly across countries. As noted in Chapter 1, genetic testing can be obtained for patients who have been diagnosed with sporadic ALS/MND, as well as presymptomatic testing of unaffected family members where there is a positive family history. Each application of testing raises difficult ethical issues and requires careful consent processes and counseling for all involved. A few countries like Israel and the United Kingdom offer genetic testing with no cost to patients, as well as presymptomatic testing for family members. However, most countries have no public support for genetic testing and some including Tunisia consider it only a research activity. Of those that do provide testing for patients free of charge like Ireland, presymptomatic testing is generally not available. It is expected that genetic testing will become more widely available in the future even in those countries where it is now considered principally a research activity.

PUBLIC SUPPORT FOR PATIENTS AND FAMILY CAREGIVERS

In all countries, the burden of care for ALS/MND patients often falls on family caregivers. The support offered for caregivers varies considerably across our countries, but many provide support in the form of financial assistance, respite care or with paid carers. As illustrated in Table 23.2, aid to patients and caregivers differs widely, frequently even within countries. In those countries where caregiver allowances are provided, they often tend to be minimal. This seems to be one area where considerable policy work is needed to ease the burden of family caregivers in most countries.

Table 23.2   Support for caregivers of patients with ALS/MND

Australia:	Financial support/access to respite care vary across states and by age
Belgium:	Direct support to carers for home care—liaison workers, home nurses
Brazil:	Highly variable policy, but good government support with immediate retirement after diagnosis with ALS
Canada:	Strong caregiver support and generous family leave but varies by province
China:	Monthly subsidy of 45 USD for ALS patients
Germany:	Broad support for caregivers
India:	No aid for caregivers
Ireland:	Highly organized care. Means-tested but 95 percent ultimately get free care, home support service 20 to 28 hours/week, caregivers and respite care allowance, but long waiting lists with gaps filled by IMNDA
Israel:	Limited government support. Most hire one or more carers at own expense
Japan:	Strong support system but varies by prefecture. Monthly cash payment of 182 USD if a family provides care at home without using insurance reimbursement
Italy:	Varies by region, but overall adequate support
Mexico:	Minimal support from GILA
Nigeria:	No aid for caregivers
Pakistan:	Very small government allowances
Poland:	Patients diagnosed with ALS have a right to a pension from social insurance
Russia:	Caregiver support from government but below minimal wage, varies by locale
South Africa:	Small caregiver allowance, USD 30/month, home nurse visits 2 to 3 times/week, great inconsistencies across regions
South Korea:	Wide range of programs of aid, home healthcare nurses. Forty-two percent of the patients hire a formal caregiver often with government subsidy
Tunisia:	No aid for caregivers
United Kingdom:	Social care means-tested, varies across local councils. A complex system of caregiver allowance from government not means-tested in last 6 months
United States:	Family Medical Leave Act; Social Security, etc.; however, need for additional direct financial support for family caregivers

ACCESS TO ASSISTIVE TECHNOLOGIES

For people living with ALS/MND, the full range of assistive technology includes aids and equipment to support comfort, independence and daily living, advanced communication technology and non-invasive ventilation to support breathing, quality and length of life. Access to a full range of resources can greatly improve the quality of life for patients with ALS/MND. Equipment is available in many countries, but accessibility can be limited by scarce public funds or by the need for patients to co-fund or completely fund measures to meet their needs. In Poland, for example, devices such as electronic communication are partially reimbursed from public resources, but the extent of compensation depends on the resources of the local social welfare agency, as well as the incomes of the patients and their families. Because the costs of electronic devices are high, patients must often rely on donations from private organizations in order to have access to them. Also, because of the rapid progression of the disease, timing is crucial. Even in highly supportive countries, such as Australia, Canada, Ireland, the United Kingdom and the United States, equipment may be available but with long delays, limiting the help offered to patients and their families.

There is a clear dividing line between HICs and LMICs where access to more than basic assisted devices including breathing apparatus is available only to those who can pay for it themselves. For example, this is the case for India, Mexico, Nigeria, Pakistan and South Africa. In China, despite some help from Oriental Rain ALS Care and the China Social Welfare Foundation, the use of invasive ventilators and the associated management costs are an unbearable financial burden to most families. Moreover, in many other countries, including Ireland, Poland and the United Kingdom, access to more sophisticated assistive technologies is means tested or can vary by locale as in Belgium. Often, charitable organizations like IMNDA in Ireland, IsrALS in Israel, LiveNow in Russia, the ALS Association of Japan and MND Associations in Australia can fill in the gaps and by-pass the bureaucracy involved in obtaining public funding.

WHERE PATIENTS WITH ALS/MND LIVE AND DIE

In all countries, most ALS/MND patients live at home at least until disease progression makes it extremely difficult. Even then, many people are cared for at home. For example, less than 5 percent of ALS patients in Israel receive institutional care and most continue to live at home through all stages of the disease, even when they are treated with invasive ventilation. In some countries including India, Mexico, Nigeria and Tunisia, there is no option because institutional care facilities are rare, but in most cases, it is a matter of personal choice or economics. It should be noted that the quality of home care varies greatly. For instance, most South African poor receive no outside formal care not already provided by family members.

Although home care is delivered in most countries by informal caregivers, mainly family members, access to respite care and caregiver support varies considerably. For instance, while Australia, Belgium, Canada, Ireland and Japan provide strong support for home caregivers, Israel provides no respite care and many families employ one or more foreign care workers for support. In South Korea, too, a large minority of the caregivers are formal paid workers. In Poland, those with no family care may be referred to nursing homes with the cost shared by the patient at 70 percent of income and by local social services, but this option is limited by a small number of beds in long-term facilities. In the United States, home-based Medicare hospice can provide several hours per week of nursing assistant caregiver support to supplement any formal care already being provided.

There is also considerable variation across these countries as to where ALS/MND patients die. In most countries reliable data are not available. Although most patients across countries and cultures indicate a desire to die at home, place of death depends on many factors. These include the ability to care for the patient at home along with the availability of adequate institutional care facilities, including hospices, cultural and social values. For example, in China issuance of a death certificate can occur only if the patient dies in a hospital.

In LMICs, including Mexico, Nigeria and Russia, 80–90 percent of ALS/MND patients die in their home. Likewise, in Italy with its strong family structure, 75 percent die at home, while in Africa, a sense of connectedness to family roots and the ancestors often determines the strong motivation not to die in institutions but close to the ancestral home. On the other hand, in Australia, the proportions dying at home vary between 25 and 34 percent, and in Belgium 25 percent. In the United Kingdom, 29 percent of patients with MND die at home, 39 percent in hospital, 17 percent in a chronic care home and 13 percent in hospice. Japan has the lowest at-home deaths with only 13 percent at home, 9.2 percent at nursing facilities and 75.8 percent in hospitals. In the United States, although 80–90 percent of people have expressed a desire to die at home, only 30 percent die at home while approximately 70 percent die in hospitals or chronic care facilities.

MULTIDISCIPLINARY CLINICS

Multidisciplinary ALS clinics (MDCs) provide comprehensive professional expertise required to assist with the management of constantly changing ALS/MND symptoms and to provide support for family caregivers.

Table 23.3 Access to multidisciplinary clinics

Widespread access	Moderate access	Limited access	No access
Belgium	Australia	China	India
Canada	Brazil	Mexico	Pakistan
Germany	Japan	Nigeria	Poland
Ireland	Italy	South Africa	Russia
Israel	South Korea	Tunisia	
United Kingdom			
United States			

MDCs are considered the gold standard for providing comprehensive care and are widely accessible throughout most of North America, the United Kingdom, Europe and other countries where their implementation has been associated with improved quality of life and possibly extension of the natural history of ALS/MND. Table 23.3 illustrates the relative availability of multidisciplinary clinics in countries represented in this book.

Even where MDCs are present, their location primarily in large cities can limit access in many countries. For instance, while Canada has a broad network of MDCs, they are all in large population centers, making access for patients living in rural areas and Northern Canada difficult. Australia, too, only has MDCs in the capital city of each state while in China and Nigeria they are found only in big cities. Similarly, although collaboration is increasing, Mexico's two current MDCs are in Mexico City, while the three MDCs in South Africa are in the main teaching hospitals. Thus, in general patients with ALS/MND residing outside of major population centers have very limited, if any, access to MDC teams.

PALLIATIVE CARE/HOSPICE

The World Health Organization (WHO) has defined palliative care as "an approach that improves the quality of life of patients and their families facing the problem associated with life threatening illness, through the prevention and relief of suffering by means of early identification and impeccable assessment and treatment of pain and other problems, physical, psychosocial and spiritual." Palliative Care affirms life and regards dying as a normal process and intends to neither hasten nor postpone death. It is a holistic approach that aims to improve the quality of life of patients with life-limiting illness where cure is no longer possible. It may

Table 23.4 Access to palliative care/hospice

Widespread	Varied	Very limited	None
Belgium	Australia	Brazil	India
Canada	Japan	China	Pakistan
Germany	Italy	Mexico	Tunisia
Ireland	Poland	Nigeria	
Israel (home)	South Korea	Russia (home)	
United Kingdom	South Africa		
United States			

exclude medical treatments, tests and procedures that can cause discomfort. Despite widespread global recognition of the importance of palliative care to reduce suffering, palliative care for ALS/MND patients is still largely inaccessible for a majority of individuals living in LMICs, and sometimes available only to a limited extent even in some more affluent countries (Table 23.4).

There are distinctions between palliative care and hospice in many countries. Hospice is often seen as palliative care provided to the patient in the terminal phase of illness, but the definition of hospice varies from country to country where it is available. For example, in the United Kingdom, where hospice care was first developed, hospices may provide palliative care at home, in hospitals and care homes or inpatient hospices. This may be not only at the end of life but earlier in the disease progression—months and even years. In contrast in the United States most hospice care is provided as home-based hospice care provided at the patient's residence, whether at home or a chronic care facility. Patients with any terminal diagnosis including ALS qualify for hospice if their life expectancy is six months or less. Most hospice care is paid for by Medicare at no additional cost to the patient. Services include care provided by a multidisciplinary team as well as medications and durable medical equipment related to the terminal diagnosis. However, in the United States families may still experience significant financial burdens relating to care of a terminally ill family member. It is likely that the financial and societal toll is even much greater in countries with more limited resources and supportive public policy.

Even in countries with active palliative care programs, they might not always be available to patients with ALS/MND. For instance, Italy, Japan and South Africa have palliative care and hospice facilities, but they may not necessarily accept ALS/MND patients. In Israel ALS patients are eligible for palliative care as provided by home-based hospice. In the United Kingdom, inpatient hospice care is widely available, and many hospices provide care for patients with MND. However, there are anecdotal reports that some hospices have limited access for patients with MND or only accept patients in the very terminal phases of their illness. It is possible that this may reflect the comprehensive high-quality care already being provided by specialized MND multidisciplinary teams, which includes palliative care.

ADVANCE DIRECTIVES (ADs)

There are opportunities earlier in the disease progression when a patient can make informed decisions regarding avoidances and preferences for future care. If these are recorded clearly through an advance directive (AD) with a proxy designated to make decisions for an incapacitated patient on their behalf, the patient's wishes can be respected. Although ADs including a living will or durable power of attorney for health care are considered legal documents in most Western countries, their implementation may vary widely. In Israel ADs are commonly used, and healthcare professionals are mandated by law to follow them. In Australia their availability varies by state. In Ireland ADs are encouraged, but are not legally binding, while in Nigeria they are generally respected. In the United States the Durable Power of Attorney for Health Care is the preferred AD document. Only an estimated 15 percent of the population has completed an AD, although it is probably lower among some minority groups.

In Pakistan there is no concept of ADs, and there is belief among many people that even discussing death might cause it to occur early. Policy changes are needed to facilitate ADs for patients with ALS/MND. Similarly, in India ADs and planning for the end of life are non-existent. In Russia there is no clear legal status of ADs. In Poland no public open debate has taken place regarding quality of life, futile care, advance directives, euthanasia or assisted suicide. Thus, it appears there is presently no perceived need for ADs.

WITHHOLDING OR WITHDRAWING CARE

In many countries there is no ethical or legal distinction between with-holding and withdrawing of life-extending care, including medical interventions such as a feeding tube or use of invasive ventilation. In other countries it is not legally permissible to withdraw treatment once it has been initiated. These approaches vary by country and often have strong religious and cultural underpinnings, which form the basis for law and public policy. For example, members of the Orthodox Jewish faith do not permit removal of a feeding tube once provided for a patient even if diagnosed with a terminal disease, such as end-stage Alzheimer's disease. In Japan it is illegal to withdraw mechanical ventilation from a patient with ALS/MND once it has been initiated. In contrast, in the United States no legal or ethical distinction is made between withholding and withdrawal of life-extending interventions.

Limiting treatments can let the disease take its natural course and support the person's comfort and dignity. If aggressive medical treatment is refused or withdrawn, a care team should still provide comprehensive physical and emotional care.

PHYSICIAN-ASSISTED SUICIDE (PAS) AND EUTHANASIA

As was discussed in Chapter 1, there is a critical distinction between PAS and euthanasia. PAS refers to a process whereby a physician licensed in a jurisdiction where it is legal can provide a prescription for a lethal dose of medication to the terminally ill patient. The patient can then use it at his/her own will in the future. Euthanasia refers to the intentional taking of a patient's life typically with lethal medications provided by injection, and is considered legal in only a few countries in the world.

There appears to be a gradual acceptance of PAS in many Western countries, even those where it is not presently legalized. In 2016 Canada federal legislation permitted PAS for patients with a "serious and incurable illness, disease, or disability" that causes intolerable suffering and as a result of which death was "reasonably foreseeable." In the Netherlands, PAS is considered legal for terminally ill patients if the physician is satisfied that the patient's request is voluntary, well-considered, well-informed and sustained. The patient must have full decision-making capacity at the time of the request, must perceive his or her situation as unbearable and be experiencing hopeless suffering.

However, PAS continues to be prohibited in many of the countries represented in this book, including China, Israel, Nigeria, Pakistan, Russia, South Korea and Tunisia. There is no legal basis for PAS in the United Kingdom and it is legal in only two Australian states, Victoria and Western Australia. In Pakistan and Tunisia, opposition to PAS is largely due to religious objections. In Chinese culture, suicide and euthanasia are contrary to moral behavior because of the concepts of strong family and integrity, and few people attempt suicide or accept euthanasia. In addition, Chinese culture is lacking in death education, and patients and their families usually avoid talking about death.

Cultural Factors That Affect ALS/MND Policy

Cultural factors and social values vary across countries and in some cases have a significant impact on ALS/MND policy. Values dominant in the West such as individual rights, personal autonomy and truth-telling in the setting of terminal illness are not universal. Moreover, there may be strong cultural and value divisions within each country that are important in understanding ALS/MND policy differences. Strongly held beliefs often exist within races, ethnic and religious groups. For instance, religious factors are especially important for death-related policies, and perhaps the single most important factor in some countries. Similarly, social structures, especially the importance of family and the role of women, can be central to the care of the terminally ill patient. In many countries, extended families and communities continue to play a central role, while in others even the nuclear family has had a diminishing role to play in care giving.

One ethical area where cultural differences are evident relates to truth-telling and disclosure to the patient. For instance, in India, Japan, China and Tunisia it is considered the responsibility of the family to protect the patients from bad news. Hence, in respecting this strongly held cultural practice, the neurologist must inform the family about the diagnosis and details of the disease rather than the patient. In Pakistan where, under Islam, disease is accepted as the will of God and a test of faith, the family and not the patient is informed, and it is left to their discretion as to how and when to tell the patient.

Another area of clear cultural differences centers on the use of life-prolonging interventions. For instance, South Africans in the terminal phase of illness strongly prefer receiving comfort care instead of extreme life-extending measures. In general, many African cultures believe that the focus should be on having a "good death" with opportunities for family reconciliation. In Tunisia most patients with ALS choose to avoid ventilation and/or tracheotomy. Similarly, Chinese patients with ALS/MND have low acceptance rates for invasive treatments. Some patients may even conceal their progressive symptoms from their doctor in order to avoid using assistive breathing apparatus for as long as possible. As a result, treatment initiation is often very late and the overall number of patients using non-invasive breathing apparatus is low.

In contrast, patients with ALS/MND in Poland have a relatively high use of interventions used to prolong life. A societal view in Poland is that life is to be highly valued and may possibly correlate with the fact that over 90 percent of Poles are Roman Catholics. A similar pattern is evident in Italy. Religious and cultural issues unique to Israel are critical factors that have shaped end-of-life policy and led to much higher use of mechanical ventilation than elsewhere, around 50 to 60 percent. Also, compared to other European countries, more Belgian patients choose mechanical ventilation. Patients place high value on patient autonomy and are actively involved in the planning for their end-of-life care.

Religious and cultural values also influence views toward medicine and health in general which, in turn, can influence the role of professional caregivers of patients with ALS/MND. For instance, in much of Africa including Nigeria, many people believe that most illnesses are due to spiritual problems and patients may prefer to present at religious centers rather than at hospitals. While most patients will consult both Western medical practitioners and traditional healers, many especially in the rural and semi-urban areas, consult with traditional healers as their preferred source for advice. During the dying process, the spiritual aspects of suffering are considered more important than the physical ones. In South Korea many patients also use Korean Oriental Medicine in combination with Western medicine.

It is important to acknowledge the impact of cultural and societal differences in understanding policy variation across countries. It is essential to take these into account when framing or implementing policy in any country. Especially as Western countries become more ethnically and culturally diverse, it will be crucial that professionals working with ALS/MND patients in multicultural environments recognize that not all cultures and ethnic groups respond the same way to the same information, particularly that related to end-of-life decision making. Therefore, care might best be provided by multidisciplinary teams with staff trained to recognize these potential differences.

SUMMARY AND FUTURE PERSPECTIVES

The discussions in these chapters have shown the wide variations in care provided to people with ALS/MND and social support for their families. There are themes that occur across many countries—the role of ALS multidisciplinary teams, the need for palliative care and the influence of cultural aspects of care on end-of-life decision making within certain regions of the world. The availability and provision of medications, medical equipment and support for patients and caregivers are highly variable. Countries should be encouraged to develop national ALS registries when possible in order to obtain accurate data related to the incidence and prevalence of ALS/MND and also to identify potential environmental risk factors.

This book encourages further international collaboration in basic and applied research, clinical trials and the continued search not only into the causes and treatment of ALS/MND but also in the clinical care and management of symptoms. Continued research into the genetic basis of ALS/MND holds great promise to develop further insights and possible meaningful treatments. The refinement of clinical guidelines would also allow for the provision of more efficient and evidence-based care and symptom management, as well as the expansion of ALS/MND multidisciplinary clinics and palliative and hospice care. We must continue to learn from each other in a way that will continue to benefit patients and their families, while providing hope for the future and the eventual conquest of this devastating disease.

CPI Antony Rowe
Eastbourne, UK
January 13, 2021